MEDICAL PHYSICS MONOGRAPH NO. 5

BIOLOGICAL RISKS OF MEDICAL IRRADIATIONS

Edited by

Gary D. Fullerton, Ph.D.
*University of Texas Health Science Center
San Antonio, Texas*

David T. Kopp, Ph.D.
*United States Air Force
San Antonio, Texas*

Robert G. Waggener, Ph.D.
*University of Texas Health Science Center
San Antonio, Texas*

Edward W. Webster, Ph.D.
*Harvard University, MGH
Boston, Massachusetts*

Manuscripts were originally prepared for AAPM Spring Symposium, "Update on the Biological Risks of Medical Irradiations," held at the University of Texas Health Science Center, San Antonio, Texas, March 26–28, 1980. The conference was co-sponsored by The American Association of Physicists in Medicine, Southwest Chapter American Association of Physicists in Medicine, and Radiology Department, University of Texas Health Science Center, San Antonio, Texas

Published for the
American Association of Physicists in Medicine
by the American Institute of Physics

Library of Congress Catalog No. 80-53864
International Standard Book No. 0-88318-279-3
International Standard Serial No. 0163-1802

Copyright © 1980 by the American Association of
Physicists in Medicine

All rights reserved. No part of this book may be
reproduced, stored in a retrieval system, or transmitted, in any form or by any means (electronic, mechanical, photocopying, recording, or otherwise) without the prior written permission of the publisher.

Published by the American Institute of Physics
335 East 45 Street, New York, New York 10017

Printed in the United States of America

Further copies of this monograph may be obtained from:

    American Institute of Physics
    Back Numbers
    335 East 45th Street
    New York, New York 10017

Price: $21, prepaid ($15 for AAPM Members, personal copy) ($2.00 billing charge if payment not enclosed)

FOREWORD

This monograph, "The Biological Risks of Medical Irradiations," is a further American Association of Physicists in Medicine (AAPM) scientific publication and the fifth in the AAPM monograph series. It has been produced under the editorship of Gary D. Fullerton, David T. Kopp, Robert G. Waggener, and Edward W. Webster and is an official project of the Biological Effects Committee, Continuing Education Committee, and Publications Committee. This monograph is a collection of manuscripts presented in an AAPM regional symposium conducted in San Antonio and differs from others published to date in that it addresses legal and social questions as well as scientific ones. It was reviewed for the Publications Committee by Ann Wright, and we are all indebted to her for her careful review and cooperation with the editors. Issuance of such monographs is one of the means that the AAPM employs to carry out its responsibility to prepare and disseminate technical information in medical physics and related fields.

John S. Laughlin, Ph.D. FACR
Chairman, Publications Committee

PREFACE

During the past few years there has been a remarkable increase in public and professional concern regarding the biological effects of radiation, particularly at low levels. While much of this concern has focussed on potential hazards to the public from the operation of nuclear reactors, a concern magnified by the accident at Three Mile Island, the public has also increasingly questioned the risks of deleterious effects which may result from the medical use of radiation in the diagnosis and treatment of disease. It is essential that personnel professionally involved with medical radiation practice should develop an understanding of those risks and the methods of minimizing them without compromising the medical benefits. Moreover, it is the responsibility of such personnel to accurately inform the public and the medical profession in these areas of concern. The present work attempts to gather together the fund of current information necessary for education and practice at this interface between medical science and the public interest. The recent authoritative reports on the biological effects of radiation by committeees of the National Academy of Sciences and the United Nations make this work particularly timely. The information here presented derives from an intensive 3-day program designed primarily for the continuing education of medical physicists and radiologists. The objectives of the course are the objectives of the book: 1) to update understanding of radiation risks, particularly with respect to cancer induction, possible effects on future generations, and risks to the child irradiated during gestation; 2) to present information on radiation dose estimation from medical procedures; 3) to review methods for reducing radiation risks; and 4) to present an overview of the laws and regulations concerning the administration of radiation to the patient, including the potential for litigation. These collected papers are published under the auspices of the Amerian Association of Physicists in Medicine, an organization dedicated to maintaining high standards of expertise in the practice of medical physics. The concept and the realization of this book owes much to the Committees on Biological Effects, on Conuinuing Education, and on Publication of the Association.

> Edward W. Webster, Chairman
> AAPM Committee on
>   Biological Effects

American Association of Physicists in Medicine
1980 Spring Symposium "Update on the
Biological Risks of Medical Irradiations"

University of Texas Health Science Center
San Antonio, Texas

July 20 - 26, 1980

Directors	Gary D. Fullerton
	David T. Kopp
	Robert G. Waggener
	Edward W. Webster
Local Arrangements Committee	Gary D. Fullerton, Chairman
	David T. Kopp
	Bhaskaran Pillai
	Karl Prado
Program Secretaries	Marilyn Rennels
	Dotti Leathers
Editorial Assistants	Nora Gerwell
	Lavonne Banse
AAPM Headquarters	Sharon Pierce
	Karen Wojdyla
	Emily Clarke
Continuing Education Committee	Guy Simmons, Chairman
Educational Council	Ed Chaney, Chairman
Publications Committee	John Laughlin, Chairman
	Ann E. Wright, Reviewer
AAPM President	Robert G. Waggener

CONTRIBUTORS

Benjamin R. Archer, M.S., Baylor College of Medicine, Houston, TX

Victor Bond, Ph.D., Brookhaven National Laboratory, Upton, Long Island, NY

Robert Brent, M.D., Thomas Jefferson University, Stein Research Center, Philadelphia, PA

Stuart Bushong, D.Sc., Baylor College of Medicine, Houston, TX

Vincent Collins, M.D., J.D., Rosewood General Hospital, Houston, TX

Michael J. Gelfand, M.D., University of Cincinnati, Cincinnati, OH

Earle C. Gregg, Ph.D., Case Western Reserve University, Cleveland, OH

James G. Kereiakes, Ph.D., University of Cincinnati, Cincinnati, OH

David K. Lacker, Director, Texas Department of Health Resources, Austin, TX

Harry R. Maxen, M.D., University of Cincinnati, Cincinnati, OH

Fred A. Mettler, Jr., M.D., M.P.H., University of New Mexico School of Medicine, Albuquerque, NM

Joseph M. Nannus, M.S., Texas Department of Health, Austin, TX

James M. Perdue, J.D., Attorney at Law, Houston, TX

William S. Properzio, Ph.D., U.S. Public Health Service, F.D.A., Rockville, MD

Liane Russell, Ph.D., Oak Ridge National Laboratory, Oak Ridge, TN

Eugene L. Saenger, M.D., University of Cincinnati, Cincinnati, OH

Paul Selby, Ph.D., Oak Ridge National Laboratory, Oak Ridge, TN

Robert J. Shalek, Ph.D., M.D. Anderson Tumor Institute and Hospital, Houston, TX

Stephan R. Thomas, Ph.D., University of Cincinnati, Cincinnati, OH

Robert G. Waggener, Ph.D., University of Texas Health Science Center San Antonio, TX

Edward W. Webster, Ph.D., Massachusetts General Hospital, Boston, MA

TABLE OF CONTENTS

I. BIOLOGICAL BASIS

   Genetic Effects of Low-Level Irradiation   1
      Paul B. Selby

   A Basis for Estimating the Risks of Low-Level   21
   Radiation
      Victor P. Bond

   Irradiation Damage to the Embryo, Fetus   33
   and Neonate
      Liane B. Russell

   Estimates of Cancer Risks from Low-Level Exposure   55
   to Ionizing Radiation: The BEIR Report 1980
      Edward W. Webster

   Update on the UNSCEAR Report   78
      Fred A. Mettler

   Discussion - Biological Basis   92

II. RISK EVALUATION AND REDUCTION

   Dose Evaluation in Diagnostic Radiology   105
      Stewart C. Bushong

   Dose Evaluation in Nuclear Medicine   125
      James G. Kereiakes, Stephen R. Thomas, Michael
      J. Gelfand, Harry R. Maxon, Eugene L. Saenger

   Dose Evaluation in Radiation Therapy   154
      Robert J. Shalek

   Risk/Benefit Considerations in Radiology   160
      Earle C. Gregg

   Methods of Risk Reduction in Diagnostic Radiology   177
      Stewart C. Bushong

   Methods of Risk Reduction in Nuclear Medicine   193
      James G. Kereiakes, Stephen R. Thomas,
      Eugene L. Saenger

   Methods of Risk Reduction in Radiation Therapy   216
      Robert J. Shalek

Radiation Teratogenesis: Fetal Risk and Abortion 223
   Robert Brent

A Radiation Risk Education Program – Local 253
   Stewart C. Bushong and Benjamin R. Archer

A Radiation Risk Education Program – National 267
   William S. Properzio

Discussion – Risk Evaluation and Reduction 275

III. MEDICO – LEGAL RESPONSIBILITIES

   State and Federal Regulation of Radiation Risk 283
      Joseph M. Nanus and David M. Lacker

   Official AAPM Response to ALARA 293
      Robert G. Waggener

   Liability from the View of the Practitioner 300
      Vincent P. Collins

   An Analysis of the Physician's Professional 309
   Liability for Radiation of the Fetus
      Jim M. Perdue

   Liability from the View of the Medical Physicist 321
      Robert J. Shalek

   Discussion – Medico-Legal Responsibilities 329

IV. INDEX 332

I. Biological Basis

GENETIC EFFECTS OF LOW-LEVEL IRRADIATION

P. B. Selby
Biology Division, Oak Ridge National Laboratory*
Oak Ridge, Tn. 37830

ABSTRACT

Recent estimates of the genetic effects of radiation by two widely recognized committees (BEIR III and UNSCEAR 1977) are based to a large extent on data collected in mice using either the (1) specific-locus method or (2) the approach of empirically determining the nature and extent of radiation-induced genetic damage to the skeleton. Both committees made use of doubling-dose and direct methods of estimating genetic hazard. Their estimates can be applied to assessments of risk resulting from medical irradiation in terms both of risk to the population at large and to the individual.

INTRODUCTION

Since H. J. Muller's discovery in 1927 that irradiation induces mutations in the fruit fly, much has been learned to permit estimation of the hazards to humans from exposure to low-level irradiation. Three recent reviews [1,2,3] of the subject present some of the information obtained in much more detail than will be possible in this paper. In spite of many scientific advances in this area, a recent editorial and a news article serve to illustrate the widespread public ignorance about effects of radiation. Thus a Washington Post editorial on December 17, 1979, stated that "the effects of low levels of radiation are simply unknown," and the Atomic Industrial Forum Press Info (No. 108, December 1979) reported that there are "no genetic effects found in mice from radiation" and that "exposure of every generation of humans since [480 B.C.] to one-third the lethal dose of radiation would have produced no noticeable effects today." None of the quotations from these sources reflect what is currently known. The purpose of this paper is to disseminate current knowledge about genetic risks from radiation.

Emphasis will be on gene mutations and small deficiencies instead of on gross chromosomal effects because the former contribute a larger part of the total risk. Also, no attempt will be made to deal with other than low-LET radiations (gamma and X rays). Experiments on mammals will be discussed almost entirely because such data are much more useful in estimating genetic risk than are those obtained on organisms more distantly related to humans.

*Research sponsored by the Office of Health and Environmental Research, U.S. Department of Energy under contract W-7405-eng-26 with the Union Carbide Corporation.

EFFECTS OF CONSIDERABLE IMPORTANCE IN ESTIMATING GENETIC RISK FOR HUMANS THAT WERE DISCOVERED BY USE OF THE SPECIFIC-LOCUS METHOD

The technique which has provided the most information about genetic effects of radiation is the specific-locus method, which was developed in the mouse by W. L. Russell [4]. It received its name because it permits the identification of recessive mutations at specific genetic loci. The mouse that is irradiated has the normal allele for both of its genes at each of seven specific loci. The irradiated wild-type mice are mated to special test-stock (T stock) mice, which are homozygous for a recessive mutation at each of these same loci. If no mutation occurs in any of these genes, all progeny of these matings will contain the normal allele from the irradiated parent and the recessive allele from the T stock parent for all seven loci. In this case, all offspring are normal in appearance. However, if a mutation occurs at one of the loci, the offspring that receives it has the new recessive allele from the irradiated parent and the recessive allele from the T stock parent, and, as a result, the easily recognized phenotype is expressed, thereby revealing the locus at which the mutation has occurred. A presumed mutant obtained in this way is submitted to a breeding test to be sure that the mutation is at the suspected locus and to learn more about it. Although other forms of the specific-locus test now exist, the vast majority of all specific-locus data collected to date have been obtained using the test stock developed by W. L. Russell in which the seven recessive mutations include six causing changes in coat color and one causing small ears. Both gene mutations and small deficiencies are recovered in mutants by this method.

Male

In the male, the germ-cell stage of overwhelming importance in risk estimation is the stem cell, the A_s spermatogonium [5]. All results discussed here, unless otherwise noted, deal with effects on this stage.

Major findings obtained using the specific-locus method are summarized below. Early risk estimates were based on the fruit fly, <u>Drosophila melanogaster</u>. Specific-locus studies suggest that the mutational response per locus per R in mouse spermatogonia is about 13 times [1,7] higher than that in fruit fly spermatogonia. This illustrates an important reason for basing risk estimates on data collected in experiments carried out on those species most closely related to humans in which mutagenesis can be studied.

Figure 1 shows the dose-response curve for acute low-LET radiation (72 to 90 R/min) and for chronic low-LET radiation (0.0007 to 0.8 R/min). The slope under chronic conditions is only 33% of that under acute conditions, or, in other words, the dose-rate correction factor is 3 in going from effects at high dose rates

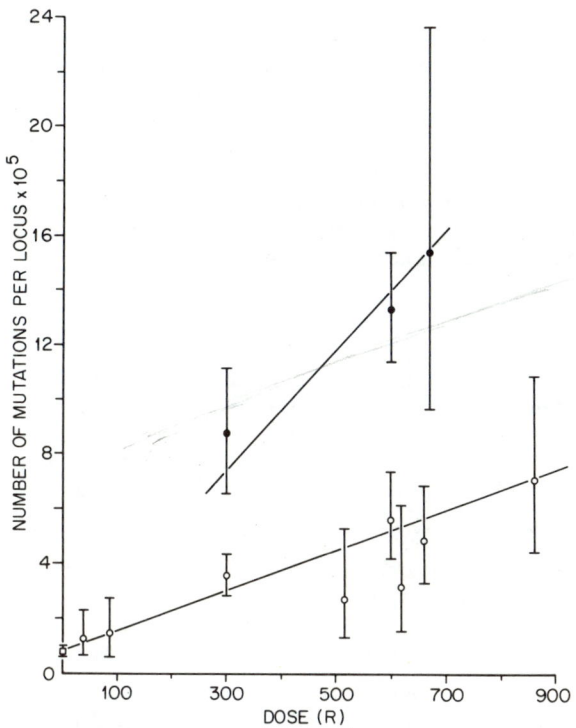

Fig. 1. Straight lines of best fit for specific-locus data obtained for mouse spermatogonia under chronic (o) and acute (●) exposure conditions [8,1]. Chronic experiments include all of those with unfractionated exposures at dose rates of 0.8 R/min and lower. Acute experiments include all of those with unfractionated exposures up to 670 R with dose rates from 72 to 90 R/min. 90% confidence intervals of data points are shown. □, control frequency. The parameters a, b_1, and b_2 in the formulas $\underline{Y}_{chronic} = a + b_1 x$ and $\underline{Y}_{acute} = a + b_2 x$ were estimated by the method of maximum likelihood. Data points at each dose, for some of which there were a few separate experiments, were combined in the figure but kept separate in computations.

to effects at low dose rates in spermatogonia [8,1]. It is of special interest that the magnitude of the dose-rate effect in the male does not change over the three-orders-of-magnitude range of exposure rates in chronic experiments. This is the basis for the belief that no matter how low the dose rate is in the male, there will be genetic effects induced by irradiation. In 1958, W. L. Russell [9] advanced his repair hypothesis to explain the dose-rate effect. He suggested that there is a repair process present in the cell which is saturated or damaged when large doses of radiation are administered at high dose rates. His hypothesis still stands as a very plausible explanation, but some alternative hypotheses cannot be ruled out.

The dose-rate effect was discovered when X rays were used for acute and gamma rays for chronic irradiation. Additional experiments have shown that the difference in response is not due to radiation quality alone, because a dose-rate effect was found for each type of radiation alone [9,10,11].

It will be noted in Figure 1 that the acute dose-response line below about 300 R is incomplete. This is because it is known that the dose response in this region is concave upward, but the exact shape of the curve is unknown. Fractionation experiments make it appear that an acute exposure of 10 R causes no more mutations than a chronic exposure of 10 R and that an acute exposure of 51 R likely induces about the same mutation frequency predicted by extending the acute line in Figure 1 downward to 51 R [12].

W. L. Russell [13] discovered that two large acute exposures to radiation, given 24 hours apart, cause an enhanced mutation frequency. Thus, for example, the induced mutation frequency following 100 R + 24 hr + 500 R of acute X irradiation is 1.9 times that found for an acute exposure to 600 R of X radiation [14]. This finding is of importance, as will be shown later, in extrapolating another type of mutation-rate data to the expected response under low-level irradiation conditions. To avoid confusion, it should be noted that this fractionation effect, by causing an enhancement of the damage, is in the opposite direction from common fractionation effects for somatic damage or from that described earlier for mutation induction with repeated acute fractions of 10 R.

One effect on a stage other than the stem cell that is of relevance to risks from medical irradiation is that the specific-locus mutation frequency is about two times higher [15] following irradiation of postspermatogonial stages with acute X radiation. In addition, there is much more radiation-induced gross chromosomal damage in some of the postspermatogonial stages [16]. For these reasons, it seems that any man whose testes were therapeutically exposed to a large dose of radiation would probably be well advised to practice strict birth control before the beginning of the long sterile period that should start by about nine weeks [17] following exposure to doses of 100 rads or more of X radiation. The sterile period would be very long, likely well over one year for exposures of 200 rad or more [17]. After the sterile period, or, if there is no sterile period, after very roughly three months (72 days for the duration of spermatogenesis [18] plus some extra time before sperm leave the body), genetic risk in men would be expected to have decreased to the lower level found for the stem cell.

Female

In the female mammal the germ-cell stage of by far the most importance in estimating genetic risk is the primary oocyte; there is no stem cell. There is, however, uncertainty over which primary oocytes in the female mouse are most relevant in estimating genetic hazard for women. Mutation induction can be most easily studied in the following three groups of mouse oocytes: (1) "mature and maturing oocytes," which are those ovulated within six weeks of irradiation of adult females, (2) "arrested oocytes," which are those ovulated more than six weeks after irradiation of adult females, and (3) those oocytes (probably pachytene and/or diplotene) that are present near the time of birth.

Figure 2 shows the weighted least-squares regression lines of specific-locus data obtained for mature and maturing oocytes in young virgin females in low-level (that is, large exposures made up of many small acute fractions or administered at a low dose rate) irradiation experiments and data points for the same oocytes irradiated with 400 R at 0.8 R/min and 90 R/min. Even though the mutation frequency of mature and maturing oocytes following acute high-dose exposure is about twice that of similarly irradiated

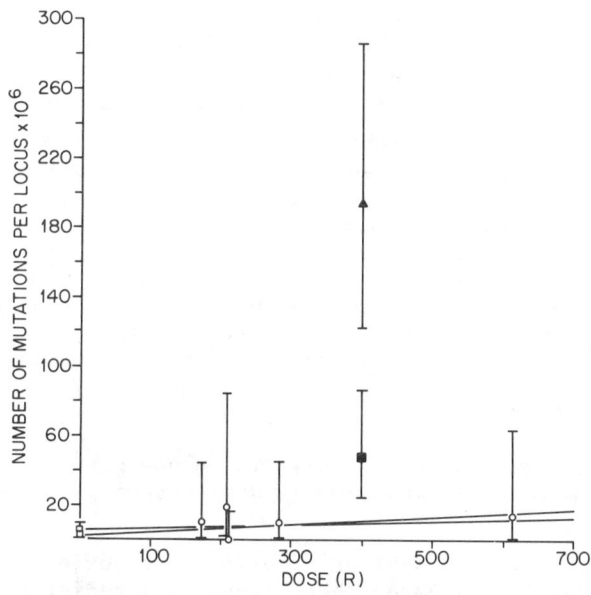

Fig. 2. Weighted least-squares regression lines of specific-locus data obtained for mature and maturing oocytes in young virgin females in low-level irradiation experiments (o) and data points for the same oocytes in experiments at 0.8 R/min (■) and 90 R/min (▲). 90% confidence intervals of data points are shown. □, control frequencies, for which there are two estimates. References 1, 11,19,20.

stem-cell spermatogonia, the dose-rate effect is clearly much more pronounced in them than it is in the spermatogonia. The mutation frequency per R continues to drop as the dose rate is lowered below 0.8 R/min, so that at 0.009 R/min there is not a statistically significant increase in the mutation frequency above that of the control[19]. The mutational response in these oocytes is also extremely low following 20 fractions of 10.6 R of acute X radiation (separated by at least 24 hours)[20]. For this fractionation, there is no suggestion that mutations are being induced by the irradiation, and the point estimate of the mutation frequency is only about one-half of the spontaneous mutation frequency in the male!

In large experiments, there is no evidence for the induction of mutations by radiation (acutely or chronically delivered) in the arrested oocytes of the adult mouse[21,19]. Also, there is no indication that mutations are induced when those oocytes present just before birth are exposed to 300 R of gamma radiation delivered at 0.8 R/min[22].

If the very conservative view is taken that the most mutable of these three groups of oocytes (the mature and maturing ones) should be used in estimating genetic risk for women, then genetic risk in women is unlikely to be any more than 44% of that in men[19], and it might be negligible. (The 44% figure is based on a regression line that includes data on old females, this line having a slope that indicates a statistically significantly higher mutation frequency than that of the control[19].)

The quotation from the Washington Post that "effects of low levels of radiation are simply unknown" is clearly incorrect as regards genetic effects. While it is true, for example, that it would not be feasible using current methodology to attempt to measure the effect of an exposure as small as 5 R (the maximum permissible exposure per generation to the general population from man-made radiation other than medical irradiation), the results of the many experiments utilizing low dose rates or small fractions give us considerable reason to be reasonably certain of what would happen even at doses much smaller than 5 R.

DOMINANT SKELETAL APPROACH IN THE MOUSE FOR ASSESSING THE MAGNITUDE OF RADIATION-INDUCED PHENOTYPIC DAMAGE

In the 1960's, U. H. Ehling[23] performed a series of experiments that strongly suggested that high-dose irradiation induces a rather high frequency of dominant mutations that cause malformations of the mouse skeleton. He demonstrated that certain classes of abnormalities were much more frequent among the F_1's of irradiated males than among those of controls. However, probably because only very few of his presumed mutants were given breeding tests to determine whether they were really mutants, his data were not used by committees in making estimates of overall genetic risk.

The approach of looking for induced phenotypic damage in the first generation, as in Ehling's experiments, was needed for evaluating genetic risk because it was extremely difficult to estimate overall genetic damage based on specific-locus data or any other genetic data then available. Thus, although the specific-locus method has been extremely useful in providing information about the physical and biological factors affecting the mutation rate (for example, dose rate, dose fractionation, sex, and cell stage), the actual mutation frequencies obtained using it cannot easily be converted to risk estimates. There is, for example, no way of knowing how representative the seven loci are of the genome as a whole. Furthermore, the specific-locus mutations are recessive mutations and almost all induced genetic disorders in the early generations following irradiation would have to be caused by dominant mutations. (Some of the specific-locus mutations have deleterious effects in heterozygotes, but the effects are difficult to measure.)

The author and his wife, working in Ehling's laboratory, performed an obvious follow-up experiment to Ehling's earlier work. Mice, of the same mouse strains used by him, were exposed to 100 R + 24 hr + 500 R of 60 R/min gamma radiation because a similar exposure regimen, although using X rays, had yielded the highest presumed dominant skeletal mutation frequency in his experiments. The important new feature of this experiment was that instead of killing the F_1's at four weeks of age, they were first raised and permitted to breed. As a result, in most cases, when an F_1 was found to have skeletal malformations that made it suspicious that a mutation was present, a sample of his offspring that could be examined to see if the anomalies were transmitted was already in existence. It was therefore possible to prove that certain abnormalities were caused by specific dominant mutations.

A total of 37 dominant skeletal mutations were found in the sample of 2646 F_1 offspring[24]. Of these 37, 31 were proved to be mutations by breeding tests[25] and 6, for which there were no progeny, were concluded to be mutations based on presumed-mutation criteria supported by the data[26]. Many of the mutations cause multiple effects, and if specific anomalies are counted, five of the 31 proved mutations caused one anomaly each, 19 caused 2-5 anomalies, five caused 6-10, and two caused 11-13. Individual dominant skeletal mutations often affect widely separated parts of the skeleton in specific ways. Effects occurred in almost all regions of the skeleton. The types of abnormalities occurring in most mutants were (1) fusions of bones or other changes in the number of separate bones, (2) gross changes in the shape of bones, or (3) shifts in the relative position of bones. Pictures of a few of the effects of two of the mutations help to show the types of damage that were detected. See Figures 4, 6, and 7.

The incomplete clavicles (Fig. 4) occur in all mice heterozygous for mutation 320, and this effect is accordingly said to have complete penetrance. In contrast, 17% of the mice with this mutation

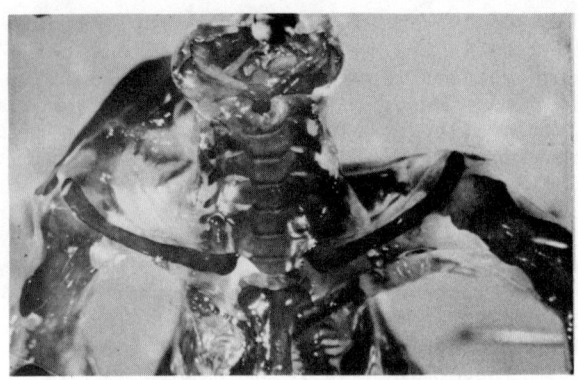

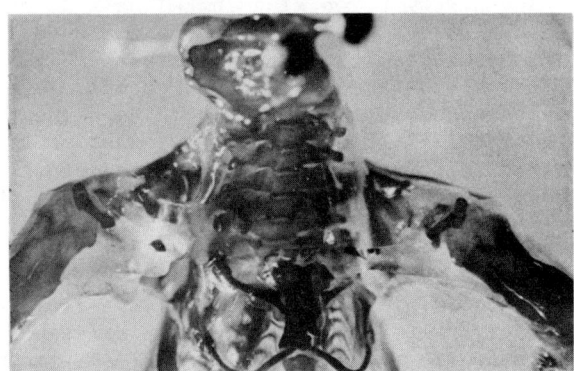

Fig. 4. Notice incomplete clavicles in mouse heterozygous for mutation 320.

have the interparietal bone completely normal, while 55%, 24%, 3%, and 1%, respectively, have this bone divided into 2 (Fig. 6), 3, 4, or 5 pieces. This subdivision of the interparietal is thus said to be a trait with incomplete penetrance. Clearly, the mutation has differing degrees of penetrance for differing degrees of severity of the syndrome. Mutation 320 causes a syndrome similar to one in humans known as cleidocranial dysplasia. The abnormalities shown in Fig. 7 are a few of the effects caused by a mutation that causes mice to have 8 additional specific bones in their skeletons.

On the basis of the 31 proved mutations, it seems to be a valid generalization that dominant mutations have incomplete penetrance for some or all of their effects. At least nine of the 31 have incomplete penetrance for every effect that they are known to cause. Mice can be greatly deformed without showing any sign of it externally. Very few dominant skeletal mutations cause any effect that is externally visible, and of those that do, most such effects occur in only a small proportion of carriers.

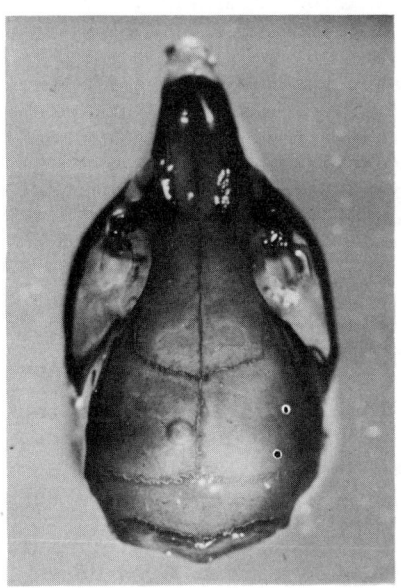

Fig. 5. Notice normal frontals and normal interparietal. Disregard air bubble in left parietal.

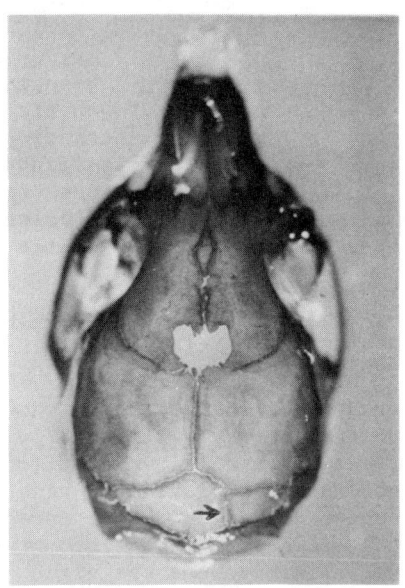

Fig. 6. Notice large frontal fontanelle and subdivision of interparietal into two pieces by a longitudinal suture (marked by arrow). Mouse is heterozygous for mutation 320.

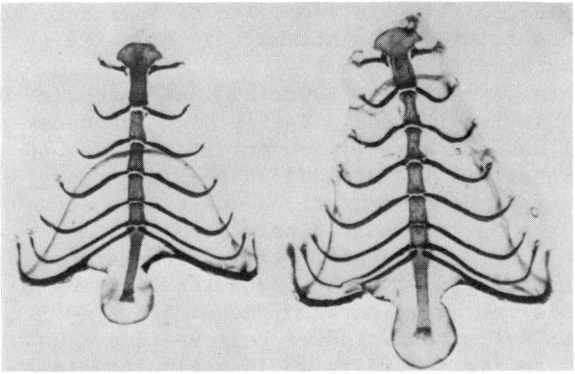

Fig. 7. Left sternum is normal. Right sternum, which is from a mouse heterozygous for mutation 565, has an additional sternebra. An additional pair of ribs is also attached to it.

FAILURE OF MULTIGENERATION IRRADIATION EXPERIMENTS TO SHOW AN ACCUMULATION OF SERIOUS GENETIC EFFECTS

Many attempts have been made to determine the extent, if any, of the accumulation of genetic effects in a population of rodents exposed to radiation generation after generation. It was reasoned that if most induced mutations have slight deleterious effects in heterozygotes, the continued accumulation of such changes, without comparable elimination by selection, would eventually cause an obvious and substantial effect on members of the population. With one exception [27], the results have been negative or equivocal [28]. The interpretation of the one positive result, which dealt with maze learning ability in rats, is not clear because it resulted from irradiation of postspermatogonial stages and a similar study using spermatogonial irradiation showed no effect [28]. Almost all of these studies have dealt with end points that are components of fitness, for example viability, fertility, and growth. Failure to find clear-cut accumulation of genetic damage in these experiments, one of which formed the basis for the quotations from the <u>Atomic Industrial Forum Press Info</u> given earlier, is now thought to result from failure to use the right sort of indicator traits. As noted by Green, one possible explanation for the negative results might have been the "relatively small sizes of the experiments so far conducted and their relative lack of power for discriminating small genetic differences in the presence of large amounts of nongenetic variability [28]." Thus, for example, the likelihood of demonstrating a slight decrease in the life span of mice (which has been attempted) seems much smaller than the likelihood of demonstrating a severalfold increase in the incidence of dominant skeletal mutations (which has not yet been attempted) following several generations of spermatogonial exposure.

The skeletal experiments described earlier have shown that high-dose irradiation induces a fairly high frequency of dominant mutations that cause skeletal abnormalities. Because most of these mutations can easily be maintained in the laboratory, there is every reason to expect that such mutations would have accumulated undetected in the earlier multigeneration experiments which were concerned with other end points. It is clear from the earlier multigeneration experiments that exposures of males to a few hundred R in each generation over scores of generations does not lead to extinction. However, such studies tell us almost nothing about the rate at which genetic disorders would accumulate in the population.

ESTIMATION OF GENETIC RISK TO HUMANS FROM RADIATION

The goal of risk estimation for genetic effects of radiation is to make a reasonable estimate of what effect a certain exposure to radiation would have upon the genetic burden of mankind. Would, for example, an exposure to one rem in 30 years cause a slight, medium, or large increase in this burden already in the first generation or, if not then, at some later time?

In order to understand genetic risk estimation, it is imperative that one have some comprehension of mankind's current genetic burden. This quantity is still imprecisely known; however, the estimate of it used by the BEIR III Committee (Committee on the Biological Effects of Ionizing Radiations of the National Academy of Sciences) in its recent report[3] is shown in Table I. The burdens for five patterns of inheritance are shown. These, when totaled, indicate that approximately 10.7% of liveborn humans can be expected to have, at some time, a serious genetic disorder. This 10.7% consists of thousands of individual disorders, most of which are extraordinarily rare and poorly understood. The last column in the Table lists a few of the more commonly known examples of these types of genetic disorders. Also shown is the number of individuals afflicted with each in the sample of 756,304 people studied in British Columbia in the major analysis[29] upon which the incidence figures are based.

Table I Current genetic burden of mankind

Type of genetic disorder	Current Incidence per million liveborn offspring[3]	Examples (number found in sample of 756,304 people studied in British Columbia[29])
Autosomal dominant	10,000	Osteogenesis imperfecta (30) Tuberous sclerosis (12)
X-linked		Hemophilia A (40)
Recessive	1,100	Cystic fibrosis (151) Albinism (28)
Irregularly inherited	90,000	Cleft palate (460) Schizophrenia (59)
Chromosomal aberrations	6,000	Down's syndrome (972)
Total	107,100	(Most are extremely rare and poorly understood.)

The risk estimates for gene mutations and small deficiencies, to be presented later, were derived using either the doubling-dose approach (also called the relative-mutation-risk approach) or the direct method of risk estimation. Because there are no human data showing that radiation induces transmitted genetic disorders, the data collected in experiments on animals must be used in estimating genetic risk. The 1977 UNSCEAR (United Nations Scientific Committee on the Effects of Atomic Radiation) Report[6] and the BEIR III

Report[3] both include estimates of genetic hazard for the first
generation following increased exposure and for genetic equilibrium.
Genetic equilibrium is what would occur many generations from now
when, theoretically, a steady-state in the incidence of genetic disorders would be reached if the mutation frequency abruptly changed
to a new level now and held constant. The UNSCEAR Committee made a
point estimate of risk, such an estimate being its best guess based
on current knowledge. In contrast, the BEIR III Committee expressed
risk as a range encompassing the degree of uncertainty that it
thought was reasonable.

Doubling-dose method

The doubling-dose approach is based on the assumption that the
likelihood of causing a disorder is, on the average, identical for
spontaneous and radiation-induced mutations. The doubling dose of
radiation is that amount expected to add as many new mutations each
generation as would occur spontaneously. A doubling of the current
incidence would not occur, however, until the doubling dose had been
applied over enough generations for equilibrium to occur between the
higher mutation frequency and selection. Even then, a doubling
would only occur for those disorders for which there is a direct
relationship between incidence and mutation frequency.

Genetic disorders are grouped into the few patterns of inheritance shown in Table I in order to make calculations less complex
and because a more sophisticated treatment is not justified by
current knowledge. The relationship between the incidence and the
mutation frequency differs among the many disorders. This relationship, which is called the mutational component, is a crucial para-
meter in applying the doubling-dose approach. Operationally, if the
mutational component of a group of disorders is 50%, this means
that at genetic equilibrium, following exposure to the doubling dose
of radiation from now until then, there would be 50% of a doubling
of the incidence of that group of disorders. For example, if there
were 10,000 per million now, there would be 15,000 per million then.
Both the BEIR III and 1977 UNSCEAR Committees assumed that the
autosomal dominants have a mutational component of 100%. The irregularly inherited disorders were assumed to have a mutational
component of 5-50% by the BEIR III Committee and of 5% by the 1977
UNSCEAR Committee. Additional assumptions about the persistence of
these classes of disorders in the population permit derivation of a
first-generation estimate from that at genetic equilibrium. For
example, if the equilibrium estimate is 100 induced disorders and
average persistence is assumed to be 5 generations, the first-
generation estimate for that category would be (100 ÷ 5) = 20
disorders.

In order to apply the doubling-dose approach, it is necessary
to have estimates, as described above, for each of the different
patterns of inheritance regarding current incidence, doubling dose,
mutational component, and, if anything besides a genetic equilibrium estimate is desired, persistence. These estimates come from

studies on humans, with the crucial exception of the doubling dose, which is based primarily, or entirely, on animal data. The estimate of the BEIR III Committee was based almost entirely on specific-locus data. The doubling dose was estimated to be 50-250 rem and 100 rad by the BEIR III and UNSCEAR Committees, respectively. Once the above estimates are in hand, calculations are easy. To illustrate with the risk estimate made by the 1977 UNSCEAR Committee for autosomal dominants and X-linked mutations combined, if the equilibrium estimate is desired for exposure of parents to 1 rad of protracted X or gamma rays, genetic risk = [(10,000 serious disorders X mutational component of 1) ÷ 100] = 100 serious genetic disorders.

Direct method

This very different approach to risk estimation is based on the author's recent determination of the extent of mutational damage occurring in the skeletons of the first-generation offspring of heavily irradiated mice. In the absence of data on this type of mutational damage following low-dose-rate exposures of spermatogonia, some of the many findings of W. L. Russell using the specific-locus method have been applied in extrapolating to expected results under low-level irradiation conditions. The estimate of genetic damage to the skeleton so obtained is expanded to what would be expected for all body systems and is restricted to that morphological damage expected to cause a serious handicap if identical effects occurred in humans.

Following a detailed discussion by V. A. McKusick and the author of the 37 individual dominant skeletal mutations found in his experiment, it was concluded that about one-half of them would, if they occurred in humans, result in a serious handicap. The other half would be expected to blend in with normal variation or be innocuous. The 1977 UNSCEAR Committee accepted this estimate, but the BEIR III Committee preferred to assume that the true value was in the range of one-quarter to three-quarters, which the author had suggested earlier[24].

In order to expand the genetic damage in the skeletal system to all body systems, thereby getting a total estimate of induced first-generation damage, the 1977 UNSCEAR Committee multiplied the frequency of dominant skeletal mutations by 10. This figure was decided upon in the following way. According to McKusick's tabulation of monogenic disorders in humans, 74 of 328 clinically important dominant disorders (about one-fifth of them) involve the skeleton[30]. This suggests that the number of skeletal mutations should be multiplied by about five to get the total number of dominant mutations. However, one-fifth is likely to be too large a fraction because of the ease of diagnosis of skeletal defects. On the other hand, it seemed unlikely that this fraction could be much lower than one-fifth because it is well known in humans and in other animals that many dominant mutations exhibit pleiotropism and affect more than one body system. In view of these considerations and of the opinions of the human geneticists, C. O. Carter and V. A. McKusick, it was felt that the factor of 10 was reasonable. The BEIR Committee assumed that the true value was in the range of 5 to 15.

At the present time, a direct estimate can be made for the first generation only. Although no data on the induction of dominant skeletal mutations in the female exist, the BEIR Committee assumed that maternal risk would not exceed 44% of that in the male based on the recent reanalysis of specific-locus data mentioned earlier [19]. The UNSCEAR Committee made a direct estimate for paternal irradiation only, but it stated that maternal risk would be expected to be low.

To illustrate the way in which the direct method calculations were made, both Committees divided the mutation frequency of 37 dominant skeletal mutations in 2646 offspring by 600 R (the exposure), by 3 (the dose-rate effect), and by 1.9 (the fractionation effect) to give the expected induced mutation frequency for 1 R of low-level spermatogonial irradiation. The remainder of the calculation, for which only the 1977 UNSCEAR version is shown, consisted of multiplying the frequency so calculated, which is 4×10^{-6} dominant skeletal mutations per R, by $\frac{1}{2}$ (the severity factor), by 10 (the factor for extrapolating to all body systems), and by 1 million (the number of progeny in which the incidence was to be estimated). The estimate is thus 20 serious genetic disorders, and it applies to (1) those conditions in humans known as autosomal dominants, (2) those conditions in humans known as irregularly inherited disorders that are caused by dominants with incomplete penetrance, and (3) any chromosomal-aberration disorders in humans that mimic dominant inheritance.

Risk estimates

Tables II and III show the genetic risk estimates agreed upon by the UNSCEAR and BEIR III Committees, respectively. The estimates for chromosomal aberrations are included even though they are not discussed in detail in this paper. The risk estimates must be compared with the current incidences, which are shown in Table I, in order to put them into perspective.

HUMAN STUDIES

As mentioned earlier, there is no clear evidence in humans of radiation-induced transmitted genetic damage. There are data, however, from men exposed in Hiroshima and Nagasaki that are on the borderline of statistical significance [31]. These data concerned mortality during the first 17 years of life among children with one or both parents exposed. From the data obtained following the atomic bombings in Japan, minimal doubling doses can be calculated. For men this value is 138 rads; for women it is over 1000 rads. The average for the two sexes is about 240 rads [31,3]. The higher the

Table II UNSCEAR 1977 risk estimates[6]

Classification of disorders	Serious genetic disorders induced by an average population exposure to 1 rad of low-dose, low-dose-rate, low-LET irradiation in a 30-year generation, per million liveborn offspring		
	First generation by doubling-dose method	First generation by direct method	Genetic equilibrium
Autosomal dominant and X-linked	20	20 in ♂, probably fewer in ♀	100
Irregularly inherited	5		45
Recessive	relatively few		very slow increase
Chromosomal aberrations	38	2–10 in ♂, probably fewer in ♀	40
Total	63	22–30 in ♂, probably fewer in ♀	185

doubling dose: the lower the risk. Accordingly, because the doubling dose based on specific-locus data in the BEIR III report is 50–250 rem, the minimal estimate in humans of 240 rem suggests that estimates of doubling doses based on mouse experiments likely lead to an overestimation of genetic risk. Nonetheless, the safe approach seems to be to base the estimates on the animal data, which come from much more controlled and numerous experiments and deal with end points more directly related to genetic hazard. It should be noted that the hint of an effect in men, but not in women, is consistent with the conclusion, based on mouse studies, that genetic risk is lower in women.

APPLICATION OF GENETIC RISK ESTIMATES TO ASSESSMENTS OF RISK RESULTING FROM MEDICAL IRRADIATION

According to the BEIR III report, the estimated annual average genetically significant dose equivalent rate of exposure to medical and dental X rays is 20 mrem/yr for patients and <0.4 mrem/yr for occupational exposures. The corresponding figures for exposure to radiopharmaceuticals is 2–4 mrem/yr for patients and <0.15 mrem/yr for occupational exposures. In contrast, background radiation amounts to 82 mrem/yr. There are several ways in which the risk

Table III BEIR III risk estimates[3]

Classification of disorders	Serious genetic disorders induced by an average population exposure to 1 rem per 30-year generation, per million liveborn offspring	
	First generation[a]	Genetic equilibrium
Autosomal dominant and X-linked	5-65	40-200
Irregularly inherited		20-900
Recessive	very few, effects in heterozygotes accounted for in top row	very slow increase
Chromosomal aberrations	less than 10[b]	only increases slightly
Total	5-75	60-1100

[a] Used direct method only.
[b] Majority of Committee feels that it is considerably closer to zero, but one member feels that it could be as much as 20.

estimates described in this paper can be applied to comprehending likely effects of medical and dental radiation. Some of these will be given, and, in all cases, the estimates of the BEIR III Committee will be applied.

It is of interest to estimate the number of individuals born in the United States each year who will at some time have a serious handicap caused by a radiation-induced mutation resulting from medical or dental irradiation of some ancestor. If, for simplicity, we assume that the annual average genetically significant exposure per person to such radiation in the United States is 22 mrem/yr, then in a generation of 30 years the average exposure per person is 0.66 rem. Further, let us assume that all medical and dental (henceforward referred to simply as medical) exposure in the USA to date is equivalent to 60 years, or 2 generations, at the above exposure rate and that 3 million babies are born alive in our country each year. The risk after two consecutive generations of exposure would be somewhat less than twice the risk after one generation of exposure, but the error when multiplying by two should lead to only a small overestimate. The BEIR III first-generation risk estimate for 1 rem is 5-75 serious genetic disorders per million liveborn offspring. Accordingly, roughly [(2) X (5-75) X (0.66) X (3 million ÷ 1 million)] or 20-300 children born in the USA each year can be expected to have, at some time, a serious genetic disorder induced by medical irradiation. If the per person exposure earlier in this century was actually much more than 0.66 rem, the above estimate is, of course, too small to an important extent. It should be kept in mind that the above estimate is more precisely the estimate of the genetic burden induced by two generations of medical exposure at current dose-equivalent rates.

If medical exposure stays constant at 22 mrem per year and if the number of births per year in the USA remains about 3 million, when genetic equilibrium occurs many centuries from now, roughly [(0.66) X (60-1100) X (3 million ÷ 1 million)] or 120-2200 children born in the USA each year would be expected to have, at some time, a serious genetic disorder induced by medical irradiation. No one knows exactly how soon genetic equilibrium would occur even in the unlikely event that exposure to radiation really stayed constant as described. It should be realized, however, that the medically induced genetic burden might begin to approach genetic equilibrium levels after only two or three centuries if the persistences and mutational components are anything like those assumed by the UNSCEAR Committee [6].

This paper does not intend to suggest that medical irradiation should not be used. However, a useful contrast for making clear the distinction between induced genetic and induced somatic effects (for example, radiation carcinogenesis and teratogenesis) of medical irradiation is provided by comparing the effects of a complete cessation of all medical exposures on the induced incidences of these different effects. It is obvious that if no more medical irradiation occurred after March 1980, no individuals born in 1981 or later would ever suffer from any somatic effects resulting from medical irradiation. In contrast, OVER ALL TIME, a total of roughly 7,200-132,000 persons in the USA would be expected to have, at some time, a serious genetic handicap resulting from mutations induced by medical irradiations before April 1980. It must be emphasized that this huge number of handicapped persons would occur in a vast, and unknown, number of offspring born over many centuries, and the incidence would not be expected to exceed 300 in any one year. This, it should be recalled, is 300 out of roughly 321,000 persons born each year in our country who will at some time have a serious genetic disorder.

The basis of the estimate just given can be understood by realizing that at genetic equilibrium exactly as many future genetic effects are induced as are selected out of the population in any one generation. It follows from this that the total of all genetic effects to be expressed <u>over all generations</u> as the result of exposure to one generation is the same as the total genetic effects found in <u>one generation</u> in the equilibrium situation. In other words, if the genetic equilibrium estimate of a class of disorders is 100 disorders per the number of children born in one generation, and if one-fifth are eliminated by selection in each generation, then, if only one generation is exposed, the first-generation incidence is 20. If no more irradiation is administered, because of transmission of the mutations induced in the first generation to later generations, the number of disorders in generations 2, 3, 4, ... n is 16, 12.80, 10.24, ... n', and the sum of the disorders over generations 1 to n is 100, which is the equilibrium estimate. In our case, for simplicity, we have assumed that medical irradiation to date is equivalent to two generations (that is, 60 years) of exposure at the annual rate of 22 mrem/yr. and that the birth rate remains 3 million offspring per year. It was shown earlier that the equilibrium estimate for this exposure rate is 120-2200 seriously handicapped individuals per year, which equals 3,600-66,000 in a 30-year generation. Thus, an OVER ALL TIME estimate for two generations of such exposure would be about twice this or 7,200-132,000 persons. This large number of handicapped persons, even though it represents only a very small increment over mankind's normal genetic burden, is a sobering reminder that medical exposures should be kept as low as possible.

The first-generation risk estimate can be used in a considerably different application to medical irradiation. To illustrate, assume that a man was exposed to 100 R of gonadal radiation as the result of therapy. This was a single exposure of gamma or X rays lasting several minutes. Five years later his wife becomes pregnant, and the couple is concerned whether or not the fetus should be aborted in view of the father's large exposure. To help answer this question, one can proceed as follows. The paternal portion of first-generation risk is 5-45 handicapped individuals (for gene mutations and small deficiencies alone) per million liveborn for each rem of protracted irradiation. Because the example deals with acute irradiation, this range must be multiplied by 3. The risk from this type of genetic damage would thus be [(100) X (15-135)] in one million or 0.15-1.35%. The risk from chromosomal aberrations for such exposure would be expected to be about 0.01-0.1% according to application of the BEIR III Report. Putting these estimates into perspective, the risk to the average man in the population that a given child will at some time have a serious genetic disorder is about 10.7% according to Table I. The risk to the average man that a given child will someday have a serious handicap of genetic, environmental, or unknown origin is about [10.7% + 0.1% + 2.7%]^{29} or 13.5%. The total risk of the irradiated man in question, assuming that no consideration is given to genetic disorders that he may or may not have, is thus about [13.5% + 0.16-1.45%] or 13.66-14.95%. In other words, an exposure this large to one individual would cause a rather small increase in his normal risk.

It must be cautioned that the assessments of risk from medical irradiation given in this section are an attempt, by using simplifying assumptions, to apply the BEIR III risk estimates to some difficult questions of concern to those in the medical profession. No attempt has been made to use precise assumptions in applying the risk estimates because there is no way precise assessments could be made in view of uncertainties as to the risk estimates themselves. The assessments made, however, should provide an understanding of the approximate effects of medical irradiation in inducing genetic

disorders. Care must be taken in extending the examples given to
other situations. For example, irradiation of different germ-cell
stages or with high-LET radiations might alter applications to
medical irradiation in ways unexpected by someone unfamiliar with
the data on which genetic risk estimates are based.

Risk estimates for genetic effects cannot easily be compared
with those for somatic effects to see which type of induced damage
is of greater importance. Not only is the time scale when somatic
and genetic effects occur very different, as explained earlier, but
it is unrealistic, for example, to equate one fatal radiation-
induced cancer at age 65 with one radiation-induced genetic disorder
that results in death after 20 years of being institutionalized for
profound mental retardation, or, alternatively, to equate one fatal
radiation-induced leukemia at an early age with one radiation-
induced late-onset genetic disorder.

It is hoped that this presentation will (1) lead to better
decisions as to the benefit-risk ratio of certain medical
irradiation procedures and (2) stimulate further efforts in
eliminating unnecessary exposures.

REFERENCES

1. P. B. Selby, The Mouse in Biomedical Research (Academic Press, N. Y., in press), chapter "Radiation Genetics" in volume 1.
2. W. L. Russell, Rochester International Conference on Environmental Toxicity, 13th, 1980, Measurement of Risks (Plenum Press, N. Y., in press), chapter "Problems and solutions in the estimation of genetic risks from radiation and chemicals."
3. Committee on the Biological Effects of Ionizing Radiations, The Effects on Populations of Exposure to Low Levels of Ionizing Radiation (National Academy Press, Washington, D. C., 1980).
4. W. L. Russell, Cold Spring Harbor Symp. Quant. Biol. $\underline{16}$, 327 (1951).
5. E. F. Oakberg, Anat. Rec. $\underline{169}$, 515 (1971).
6. United Nations Scientific Committee on the Effects of Atomic Radiation, Sources and Effects of Ionizing Radiation. A/32/40: G. A. Official Records, 32nd Session Suppl. No. 40 (1977).
7. W. L. Russell, Am. Nat. $\underline{90}$, 69 (1956).
8. W. L. Russell, E. M. Kelly, personal communication, manuscript being prepared for Proc. Natl. Acad. Sci. USA.
9. W. L. Russell, L. B. Russell, E. M. Kelly, Science $\underline{128}$, 1546 (1958).
10. W. L. Russell, L. B. Russell, E. M. Kelly, Int. J. Radiat. Biol. Relat. Stud. Phys. Chem. Med. $\underline{Suppl.}$ 311 (1960).
11. W. L. Russell, Repair from Genetic Radiation (Pergamon, Oxford, 1963), p. 205 and p. 231.
12. M. F. Lyon, R. J. S. Phillips, H. J. Bailey, Mutat. Res. $\underline{15}$, 185 (1972).
13. W. L. Russell, Proc. Natl. Acad. Sci. USA $\underline{48}$, 1724 (1962).
14. W. L. Russell, Genetics $\underline{50}$, 282 (1964).
15. W. L. Russell, J. W. Bangham, J. S. Gower, Proc. 10th Int. Cong. Genetics, Vol. 2 (Univ. of Toronto Press, 1958) p. 245.

16. W. L. Russell, Radiation Biology, Vol. 1 (McGraw-Hill, N. Y., 1954), p. 825.
17. M. J. Rowley, D. R. Leach, G. A. Warner, C. G. Heller, Radiat. Res. 59, 665 (1974).
18. E. F. Oakberg, Effects of Radiation on Meiotic Systems (Intern. Atomic Energy Agency, Vienna, 1968) p. 3.
19. W. L. Russell, Proc. Natl. Acad. Sci. USA 74, 3523 (1977).
20. M. F. Lyon, R. J. S. Phillips, Mutat. Res. 30, 375 (1975).
21. W. L. Russell, Brookhaven Symp. Biol. 20, 179 (1967).
22. P. B. Selby, S. S. Lee, E. M. Kelly, Genetics 94, s94 (1980).
23. U. H. Ehling, Genetics 54, 1381 (1966).
24. P. B. Selby, P. R. Selby, Mutat. Res. 43, 357 (1977).
25. P. B. Selby, P. R. Selby, Mutat. Res. 51, 199 (1978).
26. P. B. Selby, P. R. Selby, Mutat. Res. 50, 341 (1978).
27. H. B. Newcombe, J. F. McGregor, Genetics 50, 1065 (1964).
28. E. L. Green, Annu. Rev. Genet. 2, 87 (1968).
29. B. K. Trimble, J. H. Doughty, Ann. Hum. Genet. 38, 199 (1974).
30. V. A. McKusick, Mendelian Inheritance in Man: Catalogs of Autosomal Dominant, Autosomal Recessive, and X-linked Phenotypes, 4th ed. (The Johns Hopkins Univ. Press, Baltimore, 1975).
31. J. V. Neel, H. Kato, W. L. Schull, Genetics 76, 311 (1974).

A BASIS FOR ESTIMATING THE RISKS OF LOW-LEVEL RADIATION*

V. P. Bond
Brookhaven National Laboratory, Upton, NY 11973

Early effects of radiation (cellular or organ changes, illness and even death within hours, days or a few weeks of exposure) assume clinical significance only at doses to the whole body in excess of about 150 rads. Because such exposure levels would be expected to be encountered rarely, only a brief outline of consequences is provided here.

Radiation is similar to all other potentially hazardous and lethal agents, in that at high doses it can produce organ injury, illness and death. The principal site of action is on dividing cells in the proliferative organ systems, with delay and inhibition of mitosis, cell death, cellular depletion in vital organ systems, organ malfunction, and serious illness and possible death in the heavily exposed. The most important cellular site of action is at the stem cell level, so that the source of supply of mature functional cells is temporarily cut off with resultant impaired function of that organ and of the individual. If the individual can survive the period of severe cellular depletion, with or without treatment, then the damaged organ will spontaneously regenerate the normal complement of cells and the individual will survive. If therapeutic efforts are inadequate or regeneration cannot occur soon enough, then the individual may succumb because of the failure of the organ system.

Cellular depletion in organs can be detected at doses as low as 50 rads, and easily at doses of 100-150 rads, e.g., in the bone marrow, in the lymphopoietic organs and in the circulating lymphocyte count, and in the testis. With whole-body radiation doses in roughly the 200-400 rad range, severe bone marrow depletion leads in time to symptoms related primarily to depletion of neutrophiles and platelets in the blood. The consequent signs and symptoms are those that would be expected, i.e., infection in a variety of body locations and severe bleeding into any of a number of organs and possibly death. Death occurs mainly between 20 and 40 days after exposure. Effective treatment consists of "reverse isolation", neutrophile transfusions and large doses of antibiotics to control infection, and fresh platelet transfusions to control bleeding. Replacement of stem cells by bone marrow transfusions can be attempted at very high doses.

At doses in excess of about 1,000 rads, the "gastrointestinal syndrome" is seen, with the "central nervous system" syndrome appearing at doses in excess of about 1500 rads. Extensive descriptions of early effects may be found in several references provided[1-5].

Although a variety of late somatic effects can occur in survivors of exposure to high doses of radiation (particularly following partial body exposure in which the localized damage permits survival at very high doses), a potential increase in cancer is the principal and most serious late effect. There is no question that radiation <u>does cause</u> an increase in cancer in man at doses of the order of 100

* American Association of Physicists in Medicine, San Antonio, Texas, 26-28 March 1980.

rads (of low-LET radiation). At lower doses, it is difficult or impossible to demonstrate such an increase even in large exposed populations. Hence indirect means (interpolation or extrapolation with human data; use of animal data and models) must be employed to provide estimates of possible effects at low doses and dose rates.

Central to estimating the incidence (risk) of carcinogenic and genetic effects in man are incidence (risk) vs. exposure relationships, and their variation with exposure rate. In Fig. 1, incidence is plotted against exposure (or dose) and typical data available on the human being (e.g., for human cancer from X- or gamma-ray exposure) are represented as the hypothetical data points at relatively high doses, e.g., 100 or more rads. Of principal interest in the context of radiation protection is the very low dose and/or dose rate region, in which no excess incidence is detectable. Estimation of excess incidence at these low doses and dose rates thus must be obtained indirectly, and linear interpolation between background dose and incidence, and the data points at high doses and dose rates (curve B, slope α_L in Fig. 1) is frequently used for

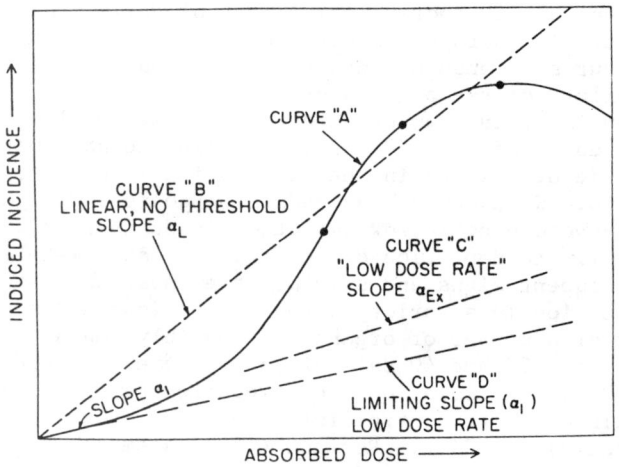

Fig. 1. Schematic curves of incidence vs. absorbed dose. The curved solid line for high absorbed doses and high dose rates (curve A) is the "true" curve. The linear, no threshold dashed line (curve B) was fitted to the three indicated experimental points and the origin. Slope α_1 indicates the essentially-linear portion of curve A at low doses. The dashed curve C, marked "low-dose rate", slope α_{Ex}, represents experimental high-dose data obtained at low dose rates. This experimental low dose rate curve may in principle, at very low dose rates, approach or become indistinguishable from the extension of the solid curve of slope α_1, the dashed curve D labeled "limiting slope (α_1), low-dose rate" in Fig. 1

the purpose. This relationship is referred to as "linear, no threshold", and is to be contrasted with the curvilinear (curve A) relationship also shown in Fig. 1. Obviously, the linear relationship predicts a greater degree of excess incidence at low doses, than does the curvilinear function.

The low-dose part of curve A in Fig. 1 in principle has the slope "α" in the formulation,

$$I = \alpha D + \beta D^2, \qquad (1)$$

in which I is the incidence of effect, D is dose and α and β are constants (an additional "cell killing" factor would have to be introduced to characterize the higher dose regions of curve A). As shown below, this function appears to represent well a large amount of relevant data in "simple" cellular systems. Curve C approximates the slope obtained experimentally at low dose rates, i.e., if the doses represented by the three solid-circle "data points" were delivered at lower and lower dose rates, the data points would move downward and approach curve C. The limiting effect of lowering the dose rate would in principle be the superposition of curve C and curve D, the extension of the low-dose α_1 slope of curve A. Thus to a very large degree, the effect of lowering the dose or the dose rate is the same, and the two are often referred to as being interchangeable. The factor by which the linear, no threshold function may overestimate the incidence at low doses and dose rates is the ratio of the slopes of curve B, to curve C (or ultimately, curve D).

Relationships among dose and dose rate can be evaluated most quantitatively in "simple" cellular systems, in which the influence of both variables can be studied in detail. For this purpose, Tradescantia data[6-8] are shown in Fig. 2, in which the incidence of pink mutant events scored in the stamen hairs is plotted against dose. A log-log plot is used to make clear the extent and nature of the data at very low doses, i.e., below 10 rads. The data (Fig. 2) indicate clearly the proportionality of dose and incidence at low doses, and the lack of a threshold for incidence of effect. The frequency of events is extremely low. The data up to about 100 or more rads can be represented well by the function $I = \alpha D + \beta D^2$ (the flattening of the curve due to "cell killing", obviously important at higher doses, is not considered here).

The effect of dose rate is seen in Fig. 3, in which are shown on arithmetic coordinates (upper curve) essentially the same data shown in Fig. 2. The two central curves with data points represent lower dose rates than used for the uppermost curve. The lower curve marked "X" represents the extension of the "αD" part of the low-dose curve in Fig. 2, corresponding to curve C (and D) in Fig. 1. The lowermost curve marked "γ" is analogous to the "X" curve in Fig. 3, and is obtained experimentally if γ- instead of X-rays are used to determine the lower part of the curve in Fig. 2[9].

The influence of average dose rate (or exposure time) is seen in more detail in Fig. 4[8]. A dose of about 80 rads was delivered at progressively lower dose rates. The incidence/80 rads is seen to

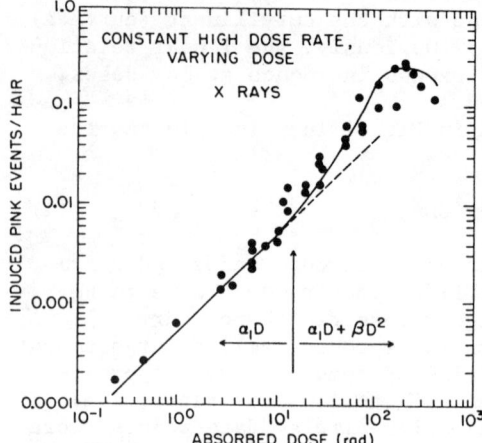

Fig. 2. X-ray dose-response curve, induced pink mutations in <u>Tradescantia</u>, on log-log plot to show detail in the low dose range. The solid circles indicate experimental points at high dose rate. Note that the low dose portion of the solid curve and its dashed-line extrapolation have a slope of unity, i.e., a linear, no threshold dose-effect relationship. The increased slope at higher doses indicates that the response in the intermediate dose range involves a higher exponent of dose (and a "cell killing" component at high doses). See text for explanation of the "$\alpha_1 D$" and "$\alpha_1 D + \beta D^2$" portions of the curve

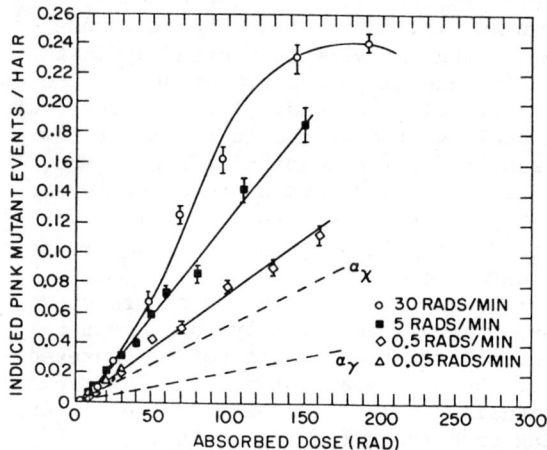

Fig. 3. Dose-response curves for pink mutant events/hair after X-irradiation at 0.05 and 0.5 rad/min (combined in one line), 5 and 30 rad/min. The dashed lines represent the alpha terms in Eq. 1, for X-rays and gamma rays

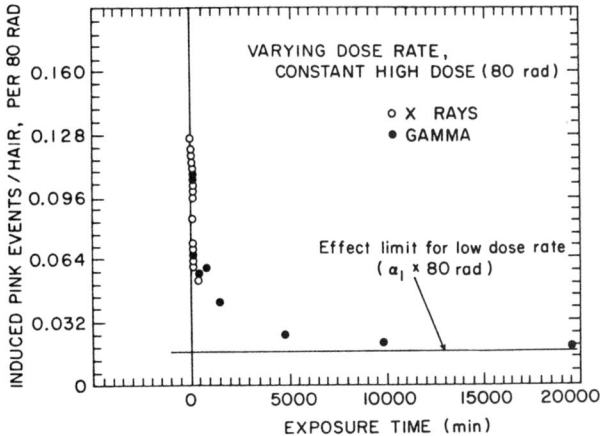

Fig. 4. Effect of dose rate on the effectiveness of a single large dose of about 80 rad, for the induction of pink mutations in Tradescantia. The horizontal line represents the expected limiting low dose rate value for 80 rad (i.e., from the linear term of Eq. 1, the value would be $2.1 \times 10^{-4} \times 80 = 0.017$). Note that the effect per 80 rad decreases appreciably as the exposure time is increased, and that the effect/80 rad at the lowest dose rates approaches asymtotically the limiting "αD" value for gamma radiation

decrease progressively as the dose rate is lowered (exposure time lengthened), and the slope (incidence/80 rads) is seen to approach asymptotically the (gamma) incidence/rad at low doses, as seen in Figs. 1 and 3. One can thus see that the lower limit of the incidence per rad (slope) at very low doses, seen in the context of a full exposure-incidence curve (Figs. 1 and 3) involving high doses and dose rates, is the same as the lower limit of the incidence/rad (slope) using high doses delivered at low dose rates.

The linear and quadratic components of incidence (Figs. 1 and 3) are thus separable equally well, by lowering either the dose or the dose rate. The two components are shown separately in Fig. 5. The "sub-effect" damage of the quadratic component can be repaired completely and at low dose rates is repaired completely before it can contribute to a visible lesion. The linear component is without threshold and shows a definite increase in incidence at small (fraction of a rad) or large doses, independent of dose rate.

These same dose-dose rate relationships appear to represent adequately a large amount of data in "higher" systems, including carcinogenesis and mutagenesis in the mammal (Figs. 6 and 7) and man[10-15]. This does not mean necessarily that the model applies literally ("models are to be used, not believed"). The relationship does, however, provide a logical, operational framework in which to consider mutagenesis and carcinogenesis.

The following points, based on the above model, are key to an adequate understanding of the risk of potential late effects of "low-level"[a] radiation exposure in man:

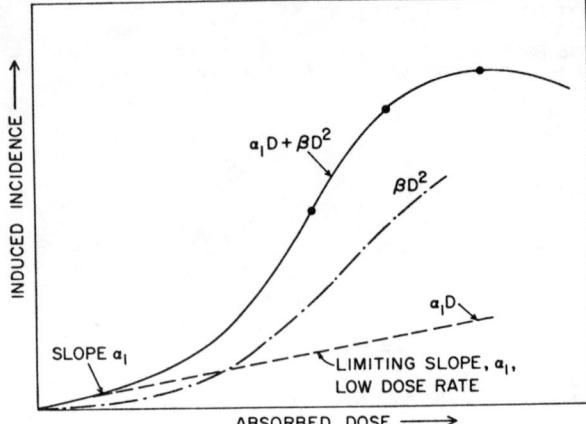

Fig. 5. The linear-quadratic dose response curve for <u>Tradescantia</u>, with the linear and squared components plotted separately (a "cell killing" factor would be needed to describe the high dose region of the curve marked "$\alpha_1 D + \beta D^2$")

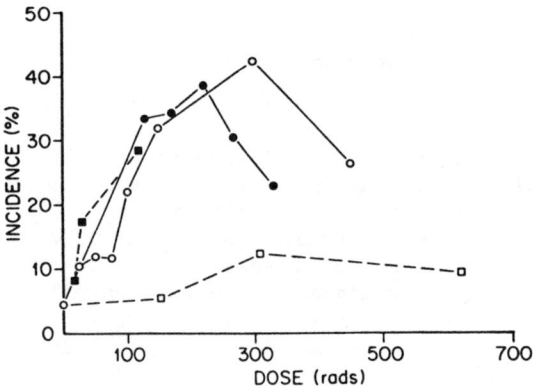

Fig. 6. Incidence of myeloid leukemia in RF male mice. Shaded symbols denote results obtained with fast neutron irradiation; open symbols denote results obtained with X-rays. Solid lines denote results obtained with acute (single) exposures; dashed lines denote results obtained with chronic (23-h, daily) exposures

1) High doses of radiation are known to cause a small increase in the background cancer rate among those exposed, and are believed to increase slightly the normal incidence of "genetic defects" in subsequent generations. Radiation carcinogenesis has been recognized since about the year 1900; genetic effects since 1927. The extent of radiation carcinogenesis became fully appreciated when the results of large scale epidemiological studies began to appear in the late 40s and in the 50s. In the Hiroshima and Nagasaki

studies, from a total of 285,000 registrants (survivors) exposed at all dose levels, 70,000 deaths from natural causes had occurred by 1974. No more than 500 of these deaths (about 0.7%) had resulted from radiation-induced cancer of any kind. No increase in genetic effects has been found to date in the first generation offspring of those exposed.

2) Radiation carcinogenesis and mutagenesis involve, to a good first approximation, randomly-induced events, and the diseases induced are indistinguishable from those occurring "naturally" or from other carcinogenic/mutagenic agents. Thus cause and effect can be related only inferentially and statistically, and not on an individual case basis. This situation contrasts with the circumstances characteristic of other common, largely by chance (random, "stochastic", or "accidental") injuries and deaths (e.g., auto accidents, electrical shock deaths, severe and/or lethal drug reactions, falls, drownings, etc.). Here, cause and effect on an individual basis is immediately evident. With carcinogenesis, however, no individual case of cancer can at present be identified, other than on a probabilistic basis, with any radiation exposure regardless of dose.

3) Radiogenic cancer is difficult to demonstrate at high doses, and essentially impossible to observe or quantify at low doses even with very large populations. The normal or background incidence of cancer is very large (about 400,000 cancer deaths/yr in the United States). Thus, although a large amount of data has been accumulated on human populations exposed to low doses of radiation, these data are all "negative" in the sense that no detectable increase in incidence has been observed. The incidence is too small at low doses to allow one to differentiate any possible increase from the large background incidence. The "signal to noise ratio" is simply too small.

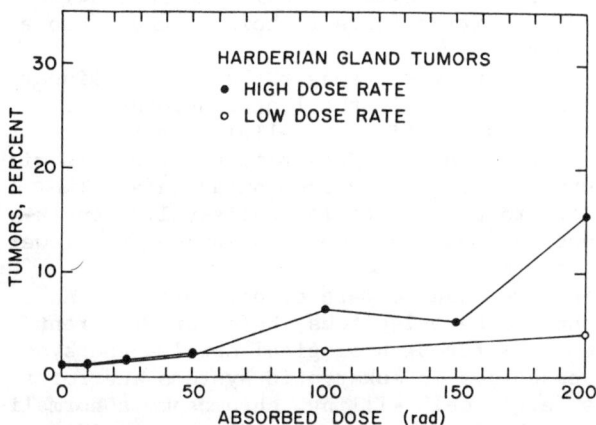

Fig. 7. Incidence of Harderian gland tumors in RFM mice after ^{137}Cs gamma ray irradiation. 45 rad/min●; 8.3 rad/day 0.

4) From radiobiological experience in lower biological systems (see foregoing) and from theory it can be reasonably postulated that there is "no threshold" for genetic effects, and for a number of induced cancers. Thus the oft-heard warning, "any amount of radiation, no matter how small, has some probability of producing harm in a population." (The phrase, "has some probability of producing" often is erroneously translated "will cause some harm".) The first statement would be equally accurate if reversed and expressed positively, i.e., "the odds are heavily in one's favor that with any given low dose of radiation, there is almost no chance at all of inducing harm of any kind in an exposed individual or in a population".

5) To estimate the potential for a given effect at low doses, it is necessary to interpolate (often mislabeled "extrapolate") over the low dose region. The process of interpolation involves the assumption of some functional relationship between increased cancer incidence and dose (see Figure 1), i.e., a curve of some shape must be drawn through the data points at high doses where positive human data exists, and zero excess effect (total incidence minus background) at zero dose (total dose minus background). The estimated incidence of effects at low doses is dependent upon the shape of the curve used and can differ substantially.

6) A major constituent of the "radiation controversy" is disagreement over the shape of the line (or curve) to be drawn to connect the data points at high doses, with zero incidence and dose. Extensive radiobiological experience with lower systems, including mutagenesis and carcinogenesis in experimental mammalian animals, indicates that the correct curve has a shape similar to that of curve A in Figure 1. The "linear hypothesis" is illustrated by the straight line no-threshold relationship depicted as curve B, Figure 1. This relationship, although held by a few scientists to be the correct function, is considered by most scientists to represent an upper limit or "worst case" situation. A very small group of scientists feel that even the linear hypothesis is unconservative. The data used to support this position fails to hold up under close scrutiny in almost every case.

7) Radiobiological data suggest strongly that a curvilinear relationship is much more likely than is the linear hypothesis. (See studies described above, using "simple" cellular systems.)

8) The carcinogenic effects of low-dose rate exposure, as with low doses, cannot be determined adequately from human data. The data simply are insufficient to permit statistically-valid conclusions to be drawn and hence one must rely on information from lower systems to address this question.

9) An enormous literature on dose rate effects exists. An effect of dose rate is found to be ubiquitous, both for different biological endpoints, and in different biological species and systems. Virtually without exception in eukaryotic systems and for a large number of endpoints (e.g., cell killing, chromosome abnormalities, acute effects such as skin erythema, mutagenesis, carcinogenesis), there is a substantial dose rate effect. If a given total dose of radiation is delivered at a low rate, when compared to the same dose delivered at a high dose rate[b] there will be a substan-

tially lower effect. The ultimate of this process as the dose rate becomes very small is the limiting slope of the "αD" or linear component, i.e., the slope of this limiting low dose rate curve D (Fig. 1) is the same as the low-dose slope α_1 of curve A.

10) High doses delivered at low-dose rates, or in small (< 10 rads) increments, are expected to have a similar low effect per rad as does a single dose (< 10 rads) exposure. Thus most exposures incurred through diagnostic X-ray, nuclear medicine techniques or occupational exposure (small increments of exposure, separated by hours or days) can be regarded, in terms of risk/rad, as constituting low-dose rate exposure.

The relationship between dose and dose rate can perhaps be more easily appreciated by use of the $\alpha D + \beta D^2$ model, "dissected" in Figure 5. In this figure, curve A of Fig. 1 is shown as being the sum of two separate curves, having αD and βD^2 components.[c] The αD or linear component is independent of dose rate over the entire curve (i.e., the effect/rad is the same at all doses, and at all dose rates). The βD^2 component, on the other hand, is highly dose and dose rate dependent, and the effect/rad decreases markedly as either the dose or the dose rate is decreased (due to repair). At sufficiently low doses (any dose rate), the βD^2 component is absent. Similarly at very low dose rates (any dose), the βD^2 contribution is negligible or absent. Hence at very low doses or dose rates, effectively all that remains of the complete curve A is the linear or αD component.

Although the $\alpha D + \beta D^2$ model may turn out to be inexact in detail, it does describe most available data. It embraces the most important concepts representing widespread current beliefs about radiation effects at low doses and dose rates; i.e., that no threshold exists for the risk of most radiogenic cancers and for genetic effects; that the upper limit of the true risk for any cancer is most unlikely to exceed that predicted using the "linear hypothesis"; and that the lower limit of risk for most cancers is unlikely to be less than the linear or "αD" component of the quadratic relationship.

11) The absolute values of radiation risks are small. For all types of cancer, the effect or risk of that effect, per rad[d] of exposure (termed variously the "risk coefficient", the slope of the dose-effect curve, or the "damage function") for all types of induced cancer, is usually taken, as an absolute upper limit, to be no more than 200 per million persons exposed to a single dose of 1 rad. That is to say, in a large population exposed to 1 rad, one would expect an upper limit of an additional 200 cancers per million people, for all time after that exposure (a risk of one in 5,000). This additional risk of the single one-rad exposure, in terms of risk per year is roughly 8 per million individuals exposed to 1 rad, for about 25 years following the exposure (an absolute risk of about 1 in 125,000 per year). If a dose magnitude and/or dose rate factor were introduced, the absolute risk values would be one-fifth to one-tenth of these risks, or lower. The risks at any dose level other than 1 rad would of course be proportionally higher or lower.

12) A comparison of exposures actually sustained by American populations from different radiation sources is shown in Table I. Note that, compared to natural background which is ubiquitous and cannot be escaped entirely, actual exposures now sustained are not large. In Table II is shown the average annual risks actually experienced by American populations, from a number of familiar sources. The average annual risk of exposure of occupational workers resulting from the upper limit value of 5 rems (average of less than 0.5 rem) per year, is small compared to the risk from other familiar sources. The risk from background radiation or from diagnostic X-rays would be substantially less than this value.

13) The risks of radiation exposure are low, compared to other risks commonly encountered (see Table II). Although the fact of public exposure to one risk does not of course justify additional exposure to other risks, a comparison of doses of radiation from different sources, or of absolute radiation risks compared to other risks commonly encountered, serves to calibrate the quantitative values of either the dose or of absolute risk in terms that are more familiar and thus meaningful. Also, comparative risks have very direct and justifiable applications, in providing an objective and defensible basis for choosing among various alternative approaches to obtaining the same benefit for either the individual or for society in general (e.g., different modes of transportation, of energy production and distribution, and of obtaining diagnostic information on patients).

U. S. Population Exposure

	Ave. Dose mrem/yr.
Natural background	100–150
Diagnostic X-ray	50–150
The "Standards"	170
weapons testing	3
jet travel, watches, color TV, etc.	1
Nuclear power plants	less than 0.001

Table I. Annual radiation doses from some of the sources to which the U.S. population is exposed. These are presented as a "calibration scale" to allow one to put a given annual exposure rate into perspective. (The "Standards" refers to the average dose for the general public). If exposure to the lungs from radon gas from sources such as masonry construction materials are included, the natural background rate would be nearly double the figure given in the table.

Chance of Serious Injury or Death-Per Year

Auto accident (disability)	1	chance in	100
Cancer, all types and causes	1	" "	700
Cancer from smoking	1	" "	2,000
Auto death	1	" "	4,000
Fire death	1	" "	25,000
The "Pill," death	1	" "	25,000
Drowning	1	" "	30,000
Electrocution	1	" "	200,000
Airplane trip, New York City-San Francisco and return	1	" "	1,000,000
Reactor Emanations; site boundary (5 to 10 mrem/yr.)	Less than 1	" "	1,000,000
Average for population within 50 miles of reactor	Less than 1	" "	10,000,000

Table 2. Annual risk rates in the U.S. population from various activities.

Footnotes

a. "Low-level" radiation exposures are arbitrarily defined here as single exposures of about 10-15 rads or less, or larger exposures delivered over periods of hours, days or more (low "dose rates"). "High-level" exposures are in the range of 25-100 or more rads, delivered within minutes to at most hours.
b. "High" and "low" dose rates are defined here arbitrarily as greater than 5-10 rads/min and less than 5 rads/yr, respectively.
c. Oversimplified, the radiation beam and the dose received from it, may be regarded as being composed of two separate components, one of high and one of low-linear energy transfer, or LET.
d. Low-LET radiation.

References

1. Hall, E. J. Radiobiology for Radiotherapists. Harper and Row, Hagerstown, MD, 1978.
2. Bond, V. P., Fliedner, T. M., and Archambeau, J. Acute Radiation Lethality; A Disturbance in Cellular Kinetics. Academic Press, New York 1965.
3. Reactor Safety Study (The "Rasmussen Report"). Appendix VI; Calculations of reactor accident consequences. Nuclear Regulatory Commission, Washington, DC 1975.
4. Langham, W. H. (Ed.) Radiobiological Factors in Manned Space Flight. NAS-NRC publication 1487, Washington, DC 1967.

5. Conard, R. A. et al. A twenty year review of findings in a Marshallese population accidentally exposed to radioactive fallout. Brookhaven National Laboratory, New York. BNL Report 50424, 1975.
6. Sparrow, A., Underbrink, A., Rossi, H.: Mutations induced in *Tradescantia* by small doses of X-rays and neutrons: Analysis of dose-response curves. Science 176, 916-921 (1972).
7. Underbrink, A., Kellerer, A., Mills, R., Sparrow, A.: Comparison of X-ray and gamma ray dose-response curves for pink somatic mutations in *Tradescantia* clones 02. Rad. Environ. Biophys. 13, 295-303 (1976).
8. Nauman, C., Underbrink, A. G., Sparrow, A. A.: Influence of radiation dose rate on somatic mutation induction in *Tradescantia* stamen hairs. Radiat. Res. 62, 79-96 (1975).
9. Bond, V. P., Meinhold, C., Rossi, H. H.: Low-dose RBE and Q for X-ray compared to γ-ray radiations. Health Phys. 34, 433-438 (1978).
10. Ullrich, R. L., Jernigan, M. C., Storer, J. B.: Neutron carcinogenesis; dose and dose rate effects in BALB/c mice. Radiat. Res. 72, 487-499 (1977).
11. Ullrich, R. L., Storer, J. B.: The influence of dose-dose rate and radiation quality on radiation carcinogenesis and life shortening in RFM and BALB/E mice. I.A.E.A. paper, I.A.E.A.-SM-224/204. Vienna 13-17 March 1978.
12. National Academy of Sciences. The "BEIR" Committee Report. Biological Effects of Ionizing Radiation. NAS/NRC, 1972 ("BEIR I"). Revised in 1979 ("BEIR III" report). Issued in draft form, Spring, 1979.
13. United Nations Scientific Committee on Effects of Atomic Radiations, "UNSCEAR" reports; 1972 and 1977 reports. Available from United Nations, New York.
14. Beebe, G. W., Kato, H., and Land, C. E. Studies on the mortality of A-bomb survivors. Mortality and radiation dose. Rad. Res. 25, 138-209, 1978.
15. Bond, V. P. Quantitative Risk in Radiation Protection Standards, Radiat. and Environ. Biophysics 17, 1-28 (1979).

IRRADIATION DAMAGE TO THE EMBRYO, FETUS, AND NEONATE*

Liane B. Russell, Ph.D.
Biology Division
Oak Ridge National Laboratory
Oak Ridge, Tennessee

INTRODUCTION

Among the somatic effects of radiation other than cancer, developmental effects on the unborn child are of greatest concern. Exposure of an embryo or fetus to relatively high doses of radiation can cause death, malformation, growth retardation, and functional impairment. Recent information from Hiroshima, most of it published since the 1972 BEIR report[1], indicates that measurable damage can be produced by doses of 10-19 rads (kerma). The effects of radiation are related to the developmental stage at which exposure occurs and corrrespondence has been demonstrated in this respect between man and other mammals. The laboratory data can therefore be used with some confidence to fill in gaps in human experience.

Where developmental effects of radiation can be measured at the cellular level, as in the case of oocyte-killing during fetal or early postnatal stages, thresholds may not be demonstrable. However, most of the perceived abnormalities produced by radiation probably result from damage to more than a single cell. It is therefore unlikely that such effects bear a linear relationship to dose. Threshold doses for some effects have, in fact, already been demonstrated, but these thresholds vary for different abnormalities. For a given total dose, decreases in dose rate generally lead to decreases in developmental effects. Because sensitive stages for many specific abnormalities are relatively short, dose protraction may result in lowering to below the threshold the portion of the total dose that is received during a particular critical period.

In comparison with the adult state, the period of early development is characterized by rapid cell proliferation, cell migration, transitions from totipotency to fixed differentiation, and (in part) association with the maternal organism. Some of these attributes are also found in some localities in the adult (e.g., in stem-cell tissues), and there is no sharp demarcation between the developing and fully formed mammal. In examining the effects of ionizing radiation on development, however, this section restricts itself to intrauterine stages (from the time of conception to the time of birth) and the early postnatal period. Both immediate and long-term effects are reviewed.

The developing organism <u>in utero</u> is potentially vulnerable to external radiation that penetrates the maternal tissues; to radionuclides that reach the conceptus after maternal ingestion, inhalation, or injection; and to indirect effects stemming from damage

* Reprinted with the permission of the National Academy of Science from the BEIR III Report.

to the mother, even when the conceptus is not itself exposed. Alterations that may be produced are morphologic abnormalities, general and local growth retardation, and functional impairments. Although work with experimental mammals has produced evidence of all these effects, it is probably incapable of revealing some of the more subtle functional changes that could be of importance in humans. However, because of the natural variability of human populations and the many other environmental influences that can act during development, it is very difficult to derive information on the effects of low-dose radiaton directly from human studies. Risk estimates must therefore be derived largely from experimental data on gross effects.

EVIDENCE FROM EXPERIMENTAL MAMMALS
CONCERNING SENSITIVITY PATTERNS

The developing organism is a dynamic system in which overall, as well as localized, conditions are ever changing with respect to cell size and type, division rate, cycle times, degree of differentiation, and association with other cell types. Nevertheless, a relatively consistent relationship has been found in different mammalian species between the developmental stage exposed to radiation and the general type of effect observed. That is, there are vastly greater similarities between the results of irradiation of different species at equivalent stages than between the results of irradiation of the same species at different stages.

Several major periods can be delineated on the basis of radiation response (Table 1). The first is the preimplantation period (cleavage, morula, and blastocyst) when radiation can lead to death of the conceptus shortly after exposure, but concepti that survive appear unimpaired with respect to morthology, size, short and long-term survival, and reproductive fitness.[2-5]. The quantitative relationship between dose and mortality was shown to be probably related to cell-cycle stage in cleavage,[6] and recent in vitro experiments[7] have discovered subtle stage-sensitivity differences within the total preimplantation period, with respect to probability and time of induced death. But in no case did embryos survive to a stage that corresponds to more than two weeks in a human pregnancy and, in a human situation, their loss would thus probably not be noted except as an apparent failure to conceive when conception was desired. In the mouse, another effect of preimplantation irradiation has been observed: exposure soon after sperm entry causes sex-chromosome loss, which can result in XO females (Turner's Syndrome in humans). The frequency of this effect is about 4% after an acute dose of 100 R of x-rays[6]. Loss of any chromosomes other than X or Y probably contributes to early death.

Shortly after implantation, the mammalian embryo begins major organogenesis when body divisions and basic organ structures are laid down. This period merges without major demarcation into the period of the fetus, during which organogenesis becomes ever more localized, and the major feature is growth. The event of birth is not a sharp dividing point in this process.

TABLE 1

Effects of 100 R of Acute X-Irradiation in Early Development of Mouse and Rat

Class of Effect	Stage of Irradiation		
	Preimplantation	Major Organogenesis	Fetal (and Early Postnatal*)
Early embryonic death	++	+	
Neonatal or early postnatal death	0	++	0
Sex-chromosome loss	+	−	−
Gross morphologic malformations	0	++	0
Localized morphologic defects or local size reduction	0	++	+
CNS defects; behavioral changes	0	++	+
Oocyte-killing	0	++	++
Induction of male sterility	0	++	+
Generalized growth retardation	0	++	+
Species	Days After Conception		
Mouse	0–4.5	7.5–12.5	13–20
Rat	0–5.5	8.5–13.5	14–32
Corresponding human stage (approx.)	0–9	14–50	51–280

Symbols as follows:

++ 100 R at almost any stage during this period produces effects. At least one stage yields incidence > 25%.
+ Effect observed from treatment of only limited number of stages during this period and/or incidence < 25%.
0 No effects observed.
− No evidence available.
* Early postnatal stages of mouse and rat correspond to human fetal stages.

As the embryo implants in the uterus and enters the period of major organogenesis, it becomes abruptly sensitive to the radiation induction of major malformations. Mortality induced by exposure during that period is no longer only of the very early prenatal type, but occurs mainly at birth or during infancy. General growth retardation can result and may be temporary or permanent. Irradiation during the fetal period can also produce localized growth retardation, as well as effects on germ-cell populations and on the central nervous system.[3-5,8-14] It is clear that although some of the radiation effects will be apparent by the time of birth, others (fertility depression, life span shortening, neuronal depletion, etc.) find expression later.[8,10,15,17-19] Among the potential delayed effects of embryonic or fetal irradiation that could be of special significance to man are neurophysiologic and behavioral changes.[20,21] However, behavior tests in experimental mammals may have little direct application to the human situation and, furthermore, are subject to a number of environmental influences whose effects are difficult to distinguish from those of the radiation history (see Brent[9] and Furchgott[22]).

Results of experiments to study mechanisms of radiation effect on the embryo and fetus have indicated that the maternal organism probably does not play a major intermediary role in the production of most radiation-induced abnormalities.[2,5,15,23] The complex chain of processes leading to the finally observed abnormal characteristic may be related by direct cellular descent to the initial developmental effect of radiation or they may be secondarily caused. In turn, an initial developmental effect results from the initial cellular effect only if the regulatory power of a process is inadequate to take care of a given amount of damage.[5] The initial cellular effect may be cell death (from aneuploidy or other causes), delay in cell division or cell migration, or interference with cell interactions. Although not all the basic mechanisms that can lead to such cellular effects have yet been identified, it is clear from the regular pattern of response observed that somatic mutation (a random process) is relatively unimportant.

The all-or-none effect of radiation during preimplantation stages was explained early by the postulated totipotency of blastomeres.[5] Recent manipulative interferences with early mammalian embryos,[24] such as cell aggregation and blastocyst injection, have amply demonstrated the great developmental plasticity of blastomeres and even of early inner-cell-mass cells and have thus confirmed the original suggestion.

Most animal experiments designed to discover critical periods in development have used relatively high, single, acute doses (100 R or greater). However, once a critical period is established, effects can be demonstrated with considerably smaller exposures. Thus, a specific skeletal change readily showed the effects of 25 R, the lowest dose tried,[25] and mitotic delay in the telencephalon could be demonstrated to have a threshold dose of less than 10 R.[26] In the case of protracted exposures, low daily doses also have produced readily measurable effects, such as reduction in female reproductive capacity after continuous irradiation at a dose rate of 0.0086 R/min (12.4 R/day),[4] various organ-weight reductions after 3 rads/day from tritiated drinking water,[27-29] and oocyte depletion with LD_{50} of only 5 rads during the sensitive period.[11] Different gross abnormalities have been found to follow different dose curves, some with high thresholds;[5,30] but where cellular effects can be directly scored, clear thresholds are sometimes absent.[31]

Protraction of the dose generally diminshes the overall incidence of gross abnormalities,[32-37] presumably because less than the threshold dose is received within the duration of many sensitive periods.[4] Fractionated acute doses are about 1.5 times more effective than continuous irradiation administered during the same intervals.[33]

A question that has been only barely touched on in experimental teratology concerns possible synergistic effects of radiation exposure and other environmental influences. A recent study on mouse embryos has shown that caffeine, at non-teratogenic concentrations, significantly increases the effect of 200 R in producing morphologic abnormalities.[38] Synergisms like this are of obvious importance in deriving risk predictions, but very few experimental results are available on which to base any quantitative estimates.

EXTERNALLY ADMINISTERED INTRAUTERINE IRRADIATION IN HUMANS

Animal experiments have clearly demonstrated the extreme importance of developmental stage, dose, and dose rate in determining the response to in utero radiation exposure. Unfortunately, one or more of these factors are usually not accurately known in cases where human concepti have been irradiated. Such cases come from two major sources: medical exposures, particularly during the early part of the century when hazards were not yet fully appreciated, and particularly therapeutic irradiations; and studies of atomic bomb survivors in Japan.

The list of human abnormalities reported after in utero irradiation is long.[39] It includes microcephaly, mental retardation, growth retardation, hydrocephaly, microphthalmia, coloboma, chorioretinitis, blindness, strabismus, nystagmus, coordination defects, mongolism, spina bifida, skull malformations, cleft palate, ear abnormalities, deformed hands, clubfeet, hypophalangism, and genital deformities. Many of these abnormalities are similar to those observed after treatment of experimental animals; and in a few human cases where stage of irradiation was accurately recorded,[40] the correspondence is remarkable.

Most commonly reported among human abnormalities are microcephaly (often combined with mental retardation), some other central nervous system defects, and growth retardation.[41-44] The Japanese bomb studies also reported these abnormalities more frequently than any others.[19,45-48] Microcephaly is particularly associated with exposure during early stages of pregnancy. At Hiroshima, for example, it resulted almost six time times more frequently when irradiation occurred before the sixteenth week of pregnancy than when it occurred in the second half of pregnancy.[45-47] A recent, more detailed followup[49] showed a 28% incidence of microcephaly after exposure (all doses combined) at some time during weeks 4-13 of the gestation period, but only a 7% incidence after exposure during the remainder of gestation. For the most sensitive interval, weeks 6-11, the incidence was 11% (2/19) for air doses of 1-9 rads, 17% (4/24) for 10-19 rads, 30% (3/10) for 20-29 rads, 40% (4/10) for 30-49 rads, 70% (7/10) for 50-99 rads, and 100% (7/7) for doses over 100 rads. In the comparable zero-dose group, the frequency was 4% (31/764).[50] Although the 11% incidence for weeks 6-11 in the lowest dose group is not significantly higher than the 6% incidence for all other stages exposed at that dose, or than the 4% control frequency, it clearly fits in as part of a dose-effect progression for the sensitive stages. In the range of 10-19 rads kerma, the average tissue dose to the fetus is estimated as 5.3 rads gamma plus 0.35 rad neutron; and in the range of 1-9 rads kerma, as 1.3 rads gamma plus 0.1 rad neutrons.[51,52]

Because some of the affected children observed in the earlier Japanese studies did not appear at the clinics for the followup,[49] it is possible that the actual effects were greater. However, it should be noted that the Nagasaki results showed no significant increase in microcephaly at kerma below 150 rads.[49] Although the total number of intrauterine exposures at Nagasaki was substantially lower than that at Hiroshima (namely, fewer than 20 during sensitive stages at kerma below 150 rads), it is clear that the effect was less in Nagasaki than in Hiroshima (only one case observed vs. seven expected if sensitivity was equal to that in Hiroshima). The differences between the cities are probably attributable to the difference in radiation quality; in the range of interest, about 20% of the kerma at Hiroshima was due to neutrons, compared with less than 1% at Nagasaki.

Deleterious effects of <u>in utero</u> radiation on body growth are clearly indicated by the Japanese data. About 80% of 1,613 children exposed <u>in utero</u> could be followed through the age of 17 (mature growth) by annual examinations.[53,54] Those who were exposed within 1,500 m of the hypocenter of the Hiroshima bomb (average kerma, 25 rads)[55] were, on the average, 2.25 cm shorter, 3 kg lighter, and 1.1 cm smaller in head circumference than those who were at least 3,000 m from the bomb.

Mental retardation was another effect found in the Japanese bomb studies. Owing to the lack of appropriate and sensitive tests for proper overall mental functioning, mental retardation must be relatively severe to be recognized in a clinical situation. In the Japanese children, the diagnosis applied only if a person was unable to perform simple calculations, to make simple conversation, or to care for himself ("profound" mental retardation), or if he was completely unmanageable or had been institutionalized. The "profound" retardation was often associated with the more severe grades of microcephaly and was not observed below 25 rads kerma of maternal exposure.[56] Other behavioral effects of <u>in utero</u> exposure have also been reported--e.g., disturbances of coordination after irradiation during the ninth to the twelfth week.[57] and retarded motor development after radiation therapy of the mother during the first two trimesters.[58]

It may be questioned why microcephaly and mental retardation figure so prominently among the array of abnormalities attributed to intrauterine irradiation. Does this represent a departure from the animal results? The answer is probably no. Head circumference has not been measured in the rodent experiments; and it would, in fact, be difficult to develop an equivalent measure. Similarly, as noted earlier, no good test to detect "mental retardation" has been developed for mice and rats. Central nervous system damage has been amply demonstrated in experimental mammals[16] and is still easily measurable at 10 R.[25] During human prenatal life, central nervous system (CNS) development occurs over a considerably longer period than does major organogenesis. However, in rodents which have a relatively much shorter fetal period than man, the two processes are much more nearly equal with respect to time occupied. Therefore, human exposure, which has been random with respect to developmental stage, is more likely to occur during some period critical for the CNS than is exposure in experimental mammals in which work has been concentrated primarily on specific stages during the period of major organogenesis. The facts that many abnormalities in systems other than the CNS have been reported in man and that stage correspondence can be good further indicate that human results are not out of line with animal data.

Histologic correspondence was noted in a report of human fetuses studied within days after exposure to radium gamma rays from maternal therapy for cervical cancer.[59] Among effects observed were destruction of proliferative and migratory brain cells and of some hematopoietic cells, necrosis of lymphoid and mesenchymal cells, and degeneration of oocytes. These observations provide a link with animal data on the CNS and, importantly, with recent observations on the extreme sensitivity of early developing oocytes.[11] The stage most exquisitely vulnerable to the latter effect in rodents is the early post-natal period, when ovarian development corresponds closely to that of a human fetus.

Because of large genetic and environmental variables encountered in human populations, it is very difficult to measure any effects that might be produced by low doses of radiation, such as those used in diagnostic radiology. It is therefore not surprising to find conflicting reports on whether the "spontaneous" incidence of malformations or growth retardation is increased as a consequence of such exposure (some authors,[60-63] report negative findings; others[64-65] positive). At present, it is impossible, on the basis of human studies alone, to determine with certainty a dose below which teratologic effects in man are not induced by exposure at sensitive stages in development. As discussed above, such thresholds do, however, probably exist and they may be higher for protracted or fractionated radiation than for acute single exposures.[4,66-67]

INTERNALLY ADMINISTERED RADIONUCLIDES DURING PREGNANCY

The effects of various radioisotopes administered to pregnant mammals have been less extensively studied than the effects of externally administered radiation. Furthermore, one cannot generaalize on the effects of administered radionuclides because, depending on the chemical form and the type and energy of the emitted radiation, they may or may not cross the placenta, they may have specific target organs, the distribution or radiation may be nonrandom, the metabolism of radioactive elements or compounds may vary greatly from person to person because of individual biologic variations or because of the disease state of a given subject, and the change in dose rate with time may be difficult to evaluate.[68] Radioisotopes administered to the mother may also affect the newborn if they are administered shortly before birth because many are excreted in the breast milk.[69,70]

In any event, before one can estimate the potential hazard of administering a radioactive nuclide or compound to a pregnant woman, one must determine with some accuracy the total dose to the fetus or a particular fetal tissue, the dose rate and how it varies with time, and the stages of gestation during which the radiation is received.

Until recently,[71] the radioactive isotopes of iodine were the radionuclides most commonly used in nuclear medicine. The two most important ones are Iodine-131 and Iodine-125. Although inorganic iodide readily crosses the placenta, iodine attached to proteins, hormones, and even radioactive rose bengal is less likely to cross. However, a significant amount of iodine usually is released from the labeled compounds and becomes available to the fetus. There is probably no radioactively labeled iodine compound that does not release some iodine to the circulation after administration.

The human fetal thyroid does not take up iodine before the twelfth week;[72,73] thereafter, however, its uptake increases and it comes to a peak in the sixth month.[73] In the mouse, there is some evidence that the fetal thyroid has a greater avidity for iodine than does the maternal thyroid.[74] Because the human fetal thyroid accumulates considerably more Iodine-131 per gram than do other fetal tissues, an inadvertent therapeutic dose to the mother of 5 mCi would deliver 6,500 rads to this organ and thereby ablate it.[75] If the dose of radioactive iodine high enough, it can even cause inhibition of growth of the underlying trachea.[71]

Pathologic effects, including thyroid destruction, have been reported in the fetus after therapeutic (ablative) doses of Iodine-131 were administered to pregnant women.[76] Tracer doses of radioactive iodine have not been reported to produce a deleterious effect on the fetus. There remains, nevertheless, a concern over the possibility of inducing thyroid cancer in susceptible people by prenatal exposure to even small amounts of radioactive iodine. If administration of radioiodine is unavoidable, it is best done before the third month of human pregnancy when the fetal thyroid has not yet developed. Even in this circumstance, the total body dose to the embryo should be estimated and considered.

Technetium-99m is a radioactive isomer that has become, in recent years, an important radionuclide for diagnostic imaging procedures. Its usefulness depends on its almost optimal gamma-ray energy (140 keV), its short half-life (6 h), its rapid excretion, and the fact that it emits no beta rays. Although radiation doses to the embryo or fetus would thus presumably be lower from technetium-99m than from some other diagnostically-used radioisotopes, there have been no direct studies on the effects of technetium-99m on intrauterine development.

Inorganic radioactive potassium, sodium, phosphorus, cesium, and strontium cross the placenta readily. Experiments with radioactive phosphorus and strontium have indicated that if the dose is large enough, embryonic pathology and death can be induced.[77,78]

Because tritium (hydrogen-3) is a potential pollutant from nuclear-energy production, its effect on development has been the subject of a number of studies. Tritiated water (HTO) is a common chemical state of tritium and it has easy and rapid access to living cells, including those of the embryo or fetus. HTO administered in the drinking water to rats throughout pregnancy produced significant decreases in relative weights of brain, testes and probably ovaries[27], and increases in norepinephrine concentration[26] at doses of 10 μCi/ml (estimated at 3 rads/day) and produced weight decreases in a number of organs at higher doses.[27] Because the length of the critical period for various organs is not known, the total damaging dose cannot yet be estimated. Relative brain weight was found to be reduced at only 0.3 rad/day (1 μCi/ml of drinking water) when exposure began at the time of the mother's conception.[19,28] Even lower exposures (0.003 rad/day and 0.03 rad/day) have been implicated in the induction of behavioral damage, such as delayed development of the righting reflex and depressed spontaneous activity.[19] However, because the data fail to show a clear dose dependence, there is some doubt about the validity of this suggestion.

Tritiated drinking water has been used to study the effects of radiation on development of a sensitive cell type, the oocyte. Oocyte counts were made in serial sections of exposed and control animals. In squirrel monkeys continuously exposed from conception to birth, the LD_{50} was 0.5 μCi/ml of body water, giving a fetal dose rate estimated at 0.11 rad/day. Because the sensitive period for development is probably the last trimester, the LD_{50} calculated to be 5 rads.[11] In the mouse, the sensitive period occurs during the first two weeks after birth and by a similar calculation, the LD_{50} from tritiated drinking water at that time is slightly below 5 rads.[30]

DEVELOPMENTAL EFFECTS OF BACKGROUND AND FALLOUT RADIATION

The average abdominal exposure for the U.S. population from background radiation is probably around 80 mrems/yr. It is assumed that the embryo and fetus also are exposed to natural background radiation at about the same dose rate. Radiation from remaining fallout (at present) adds less than 4% of the background dose rate; and contributions from other man-made sources (excluding medical irradiation), such as nuclear and coal-fired power plants and consumer products, add less than 1%.

It appears, therefore, that the average American receives a dose of about 60 mrads during intrauterine life, or about 0.2 mrad/day. It has been suggested that the frequency of neonatal deaths from congenital malformation is highly correlated with the background radiation resulting from geomagnetic conditions and altitude.[79] However, this claim is not supported by the experimental data on low-dose-rate irradiation of developing mammals. Where a clear correlation with altitude does exist in the human data, it has been attributed instead to effects of hypoxia on intrauterine development.[80] In general, the natural and man-made background radiation during gestation is so low in total magnitude and dose rate that it is not thought to be a factor in the normal incidence of congenital malformations, intrauterine or extrauterine retardation, or embryonic death.

POSTNATAL IRRADIATION EFFECTS

Numerous reports have indicated that radiation exposure of the neonate, infant, or child can result in growth retardation.[81-88] Followup studies on children exposed in Hiroshima, Nagasaki, or the Marshall Islands to atomic bomb or fallout radiation indicated that the younger children were more susceptible to these growth-retarding effects than the older ones. The most conclusive evidence on postnatal radiation effects comes from a multivariate analysis of anthropometric data on children exposed to the Hiroshima bomb and examined periodically up to 8 years later.[89] As radiation exposure increased, there were small but statistically significant decreases in body measurements and growth rates in those who had received kerma of 100 rads or more.

Among the Rongelap children exposed to radioactive fallout, two boys who were infants at the time of exposure developed atrophy of the thyroid before puberty. The resulting hypothyroidism led to retarded body growth and sluggishness of behavior. It was estimated that the whole-body dose from externally deposited fallout was 175 rads and the thyroid dose resulting from concentration of radioiodines between 700 and 1,400 rads.[87,90,91]

Individual case reports of children who received radiation therapy have also indicated that localized irradiation can result in local retardation, especially if growth centers (such as open epiphyses) or tissues with some growth potential are exposed. These effects are more obvious when irradiation is unilateral.

It is difficult to determine whether exposures to diagnostic radiation can produce growth retardation in growing children, inasmuch as any infant or child who receives significant exposures to diagnostic radiation is likely to have an illness that in itself could be responsible for growth retardation. Animal data support the belief that whole-body or partial-body irradiation in the diagnostic dose range probably does not affect the growth of infants or children.[31,35,92]

Early postnatal exposures of rodents can have devastating effects on female fertility. The great bulk of oocyte destruction caused by continuous exposure from conception to 14 days of age is the result of irradiation received after birth. Continuous gamma radiation at the rate of 8.4 R/day from birth to weaning totally sterilized female mice but had no effect on males.[34] The LD_{50} for oocyte-killing in the mouse during the first two postnatal weeks is about 5 rads.[11] For acute irradiation, Oakberg[93] found the LD_{50} of Stage I oocytes in ten-day-old mice to be 8.4 R. It is likely that in primates, including humans, the corresponding stage in ovarian development occurs during the third trimester of intrauterine environment.[11] For some other organ systems, as well, it is probable that the first two postnatal weeks of rodent development correspond to the latter part of human pregnancy.

ESTIMATE OF RISK FROM INTRAUTERINE AND EARLY POSTNATAL IRRADIATION

At relatively high doses and dose rates, it can be established that there is, in general, good correspondence between results obtained from work with experimental mammals and those available for man. This correspondence obtains for developmentally (but not chronologically) equivalent stages of irradiation; because of it, one may gain confidence in the extrapolation of animal data to the human situation. This is fortuante because available results in man fail, for a number of reasons, to provide direct information on the magnitude of risk at low exposures. The genetic and environmental variability in human populations makes the measurement of small increments in a miscellany of structural or functional impairments next to impossible to measure. There are, furthermore, no good tests for some of the subtle depressions in physical or mental performance or general fitness that could conceivably result from low-level irradiation during development, especially in view of the fact that the CNS in man is vulnerable for an extended period. Finally, the random exposures that are encountered in most epidemiologic studies fail to provide sufficiently large samples for any specific sensitive period during development.

The animal data leave no doubt that readily measurable damage can be caused by doses well below 10 R applied at stages that are sensitive to the specific effect being studied (Table 2). Examples are oocyte-killing in primates with an LD_{50} of only 5 rads,[11] CNS damage in the mouse, with a threshold dose below 10 R,[25] and brain damage and behavioral damage in the rat from doses that are less than 6 rads over the whole intrauterine period and, presumably, only a fraction of this for the sensitive period.

The Japanese atomic bomb data for small head circumference indicate that the human embryo is sensitive down to a few rads of mixed gamma and neutron radiation, in that air kerma of 10-19 rads (i.e., fetal doses averaging 5.3 rads gamma plus 0.35 rad

TABLE 2

Reports of Early Development Studies
Using Total Doses Less Than 10 Rads or Rates Less Than 10 Rads/Day

Organism	Source of Radiation	Dose Yielding Effect	Stage*	Effect	Reference
Single Exposure					
Mouse	X-Ray	Threshold < 10 R	13†	Mitotic delay in telencephalon	26
Human	Hiroshima bomb (80% 20% neutron)+	< 5 Rads+ 5-10 Rads+	wk 6-11† wk 6-11†	11% Microcephaly 17% Microcephaly	49
Mouse	X-Ray	LD_{50} = 8 R	29†	Oocyte-killing	93
Protracted Exposure					
Mouse	HTO^d	LD_{50} 5 Rads	19-33†	Oocyte-killing	31
Monkey	HTO	LD_{50} = 5 Rads	Last trimester	Oocyte-killing	12
Rat	HTO	3 Rads/day 6 Rads/day	0-Term 0-Term	Reduced brain, testes, ovary wts. Ditto; also spleen and overall———	28
Rat	HTO	3 Rads/day 0.3 Rads/day	0-146 0-146	30% reduction in testes wt——— Decreased brain wt in "F_2"———	29
Rat	HTO	0.3 Rad/day	0-Term	Decreased brain wt in "F_2"	28
Rat	HTO	3.3 Rads/day	0-Term	Decreased brain wt, increased norepinephrine	27
Rat	HTO	3.3 Rads/day	0-Term	No effect on lifespan	94
Rat	Cobalt 60	2.5 R/day	0-Term	Prenatal and postnatal mortality	37
Mouse	Cesium-137	8.4 R/day	20-40	Complete sterility in females	35
Mouse	X-Ray	2.5, 5, or 10 R/day	0-18	No effect	34

* Days after conception, except where otherwise indicated. Some post-conception intervals listed occur after birth.
0 Indicates exposures started within hours after conception
† Critical period. Where this ntation appears, effects apply to this stage only.
+ Estimated dose of gamma rays plus neutrons received by embryo.
d HTO = Tritiated drinking water.

neutrons) produced a clearly significant increase in incidence at Hiroshoma,[49] and there are indications that air kerma of 1-9 rads was also damaging to embryos that were in sensitive stages of development at the time of the bombing. Part of the effect is presumably attributable to the fast-neutron dose, inasmuch as no significant increase in microcephaly was detectable below 150 rads kerma in the much smaller Nagasaki sample. It may be noted that microcephaly is a gross abnormality and that it is possible that more subtle changes could have gone undetected.

Where cell-killing effects can be directly measured, as in oocyte-killing, there does not appear to be any clear threshold doses under some conditions.[30] For morphologic malformations, however, a generalized straight-line extrapolation from the results of acute irradiation at high or moderate doses is probably not valid. Because it is unlikely that any perceived developmental abnormality results from damage to a single target, there are probably threshold doses for all such abnormalities. Furthermore, for a given total exposure, lowering of dose rate has been shown to diminish the effect because, with protraction, only a portion of the dose is received during a given critical period. It is therefore likely that low-dose-rate exposures (0.01 R/min or less) at total doses of less than 1 R would not have widespread effects, even though specific damage, such as oocyte-killing, could presumably still occur. Radiation at such doses in medical practice can have clear benefits to the health of individual mothers, so one must balance these benefits against the small risk to the conceptus. However, even at such low doses, indiscriminate exposures of larger populations of embryos or fetuses should be avoided. The possibility that a pregnancy exists should always be considered before women of child-bearing age are exposed to radiation appreciably above background.

Until more is known about synergisms between radiation and other environmental agents, the possibility of such interactions (as shown in the case of caffeine[37]) should add a cautionary element to risk estimates.

SUMMARY AND CONCLUSIONS

Developing mammals, including man, are particularly sensitive to radiation during their intrauterine and early post-natal life. The effects prduced are strongly related to the developmental stage at which radiation is received and, at moderate to high doses, close correspondence has been demonstrated in this respect between man and various experimental species. The experimental data can therefore be used with some confidence to fill in gaps in the human experience, particularly with respect to extrapolations to low exposure levels, where it is difficult to obtain direct evidence in genetically and environmentally heterogeneous human populations.

Radiation during preimplantation stages probably produces no abnormalities in survivors, owing to the great developmental plasticity of very early mammalian embryos. Radiation at later stages may, however, produce morphologic abnormalities, general or local growth retardation, or functional impairments if doses are sufficient. Obvious malformations are particularly associated with irradiation during the period of major organogenesis which in man extends approximately from week two through week nine after conception. More restricted morphologic and functional abnormalities and growth retardations dominate the spectrum of radiation effects produced during the fetal and early post-natal periods. Some of these effects can be apparent at birth and others may show up later; subtle functional damage cannot be adequately measured with available techniques. Because the central nervous system is formed during a relatively long period in human development, such abnormalities as microcephaly and mental retardation figure prominently among the list of radiation effects reported in man.

Animal data indicate that readily measurable damage can be caused by doses well below 10 R of acute irradiation applied at stages that are sensitive to specific effects being studied (CNS injury and oocyte-killing). Atomic-bomb data for Hiroshima show that microcephaly was induced by acute air doses in the 10-19 kerma range (average fetal dose, 5.3 rads gamma plus 0.4 rad neutrons) received during the sensitive period and suggest that it was also increased in the 1-9 kerma range (average fetal dose, 1.3 rads gamma plus 0.11 rad neutrons). However, it is likely that there are threshold doses for most maldevelopments and that these are of a variety of magnitudes. Lowering of the dose rate diminishes the damage. Until an exposure has been clearly established below which even subtle damage does not occur, it seems prudent not to subject the abdominal area of women of child-bearing age to quantities of radiation appreciably above background, unless a clear health benefit to the mother or child from such an exposure can be demonstrated. Considerably more research is also needed to explore possible synergistic interactions between radiation and other environmental agents.

1. National Research Council, Advisory Committee on the Biological Efects of Ionizing Radiations. The Effects on Populations of Exposure to Low Levels of Ionizing Radiation. Washington, D.C.: National Academy of Sciences, 1972.

2. Brent, R.L. and B.T. Bolden. The indirect effect of irradiation on embryonic development. III. The contribution of ovarian irradiation, uterine irradiation, oviduct irradiation, and zygote irradiation to fetal mortality and growth retardation in the rat. Radiat. Res. 30:759-773. 1967.

3. Russell, L.B. X-ray-induced developmental abnormalities in the mouse and their use in the analysis of embryological patterns. I. External and gross visceral changes. J. Exp. Zool. 114:545-602, 1950.

4. Russell, L.B., S.K. Badgett, C.L. Saylors. Comparison of the effects of acute, continuous, and fractionated irradiation during embryonic development; pp. 343-359. In A.A. Buzzati-Traverso, Ed., Special Supplement to International Journal of Radiation Biology. Immediate and Low-Level Effects of Ionnizing Radiation Conference held in Venice. London: Taylor & Francis, 1960.

5. Russell, L.B. and W.L. Russell. An analysis of the changing radiation response of the developing mouse embryo. J. Cell. Comp. Physiol. 43:103-149, 1954.

6. Russell, L.B. and C.S. Montgomery. Radiation sensitivity differences within cell-division cycles during cleavage. Int. J. Rad. Biol. 10:151-164, 1966.

7. Goldstein, L.S., A.I. Spindle, R.A. Pedersen. X-ray sensitivity of the preimplantation mouse embryo in vitro. Radiat. Res. 62:267-287, 1975.

8. Brent, R.L. Effects of radiation oon the fetus, newborn and child; pp. 23-60. In R.M. Fry, D. Grahn, M.L. Griem, and J.H. Rust., Eds., Late Effects of Radiation. London: Taylor & Francis, Ltd., 1970.

9. Brent, R.L. Environmental factors, Radiation, pp. 179-197. In R.L. Brent and M. Harris, Eds. Prevention of Embryonic, Fetal, and Perinatal Disease. Vol. 3. Department of Health, Education, and Welfare Publication No. (NIH) 76-853, 1976.

10. Brent, R.L. Irradiation in pregnancy; pp. 1-32, In J.J. Sciarra Ed. Davis' Gynecology and Obstetrics. Vol. 2. New York: Harper & Row, 1972.

11. Brent, R.L. and R.O. Gorson. Radiation Exposure in pregnancy; pp. 1-48. In R.D. Moseley, Jr., D.H. Baker, R.O. Gorson, A. Lalli, H.B. Latourette, and J.L Quinn, III, Eds. Current Problems in Radiology. Vol. 2; Chicago: Year Book Medical Publishers, Inc., 1972

12. Dobson, R.L., C.G. Koehler, J.S. Felton, T.C. Kwan, B J. Wuebbles, and D.C.L. Jones. Vulnerability of female germ cells in developing mice and monkeys to tritium, gamma rays, and polycyclic hydrocarbons. In Proceedings of Symposium on Developmental Toxicology of Energy-Related Pollutants. U.S. Department of Energy Symposium Series. (In press).

13. Rugh, R. Major radiobiological concepts and effects of ionnizing radiation on the embryo and fetus; pp. 3- 26. In T.J. Haley and R.S. Snier, Eds. Response of the Nervous System to Ionnizing Radiation. New York: Academic Press, 1962.

14. Russell, L.B. X-ray-induced developmental abnormalities in the mouse and their use in the analysis of em bryological patterns. II. Abnormalities of the vertebral column and thorax. J. Exp. Zool. 131:329-395, 1956.

15. Brent, R.L. and B.T. Bolden. Indirect effect of x-irradiation on embryonic development. V. Utilization of high doses of maternal irradiation on the first day of gestation. Radiation Res. 36:563-570, 1968.

16. Cowen, D. and L.M. Geller. Long-term pathological effects of prenatal x-irradiation on the central nervous system of the rat. J. Neuropathol. Exp. Neurol. 19:488-527, 1960.

17. Hicks, S.P. and C.J. D'Amato. Effects of ionizing radiations on mammalian development, pp. 196-250. In D.H. Woollam, Ed. Advances in Teratology, Vol. 1. London: Logos Press, Ltd., 1966.

18. Murphree, W.T. and H. Pace. The effects of prenatal radiation on postnatal development in rats. Radiat. Res. 12:495-504, 1960.

19. Rugh, R. and M. Wohlfromm. X-irradiation sterilization of the premature female mouse. Atompraxis 10:511-518, 1964.

20. Cahill, D.F., L.W. Reiter, J.A. Santolucito, G.I. Rehnberg, M.E. Ash, J. Favor, S.J. Bursian, J.F. Wright, and J.W. Laskey. Biological assessment of continuous exposure to tritium and lead in the rat. In Biological and Environmental Effects of Low-Level Radiation. Vol.2. Vienna: International Atomic Energy Agency, 1976.

21. Piontkovskii, I.A. Certain properties of the higher nervous activity in adult animals irradiated prenatally by ionizing radiations. The problem of the effect of ionizing irradiation in offspring. Byull. Eksp. Biol. Med. 46:77-80, 1958 (in Russion).

22. Furchtgott, E. Behavioral effects of ionizing radiations. Psychol. Bull. 60:157-200, 1963.

23. Brent, R.L. and B.T. Bolden. The indirect effect of irradiation on embryonic development. IV. The lethal effects of maternal irradiation on the first day of gestation in the rat. Proc. Soc. Exp. Biol. Med. 125:709-712, 1967.

24. Herbert, M.C. and C.F. Graham. Cell determination and biochemical differentiation of the early mammalian embryo. Current Topics in Develop. Biol. 8:151-178, 1974.

25. Russell, L.B. Effects of low doses of x-rays on embryonic development in the mouse. Proc. Soc. Exp. Biol. Med. 95:174-178, 1957.

26. Kameyama, Y., K. Hoshino, and Y. Hayashi. Effects of low-dose x-radiation on the matrix cells in the telencephalon of mouse embryos. In Proceedings of Symposium on Developmental Toxicology of Energy-Related Pollutants. U.S. Department of Energy Symposium Series. (In press).

27. Bursian, S.J., D.F. Cahill, and J.W. Laskey. Some aspects of brain neurochemistry after intrauterine exposure to tritium. Int. J. Radiat. Biol. 27:455-461, 1975.

28. Cahill, D.F. and C.L. Yuile. Tritium. Some effects of continuous exposure in utero on mammalian development. Radiat. Res. 44:727-737, 1970.

29. Laskey, J.W., J.L. Parrish, and D.F. Cahill. Some effects of lifetime parental exposure to low levels of tritium on the F_2 generation. Radiat. Res. 56:171-179, 1973.

30. Russell, L.B. and M.H. Major. Radiation-induced presumed somatic mutations in the house mouse. Genetics 42:161-175, 1957.

31. Dobson, R.L. and C. Kwan. The tritium RBE at low level exposure--variation with dose, dose rate, and exposure duration. Current Topics in Rad. Res. Quart. 12:44-62, 1977.

32. Coppenger, C.J. and S.O. Brown. Post-natal manifestations in albino rats continuously irradiated during pre-natal development. Texas Rep. Biol. Med. 23:45-55, 1965.

33. Konermann, G. Die Keimesentwicklung der Maus nach Einwirkung kontinuierlicher Co60-Gammabestrahlung wahrend der Blastogenese, der Organogenese und der Fetalperiode. Strahlentherapie 137:451-466, 1969.

34. Kriegel, H. and H. Langendorf. Wirkung einer fraktionierten Rontgenbestrahlung auf die Embryonalentwicklung der Maus. Strahlentherapie 123: 429-437, 1964.

35. Ronnback, C. Effects of continuous irradiation during gestation and suckling periods in mice. Acta Radiol. 3:169-176, 1965.

36. Stadler, J. and J.W. Gowen. Observations on the effects of continuous irradiation over 10 generations on reproductivites of different strains of mice. In W.D. Carlson and F.X. Gassner, Eds. Proceedings of an International Symposium on the Effects of Ionizing Radiation on Reproductive Systems. New York: Pergamon Press, 1964.

37. Vorisek, P. Einfluss der kontinuierlichen intrauterinen Bestrahlung auf die perinatale Mortalitat der Frucht. Strahlentherapie 1127:112-120, 1965.

38. Yielding, L.W.; T.L. Riley; K.L. Yielding. Preliminary study of caffeine and chloroquine enhancement of x-ray-induced birth defects. Biochem. Biophys. Res. Commun. 68:1356-1361, 1976.

39. Russell, L.B. and W.L. Russell. Radiation hazards to the embryo and fetus. Radiology 58:369-376, 1952.

40. Feldweg, P. Ein ungewohnlicher Fall von Fruchtschadigung durch Rontgenstrahlen. Strahlentherapie 26:799-801, 1972.

41. Dekaban, A.S. Abnormalities in children exposed to x-irradiation during various stages of gestation. Tentative timetable of radiation injury to human fetus. J. Nucl. Med. 9:471-477, 1968.

42. Goldstein, L. and D.P. Murphy. Etiology of ill health in children born after maternal pelvic irradiation. II. Defective children born after postconceptional maternal irradiation. Amer. J. Roentgenol. 22:322-331, 1929.

43. Goldstein, L. and D.P. Murphy. Microcephalic idiocy following radium therapy for uterine cancer during pregnancy. Amer. J. Obst. Gynecol. 18:189-195, 281-283, 1929.

44. Zappert, J. Uber roentgenogene fetale Microcephalie. Montasschr. Kinderheilk. 34:490-493, 1926.

45. Miller, R.W. Delayed radiation effects in atomic bomb survivors. Science 166:569-574, 1969.

46. Wood, J.W., K.G. Johnson, and Y. Omori. In utero exposure to the Hiroshima atomic bomb. An evaluation of head size and mental retardation: 20 years later. Pediatrics 39:385-392, 1967.

47. Wood, J.W., K.G. Johnson, Y. Omori, S. Kawamoto, and R.J. Keehn. Mental retardation in children exposed in utero to the atomic bomb in Hiroshima and nagasaki. Amer. J. Public Health 57:1381-1390, 1967.

48. Yamazaki, J., S. Wright, and P. Wright. Outcome of pregnancy in women exposed to the atomic bomb in Nagasaki Amer. J. Dis. Child. 87:448-463, 1954.

49. Miller, R.W. and J.J. Mulvihill. Small head size after atomic irradiation. Teratology 14:355-357, 1976.

50. Blot, W.J. Growth and development following prenatal and childhood exposure (to atomic radiation). J. Radiat. Res. (Tokyo) 16(Suppl.):82-88, 1975.

51. Beebe, G.W., H. Kato, and C.E. Land. Life Span Study Report 8. Mortality Experience of Atomic Bomb Survivors 1950-74. Radiation Effects Research Foundation Technical Report TR 1-77. Hiroshima: Radiation Effects Research Foundation, 1978.

52. Kerr, G.D. Organ Dose Estimates for the Japanese Atomic Bomb Survivors. ORNL-5436. Springfield, Va.: National Technical Information Service, 1978. 46 pp.

53. United Nations Scientific Committee on the Effects of Atomic Radiation. General Assembly Document, 24th Session, Suppl. No. 13 (A/7613). New York: United Nations, 1969.

54. Wood, J.W., R.J. Keehn, S. Kawamoto, and K.G. Johnson. The growth and development of children exposed in utero to the atomic bomb in Hiroshima and Nagasaki. Amer. J. Public Health 57:1374-1380, 1967.

55. Beebe, G.W., H. Kato, and C.E. Land. Life Span Study Report 9 Mortality and Radiation Dose. October 1950-September, 1966. p. 90. Atomic Bomb Casualty Commission Technical Report TR 11-70. Hiroshima: Atomic Bomb Casualty Commission, 1970.

56. Blot, W.J. and R.W. Miller. Mental retardation following in utero exposure to the atomic bombs of Hiroshima and Nagasaki. Radiology 106:617-619, 1973.

57. Stettner, E. Ein weiterer Fall Einer Schadingung einer menschlichen Frucht durch Rontgen Bestrahlung. Jahrb. Kinderheikd. Phys. Erzieh. 95:43-51, 1921.

58. Scharer, K., J. Muhlethaler, M. Stettler, and H. Bosch. Chronic radiation nephritis after exposure in utero. Helv. Paediatr. Acta 23:489-508, 1968.

59. Driscoll, S.E., S.P. Hicks, E.H. Copenhaver, and C.L. Easterday. Acute radiation injury in two human fetuses. Arch. Path. 76:113-119, 1963.

60. Kinlen, L.J. and E.D. Acheson. Diagnostic irradiation, congenital malformations, and spontaneous abortion. Brit. J. Radiol. 41:648-654, 1968.

61. Nokkentved, K. Effect of diagnostic radiation upon the human foetus. Copenhagen: Munksgaard, 1968.

62. Tabuchi, A. Fetal disorders due to ionizing radiation. Hiroshima J. Med. Sci. 13:125-176, 1964.

63. Tabuchi, A., S. Nakagawa, T.Hirai, H. Sato, I. Hori, and M. Matsuda; K. Yano; K. Shimada; Y. Nakao. Fetal hazards due to x-ray diagnosis during pregnancy. Hiroshima J. Med. Sci. 16:49-66, 1967.

64. Heinonen, O.P., D. Slone, and S. Shapiro. Birth Defects and Drugs in Pregnancy. Littleton, MA: Publishing Sciences Group, Inc., 1977.

65. Jacobsen, L and L. Mellembaard. Anomalies of the eyes in descendants of women irradiation with small x-ray doses during age of fertility. Acta Ophthal. 46:352-354, 1968.

66. Brent, R.L. The response of the 9 1/2-day-old rat embryo to variations in dose rate of 150 R x-irradiation. Radiat. Res. 45:127-136, 1971.

67. Brizzee, K.R. and R.B. Brannon. Cell recovery in fetal brain after ionizing radiations. Int. J. Radiat. Biol. 21:375, 1972.

68. Cloutier, R.J., S.A. Smith, and E.E. Watson. Dose to the fetus from radionuclides in the bladder. Health Phys. 25:147-161, 1973.

69. Berke, R.A., E.C. Hoops, J.C. Kereiakes, and E.L. Saenger. Radiation dose to breast-feeding child after mother has 99m-MAA lung scan. J. Nucl. Med. 14:51-52, 1973.

70. Wyburn, J.R. Human breast milk excretion of radionuclides followimg administration of radiopharmaceuticals. J. Nucl. Med. 14:115-117, 1972.

71. Sikov, M.R., D.D. Mahlum, and E.B. Howard. Effect of age on the morphologic response of the rat thyroid to irradiation by Iodine 131I. Radiat. Res. 49:233-244, 1972.

72. Chapman, E.R., G.W. Corner, Jr., D. Robinson, and R.D. Evans. The collection of radioactive iodine by the human fetal thyroid. J. Clin. Endocrinol. 8:717-720, 1948.

73. Evans, T.C., R.M. Kretzschmar, R.E. Hodges, and C.W. Song. Radioiodine uptake studies of the human fetal thryoid. J. Nucl. Med. 8:157-165, 1965.

74. Jacobsen, A.G. and R.L. Brent. Radioiodine concentration by the fetal mouse thyroid. Endocrinol. 65:408- 416, 1959.

75. Dyer, N.C., A.B. Brill, S.R. Glasser, and D.A. Goss. Maternal-fetal transport and distribution of 59Fe and 131I in humans. Amer. J. Obst. Gynecol. 103:290-296, 1969.

76. Green, H.G., F.J. Gareis, T.H. Shepard, and V.C. Kelley. Cretinism associated with maternal sodium iodine I131 therapy during pregnancy. Amer. J. Dis. Child. 122: 247-249, 1971.

77. Frolen, H. Genetic effects of ^{90}Sr on various stages of spermatogenesis in mice. Acta Radiol. 9:596-608, 1970.

78. Sikov, M.R. and T.R. Noonan. Anomalous development induced in the embryonic rat by the maternal administration of radiophosphorus. Amer. J. Anat. 103: 138-162, 1958.

79. Wesley, J.P. Background radiation as the cause of fetal congenital malformation. Int. J. Rad. Biol. 2: 97-112, 1960.

80. Grahn, D. and J. Kratchman. Variation in neonatal death rate and birth weight in the United States and possible relations to environmental radiation, geology, and altitude. Amer. J. Hum. Gen. 15:329-352, 1963.

81. Conard, R. and A. Hicking. Medical findings in Marshallese people exposed to fallout radiation. JAMA 192:457, 1965.

82. Dawson, W.D. Growth impairment following radiotherapy in childhood. Clin. Radiol. 19:241-256, 1968.

83. Miller, R.W. Effects of ionnizing radiation from the atomic bomb on Japanes children. Pediatrics 41:257-263, 1968.

84. Murphy, W.T. and D.L. Berens. Late sequelae following cancericidal radiation in children. A report of 3 cases. Radiology 58:35-42, 1952.

85. Reynolds, E.L. Growth and Development of Hiroshima Children Exposed to the Atomic Bomb. Three-Year Study (1951-1953). Atomic Bomb Casualty Commission Technical Report TR 20-59. Hiroshima: Atomic Bomb Casualty Commission, 1959.

86. Shurygin, V.P. Changes in the long bones of children after radiotherapy. Med. Radiol. (Moskva) 12:37-42, 1967.

87. Sutow, W.W., R.A. Conard, and K.M. Griffith. Growth status of children exposed to fallout irradiation on Marshall Islands. Pediatrics 36:721-731, 1965.

88. Vaughan, J. The effects of skeletal irradiation. Clin. Orthoped. 56:288-303, 1968.

89. Nehemias, J.V. Multivariate analysis and the IBM 704 computer applied to ABCC data on growth of surviving Hiroshima children. Health Physics 8:165-183, 1962.

90. Conard, R.A. Medical survey of the people of Rongelap and Utirik Islands, thirteen, fourteen, and fifteen years after exposure to fallout radiation (March 1968, March 1969). BNL 50220 (T-562). New York: Brookhaven National Laboratory, 1970.

91. Sutow, W.W. and R.A. Conard. The effects of fallout radiation on Marshallese children; pp. 661-672. In M.R. Sikov and D.D. Mahlum, Eds. Radiation Biology of the Fetal and Juvenile Mammal. Ninth Annual Hanford Biology Symposium. U.S. Atomic Energy Commission Series. No. 17. CONF-690501. Richland, Washington, 1969.

92. Billings, M., J. Yamazaki, L. Bennett, and B. Lamson. Late effects of low-dose whole-body x-irradiation of four-day-old rats. Pediatrics 38:1047-1056, 1966.

93. Oakberg, E.F. Gamma-ray sensitivity of oocytes of immature mice. Proc. Soc. Exp. Biol. Med. 109: 763-767, 1962.

94. Cahill, D.F., J.F. Wright, J.H. Godbold, J.M. Ward, J.W. Laskey, and E.A. Tompkins. Neroplastic and life-span effects of chronic expousre to tritium. II. Rats exposed in utero. J. Nat. Cancer Inst. 55:1165-1169, 1975.

ESTIMATES OF CANCER RISKS FROM LOW-LEVEL EXPOSURE TO IONIZING RADIATION: THE BEIR REPORT 1980

Edward W. Webster, Ph.D.
Massachusetts General Hospital, Boston, Ma. 02114

ABSTRACT

This paper summarizes the significant conclusions of the National Academy of Sciences 1980 report on the carcinogenic effects of low levels of ionizing radiation. The dearth of epidemiological data on the effects of doses in the range 1 to 20 rads makes it necessary to assume a theoretical relation between radiation dose and the likelihood of cancer induction, so that predictions of low-dose effects can be made on the basis of relatively well-defined high-dose observations in man. The BEIR Committee has been guided by radiobiological data on cellular and animal effects and by the statistically weak data on human cancer induction by low doses, primarily the Japanese A-bomb survivor data, to derive an envelope of risk estimates based on three dose/effect relations. Employment of a linear-quadratic relation derived from cancer mortality of the survivors in the period 1950-74 has provided the basis for the preferred set of risk estimates for whole-body exposure to low LET radiation. No allowance has been made for dose-rate effects. The best estimate of increased cancer mortality risk for 1 rad/year of whole-body low LET radiation received between ages 20 and 65 is about 2% of the normal expectation of death from cancer. The increase in the risk of cancer occurrence is similar. For estimating risks from partial body exposure to specific internal organs, the predominance of high-dose data has led to the adoption by default of a linear dose/effect relation except for leukemia and bone cancer. The continuing uncertainty regarding increased sensitivity of the fetus to the carcinogenic effects of radiation is noted. The Report expresses skepticism regarding several recent claims of increased cancer in limited populations exposed to doses of the order of 1 rad.

INTRODUCTION

The BEIR Report of 1980 (sometimes known as BEIR III)[1] is a revision of the first review entitled "The Effects on Populations of Exposure to Low Levels of Ionizing Radiation" (BEIR I) published by the National Academy of Sciences in 1972[2]. Like its predecessor, the review is concerned with genetic effects and somatic effects with major emphasis on the latter, and discusses not only the induction of malignancies but also other somatic effects such as developmental abnormalities following fetal irradiation, growth retardation, cataracts and effects on fertility. This commentary will not cover these latter topics or genetic effects (which are discussed by others in these proceedings), but, consonant with the 1980 Report, will give major emphasis to the cancer risks incurred by adult populations.

Low doses may be defined as those in the range of 1 to 10 rads;

that is, the range of doses received in occupational exposures or in diagnostic radiological procedures. As in the BEIR I Report, it is explicitly recognized by the BEIR III Committee that it is <u>not</u> known whether doses in this range, such as those due to continued background exposure (approximately 0.1 to 0.5 rad/year) or single doses of the order of 1 rad, have any deleterious effect. Investigations of populations living in high background areas have not shown any increased incidence of somatic effects. It is contended that such effects, if they are real, are so small as to be hidden by the normal variability of these effects which are also produced by other environmental and genetic factors, and will therefore continue to escape recognition.

There are, therefore, in the low dose range few direct human observations to provide guidance concerning risks. Those studies which have sought deleterious effects are either negative, equivocal, or when positive, subject to serious methodological criticisms or offset by equally valid negative studies. An important reason for this situation, recognized by the BEIR Report, is the large statistical requirement for a positive study. This requirement is illustrated by the following example.

Let us assume that the incidence of radiation-induced breast cancer in women is linear with dose and that the risk in an adult exposed female population, after a latent period of about 15 years is 5 cases per million per year per rad. Then in a population of 100,000 women receiving 20 rads one would expect to find eventually 10 excess cases of radiogenic breast cancer per year; and over a risk period of 20 years following the latent interval, about 200 excess cases. In an unirradiated control population of 100,000 the normal expectation in the USA of breast cancer over the total 35 year period would be about 7,000 cases. The standard deviation of this number is about 84. There is only about 1 chance in 20 that an observed excess of 200 beyond the normal expectation of 7,000 can occur fortuitously, and we might reasonably conclude that the excess was radiation-induced. However, to demonstrate such an effect confidently at 10 rads, the study population (both the exposed and the unexposed control) must be increased by a factor of 4 to 400,000 each, and to demonstrate the effect at 5 rads would require populations each of 1.6 million. Note that the largest exposed population studied to date for radiogenic breast cancer with doses above and below 10 rads, the Japanese A-bomb survivors, contained only about 60,000 women[3]. The breast is believed to be one of the most radiosensitive organs.[1]

DOSE/EFFECT MODELS

In the absence of human or even animal data on the effects of low LET radiation doses of about 1 rad, the effects of such doses must be estimated on the basis of data for higher doses. These estimates depend primarily on the assumptions made regarding the shape of the dose/effect curve rather than on any actual observations at low doses in human populations. Although there are innumerable mathematical models which may be used for projection into the low dose

range, the main contenders are the following three, which are illustrated in Figure 1.
1. The linear, no-threshold model or L model, which was used in the BEIR Report 1972;
2. The linear-quadratic or LQ model, with a linear relation at the lowest doses, curving upward at the higher doses;
3. The pure quadratic (dose-squared) model or Q model, where there is zero slope at zero dose and a continuously increasing risk per rad, i.e. slope.

The choice of model between these three can change the risk estimate by one or two orders of magnitude for doses in the 1 to 10 rad range and therefore vitally affects opinion and policy regarding low level radiation risks. For example,

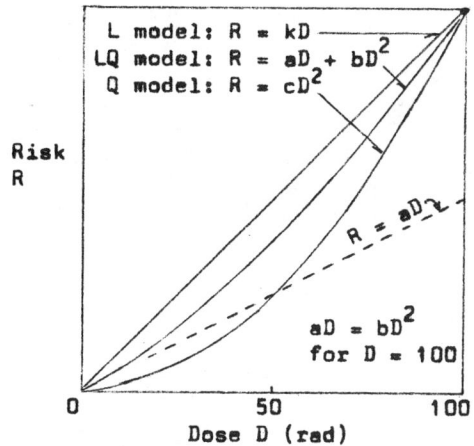

FIGURE 1 Dose/effect models projected from common point at 100 rad.

suppose the risk R is established at a dose D = 100 rads as in Fig. 1. Suppose also that in the linear-quadratic model, the linear and square-law terms are equal at 100 rads as in Fig. 1; i.e. a/b = 100. Then at a dose of 10 rads, the risks relative to the L model would be 0.55 for the LQ model and 0.1 for the Q model, while at a dose of 1 rad the risks relative to the L model would be 0.505 for the LQ model and 0.01 for the Q model. On the other hand if a/b = 10 in the LQ model, then at 10 rads the risks relative to the L model are only 0.18 for the LQ model and 0.1 for the Q model. The risks at low doses in the LQ model are clearly sensitive to the value chosen for the ratio a/b. Guidance concerning the validity of these models is obtained in the general radiobiologic arena, that is from data on radiation damage to cells and cell components and data on cancer induction in irradiated animal populations. The BEIR Report, however, does not discuss in detail the results of cellular and animal experiments. Considerably more detail is provided in the UNSCEAR Report 1977[4]. In addition a powerful line of reasoning derives from the differences in response caused by two different kinds of radiation: a) those depositing low concentrations of energy in the sensitive volumes of cells (such as DNA molecules), i.e. x rays, gamma rays and beta rays, the so-called <u>low LET radiations</u>; and b) those depositing high concentrations, i.e. fast neutrons and alpha rays, the so-called <u>high LET radiations</u>.

CHROMOSOMAL ABERRATIONS

There is a large body of data which indicates that for many biological effects occurring <u>in vitro</u> the dose/effect relation for low LET radiation is of the linear quadratic form. A good example is the frequency of dicentric chromosomes induced in cultures of human lymphocytes exposed to gamma rays[5] (Figure 2). The two curves relate to two different dose-rates (400 rads/hour and 10 rads/hour). The smaller numbers of dicentrics at the lower dose-rate is attributed to repair of individual lesions in the chromosome threads. Both relations are curved upwards. In contrast irradiation by alpha rays (high LET) shows linearity of the dose/effect curve over the same range of lesion frequency per cell and a much greater effect per rad[6] (Figure 3). The comparison in Figure 4 of five different types of radiation (high LET and low LET) is revealing: linear relation for neutrons and alpha rays and a non-linear relation for x rays and gamma rays, and a large value for the RBE (the ratio of doses for the same effect)[6]. This value increases steadily as the absorbed dose falls and reaches more than 100 for alpha rays in comparison with Co-60 gamma rays at the 1 rad level.

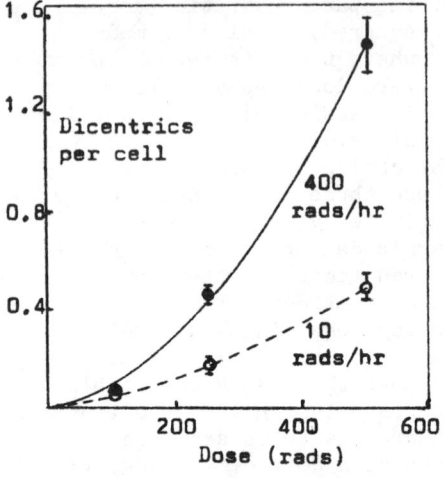

FIGURE 2 Dicentrics induced in human lymphocyte cultures by Cesium-137 gamma rays.

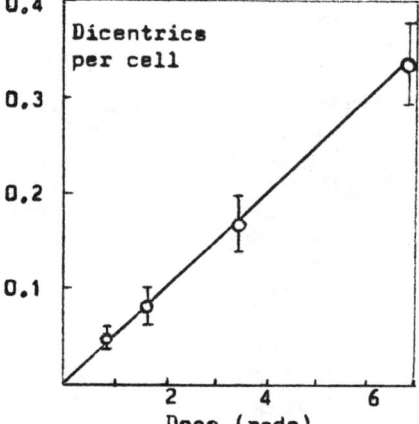

FIGURE 3 Dicentrics induced in human lymphocyte cultures by alpha radiation. (Redrawn from DuFrain et al[6])

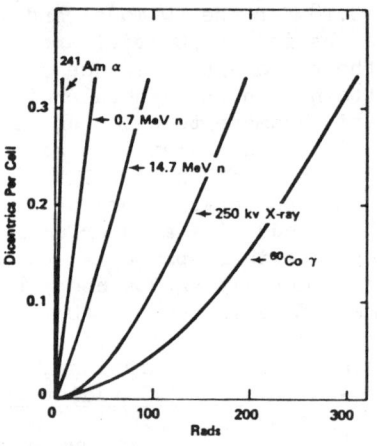

FIGURE 4 Dose response curves for dicentric chromosome induction for high and low LET radiation (courtesy of Health Physics)[6]

CANCER INDUCTION IN ANIMALS

Typical of the results of animal experimentation to induce tumors by ionizing radiation are those of Ullrich and his collaborators at Oak Ridge National Laboratory[7]. This group has examined the induction of eight different types of cancer in female mice by gamma radiation and fast neutrons. Typical of the dose response relationships observed are those for thymic lymphoma (Figures 5 and 6). The lowest dose point for gamma irradiation in Figure 5 is 10 rads. The number of animals used in these experiments was large enough to define the response quite precisely: the standard error of the excess incidence is shown in the figures and for the gamma ray data at zero and 10 rads is within the size of the actual plotted points. At the lowest doses the incidence is not linear with gamma ray dose and in fact fits a dose-squared law. In contrast, the fast neutron response up to about 40 rads is linear. Figure 6 shows, as is usual with high LET radiation, that there is very little dose-rate effect (5 rads/min. vs. 1 rad/day). A more recent example from the same group is given by the lung cancer results[8] reproduced for x-ray and fast neutron exposure in Figure 7. Again the cancer incidence as a function of low LET radiation dose is highly curvilinear, being essentially flat up to 250 rads, whereas it is linear with dose for fast neutron irradiation.

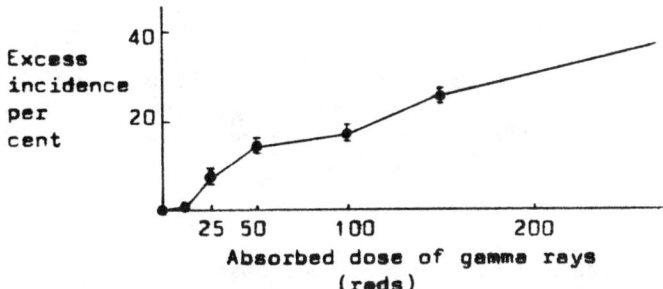

FIGURE 5 Incidence of thymic lymphoma in female RFM mice irradiated with gamma rays (after Ullrich et al)

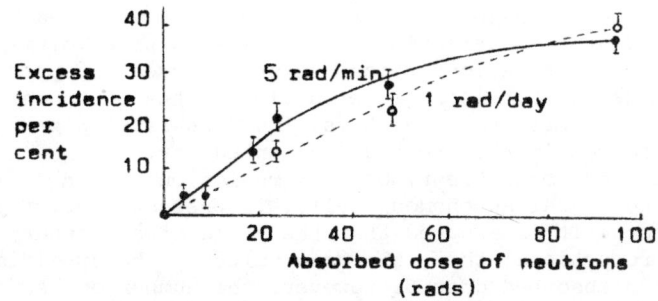

FIGURE 6 Incidence of thymic lymphoma in female RFM mice irradiated with fast neutrons (after Ullrich et al)

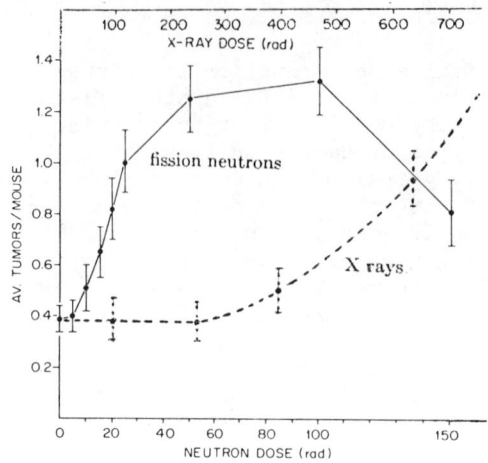
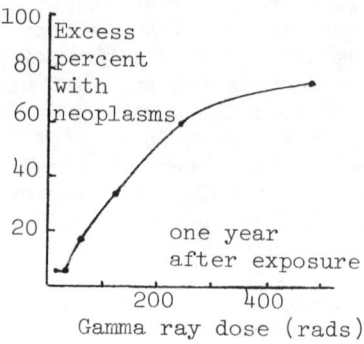

FIGURE 7 Lung cancer in RFM mice as functions of radiation dose after exposure to x-rays and fast neutrons (after Ullrich et al)

FIGURE 8 Mammary neoplasms in Sprague-Dawley rats after total-body Co-60 irradiation (control incidence subtracted). (After Shellabarger et al., 1969)

Almost all of the experimental dose/effect curves in the literature for cancer in animals induced by low LET radiation are concave upwards at low doses. An exception (Figure 8) is provided by the induction of mammary cancer in Sprague-Dawley rats, a strain in which the normal incidence approaches 100% and irradiation effectively advances the time of appearance. In this case there is evident linearity down to about 25 rads[9].

THEORETICAL CONSIDERATIONS

The curvature and dose-rate effect observed generally for low LET radiation in contrast to the linear response and minimal dose-rate effect observed for high LET radiation led Kellerer and Rossi[10] in 1972 to propose a generalized two-hit model for permanent damage. This model employs the known facts concerning the micro-distribution of energy deposited in cells and postulates that the great majority of low LET radiation interactions in small sensitive volumes produce highly reparable sub-lesions which are transformed into permanent lesions if a second hit is registered closely spaced in both time and distance. The effects of high vs. low dose-rate, high vs. low doses, and changes in LET are thus accounted for.

The Kellerer-Rossi theory of dual radiation action as it applies to individual <u>autonomous</u> cells, is presented briefly in the BEIR III Report. It is assumed that the yield of elementary sub-lesions is proportional to $\bar{z}$, the mean value of the specific energy z; i.e. to the absorbed dose D. However, the number of lesions (i.e. size of effect) produced by the combination of two sub-lesions is proportional to the mean value of the square of the specific energy, i.e., $\overline{Z^2}$. It can be shown that $\overline{Z^2}$ is a quadratic function of D, leading to the relation:

$$E = K (\zeta D + D^2)$$

Microdosimetric theory indicates that for a 1 μm site of energy deposition, the value of ζ for low LET radiation is about 20 rads, but for high LET radiation the value is typically 2000 rads. In the above equation the D^2 term dominates when D is greater than ζ and therefore for a 1 μm site the dose-effect relationship should be approximately linear only up to about 10 rads for low LET radiation, but up to much higher values for high LET radiation. It also follows that at low doses, the RBE for high LET radiation will approach the ratio of the linear term coefficient ζ for high and low LET radiation (about 100) and fall for higher dose values according to the inverse square root of the high LET dose. If carcinogenesis requires the establishment of a lesion in more than one contiguous cells, then the dose/effect curve would not be linear even at very low doses.

Rossi[11] has analyzed the results of a number of carefully performed radiobiological experiments which employed both low LET and high LET radiations over wide ranges of dose in order to examine the variation of RBE as a function of dose. The log-log plots of RBE versus neutron dose in Figure 9 show that the predicted relationship is followed by a wide variety of biological effects (including lens opacification in the mouse, chromosome aberrations in human lymphocytes, plant mutation, cell survival, mammary cancer in the rat, and human leukemia in the Japanese A-bomb survivors), although the proposed rule may not be universal. The significance of the inverse variability of the RBE if it applies to carcinogenesis is that if the high LET response for a given type of malignancy is linear, then the low LET response must be non-linear with positive (upward) curvature.

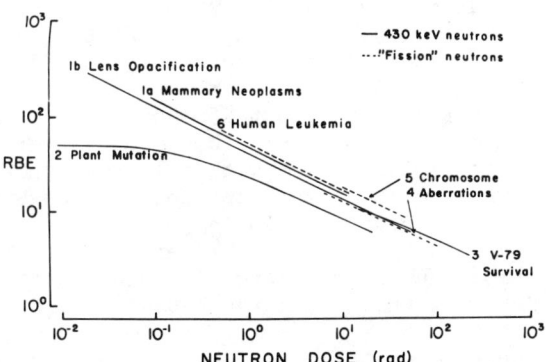

FIGURE 9 Variation of RBE according to $D_n^{-\frac{1}{2}}$ where D = fast neutron dose, for 6 biological end-points (after H. H. Rossi[11])

DOSE/EFFECT MODELS UTILIZED

WHOLE-BODY EXPOSURE

The above considerations led the Somatic Effects Sub-Committee of the BEIR III Committee to adopt the linear-quadratic dose/effect relationship (LQ) as the preferred model for estimating the total cancer risks from whole-body exposure to low LET radiation. This position was importantly supported by epidemiologic evidence of a non-linear dose/effect relation for human leukemia and some bone cancer, as discussed below. Nevertheless, the adoption of this model is subject to reservations by some members of the sub-committee. The reasons are primarily related to the present state of epidemiologic knowledge and include the following points which are discussed in more detail later.

1. The existing human low-dose data, primarily the results of follow-up of the Japanese A-bomb survivors, is statistically weak in the dose region below 100 rads, so that it does not clearly discriminate between competing linear and non-linear responses. This is particularly so for the Nagasaki data which is more relevant to the estimation of low LET radiation risks since the radiation field in Nagasaki (unlike Hiroshima) was almost devoid of neutron contamination. Moreover there are two sources of survivor data in Nagasaki, namely the death certificate data from the Life Span Study and the Tumor Registry data which records tumor incidence. The incidence vs. dose data for solid tumors appears to be fitted best by a linear relationship (but see later section on total cancer mortality in Nagasaki).
2. There is a belief that all types of cancer may not follow the same dose/effect relation. For example, cancer of the breast is often cited as following a linear dose/effect relation[12] for low LET radiation. The human data at low doses is weak in all studies of mammary cancer and in some studies there are no data below 100 rads. In Nagasaki where the data extends to the 0 to 50 rad range the data is consistent with linearity (but also with other relationships). On the other hand the largest body of animal data on mammary cancer induced by low LET radiation is that for the Sprague-Dawley rat, which, as noted earlier, appears to be linear down to about 25 rads.
3. There are some human data which, although controversial, indicate levels of effect consistent with a linear hypothesis down to a few rads. The two important examples are the study by Modan of late thyroid cancer following 6 rad doses to the thyroid gland[13] received by Israeli children during x-ray therapy for tinea capitis; and the retrospective studies of Stewart[14] and others which show an association between childhood cancer and irradiation at the 1 rad level in utero. Although remaining controversial neither of these studies can be completely discounted.

PARTIAL-BODY EXPOSURE

The problem of the "best model" is particularly acute in estimating cancer risks for specific organs following partial-body irradiation. Most of the human data in this context relate to persons who were irradiated therapeutically with relatively high doses. Typical is the ankylosing spondylitis study in England where spinal irradiation of the order of 2000 R in air was delivered (organ doses 50 to 2000 rads for a single course of therapy). In these situations there is no direct guidance concerning the dose-effect curve and therefore the most conservative linear relationship was implicitly adopted for all organs except the blood-forming organs, bone and skin. This adoption is inherent in any expression of risk which is given on a "per rad" basis.

WHOLE BODY IRRADIATION AND TOTAL CANCER RISK

In the occupational and environmental areas an assesment of the total cancer risk is necessary, mainly for low doses of low LET radiation. Because of the differences in latent period between leukemia and solid cancer (assumed to be two years and ten years respectively), risk estimates were made separately in the BEIR Report for these effects. The estimates rely heavily on the data for the Japanese A-bomb survivors[15], which is the only large population to have received whole-body irradiation over a wide dose range.

LEUKEMIA

Figure 10 shows as heavy lines for both Hiroshima and Nagasaki the relative risks of leukemia mortality as a function of kerma, based on the Life Span Study sample of the bomb survivors over the period 1950-74. It is notable that the Nagasaki response is markedly non-linear. Recent analyses of dose/effect relationships for these data have been prepared by Ishimaru et al[16] and by Land et al[17]. In both analyses a linear dose response was assumed for the fast neutron dose component. The Ishimaru analysis shows that the data for both cities and for all types of leukemia is slightly better fitted by a dose-squared response to gamma rays than by a linear response. The Land analysis tests additionally a linear-quadratic dose response for gamma ray dose (to the bone marrow), and shows that this relation fits the data marginally better than the linear or dose-squared responses. For the LQ model the dose-squared term is equal to the linear term at 116 rads and the RBE for 1 rad of fast neutrons is 23. On the other hand these analyses are based on only 35 deaths in Nagasaki, eleven of which occurred for kermas below 100 rads, so that the curvilinearity in the LSS study may be due to large sampling errors. Beebe et al[15] therefore computed the relative risks as a dose function for the much larger number of leukemia cases contained in the Leukemia Registry for Hiroshima and Nagasaki over the period 1946-74, assuming that the dose distribution enumerated for survivors in the 1950 census was applicable to all these cases. However, uncertainty in the validity of this assumption arises from the effects of migration into and out of the cities. The dose responses for the entire Registry are included in Figure 10 as dotted lines. It is evident that in Nagasaki the dose response is much less curvilinear than for the Life Span Study. As noted earlier the Committee preferred the LQ model for the gamma ray response and the absolute risk for this model was computed as 1 case per year per million persons exposed to a whole body dose of 1 rad, starting 2 years after the exposure and continuing for 25 years; that is, a total risk of 25 cases per million.

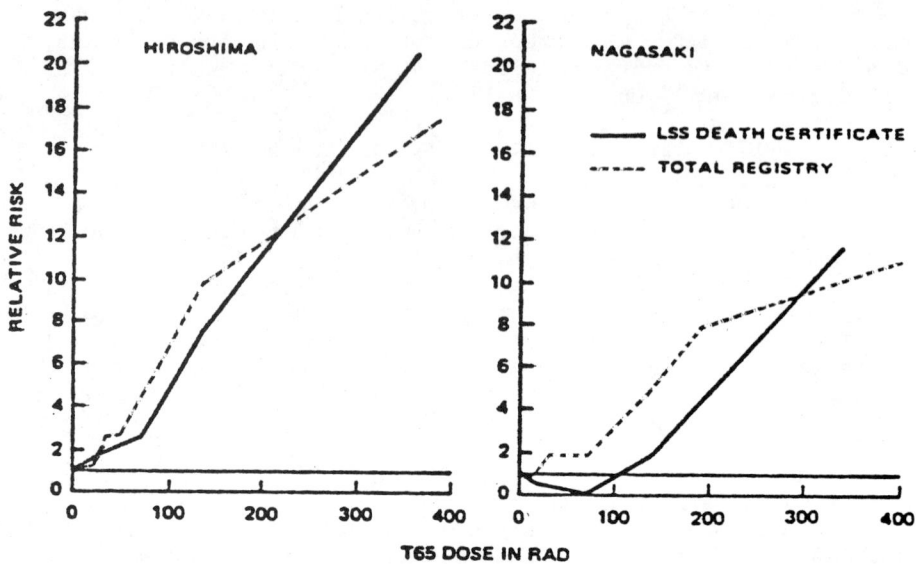

FIGURE 10 Leukemia in Japanese A-bomb survivors as function of total kerma. LSS death certificates 1950-74.
Total Leukemia Registry 1946-74

SOLID CANCER

The mortality from solid cancer excluding leukemia in the Nagasaki A-bomb survivors shows no significant excess over the period 1950-74 for the 1-100 rad group compared with the zero dose group as a control. The data shown in Figure 11 is statistically weak and will support linear, linear-quadratic, and quadratic relationships to dose. The preferred function based primarily on non-human biological experimentation is the linear-quadratic even though the other functions cannot be ruled out. The slope of the best linear fit (regression coefficient) for the gamma ray response based on both the Hiroshima and Nagasaki data is 1.4 deaths/million persons per year per rad after a 10 year latent period. A linear-quadratic fit to the data was obtained based on the assumption of equal linear and dose-squared components of risk at 116 rads (as for leukemia) and this yielded a linear coefficient of 0.4 deaths/10^6 person-year-rad. However, this value was discarded because the RBE for fast neutrons at 1 rad was then about 90 and the ratio of solid cancer to leukemia produced by gamma rays was about 0.4 (a preconceived ratio of about 5 based on the ankylosing spondylitis study was thought to be more appropriate). For these reasons an

RBE for fast neutrons corresponding to that for leukemia was introduced as a further constraint, leading to a linear coefficient in the LQ model of 1.4 deaths/10^6 person-year-rad. This further constraint likewise increased the gamma dose coefficient in the linear model from 1.4 to 3.47 deaths/10^6P-Y-rad, which represents an increase in the risk estimate by a factor of 2.5 over the best-fitting linear regression based primarily on the Nagasaki data.

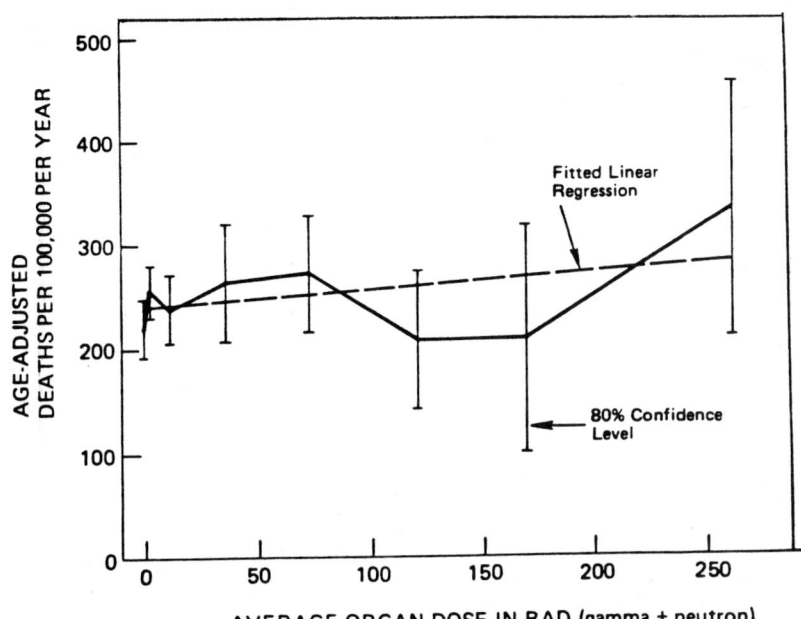

FIGURE 11 Deaths from all cancers except leukemia in Nagasaki 1955-74 and fitted linear dose response

These final risk estimates are considerably greater than an estimate which has been derived by Webster[18] based on the total cancer mortality in Nagasaki employing data from Reference 15 for solid cancer over the period 1955-74 and for leukemia over the period 1950-74. These data uncorrected for age are shown in Figure 12 and are consistent with both a dose-squared and a linear-quadratic relationship. They are also similar to those contained in a BEIR III minority report by H.H. Rossi. The coefficient for the linear low dose segment of Figure 12 (Nagasaki data) is 0.25 deaths /million-year-rad (kerma) or 0.5 deaths/million-year-rad (average organ dose). It must also be noted that the total cancer incidence in Nagasaki over the period 1959-70 based on data from the Nagasaki Tumor Registry[15], is consistent with linearity but indicates a considerably higher risk per rad than is consistent with the best fit to the mortality data. The two sets of data are compared in Figure 12.

There is more reason to doubt the accuracy of the Tumor Registry data than the Life Span Study mortality data.

The BEIR III Committee agreed that the incidence of radiogenic cancer was more significant than mortality from cancer as a measure of social harm produced by radiation exposure. Accordingly the risk estimates of mortality, for which a stronger data base exists, have been supplemented by risk estimates for cancer incidence using three different approaches. In the first and preferred method, the mortality estimates derived from the Japanese A-bomb survivors have been expanded by applying an incidence vs. mortality ratio derived from U.S. cancer statistics, weighted according to the radiosensitivity of the principal cancer sites. The second approach uses the Japanese Tumor Registry data which, as noted above, indicates a level of excess cancer cases greater than those derived from mortality. In the third approach, total incidence from whole-body irradiation is derived by summing the separate incidences of cancer at the many sites reviewed in the Report (Table 3). This approach, the reliability of which is criticised in the Report, intrinsically assumes a linear dose response, but because of presumed over-estimates of the risks to specific organs leads to whole-body risk estimates well above those obtained in the other approaches. Specifically, the summed sites approach leads to linear risk estimates about four times greater than the LQ estimates based on expanded mortality or Tumor Registry data.

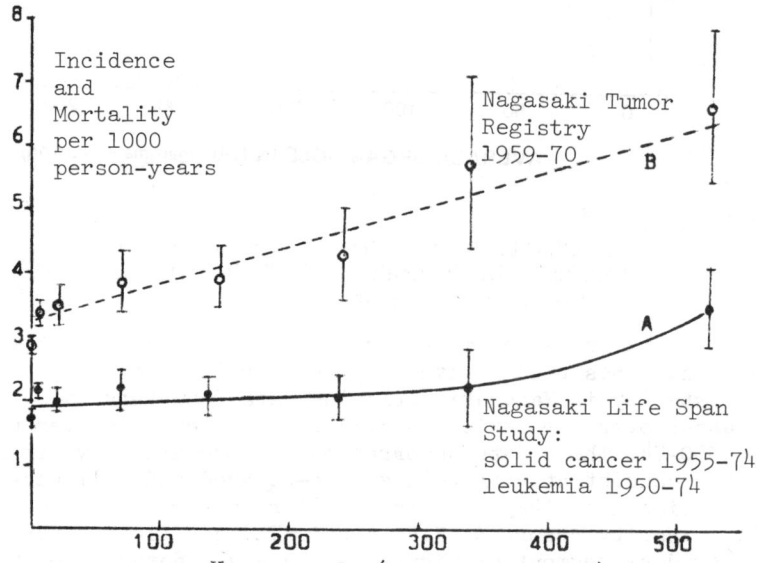

FIGURE 12 Dose response curves for total cancer mortality (Curve A, Life Span Study) and total cancer incidence (Curve B, Tumor Registry) in Nagasaki. Error bars are one standard deviation.

It is of great significance that the major difference between an earlier draft of the Report (which was withdrawn in May 1979 after repudiation by a majority of the Somatic Effects Sub-committee), and the final 1980 version, was the substitution of the LQ model applied to the Japanese A-bomb survivors as the basis for the preferred set of whole-body risk estimates, instead of the estimates based on the sum of the site risks, a position still strongly supported by E. P. Radford in his minority opinion. The coefficient for the LQ mortality model 1.4 x 10^{-6}/person-year-rad) is more than 10 times lower than the risk coefficient for the linear summed sites model (18×10^{-6}).

ESTIMATION OF LIFETIME RISKS

Because human populations have been followed for only a limited time after irradiation, the total cancer risk over a 40-50 year period is not known. It is therefore necessary to make assumptions about the duration of the risk and its magnitude as a function of age. Two methods have been used:
a) the absolute risk method and b) the relative risk method.
These are illustrated in Figure 13. The absolute risk method assumes a constant annual yield of cancer beyond the latent period irrespective of time or age. The relative risk method assumes that radiation-induced cancer is a constant fraction of the normal cancer rate, and therefore the excess generally increases as a function of age. Thus, whether the expression time is limited or endures for the remaining life span, the relative risk method generally predicts a greater excess of cancer, typically by a factor of about 3.

APPLICATION OF RISK FACTORS TO SPECIFIC POPULATIONS

In the Report the absolute and relative risk extrapolations are applied to several populations of interest. These are represen-

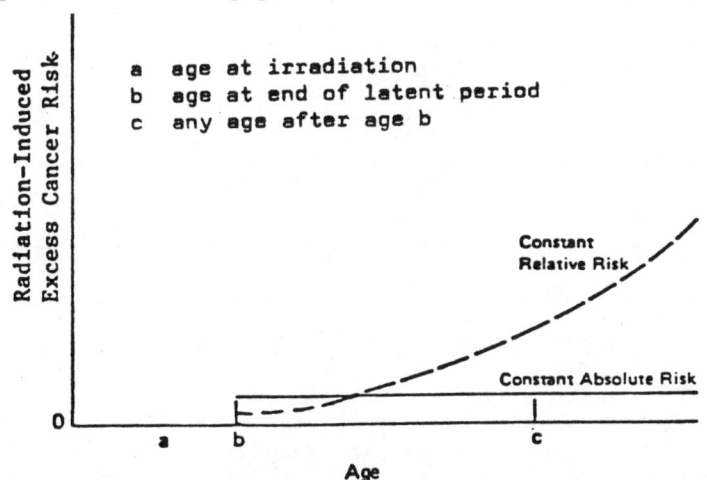

FIGURE 13 Carcinogenic risk following radiation: absolute and relative risk models.

tative of a general population exposed either to a single whole-body low LET dose or to a chronic low level dose throughout life. A single dose of 10 rad was chosen bacause the Committee had little confidence that the estimated risks would pertain at lower doses such as 1 rad. Occupational groups starting at one age and ending at a later age are also considered.

Table 1 reproduces the lifetime mortality risks using the absolute risk projection to a life table population of 1 million receiving a <u>single dose of 10 rads</u>. According to the preferred LQ model, the normal cancer expectation of 164,000 would be increased by about 0.5% of that expectation. Table 2 reproduces lifetime mortality risks again using the absolute risk projection, to a population of 1 million receiving <u>1 rad/year between the ages 20 and 65</u>. According to the preferred LQ model the normal cancer mortality expectation of 171,500 would be increased by about 2% of that expectation.

These new estimates do not differ significantly from those in the preceding BEIR and UNSCEAR Reports. However, the consideration given to the "less-than-linear" dose response relations is new and potentially can change risk estimates substantially in a downward direction depending on the particular non-linear model employed.

Table 1 Lifetime mortality risks per million from 10 rads single dose to lifetable population for absolute risk projection model

Model	Excess cancer deaths				
	Leukemia	bone	Other solid	Total	% of normal ca. expected
Quadratic	30		65	95	0.058
Linear-quadratic	230		536	766	0.47
Linear	475		1196	1671	1.0

Table 2 Lifetime mortality risks per million from 1 rad per year to population starting at age 20 and ending at age 65 for absolute risk projection model

Model	Excess cancer deaths				
	Leukemia	bone	Other solid	Total	% of normal ca. expected
Linear-quadratic	837		2466	3303	1.9
Linear	1888		6090	7978	4.65

RISK ESTIMATION FOR SPECIFIC ORGANS

a) <u>Leukemia</u>. The Japanese data and the likely linear-quadratic dose response have been discussed earlier. In the most recent follow-up of the ankylosing spondylitis cases who received one course of treatment with a mean marrow dose of about 300 rads the excess leukemia risk was estimated at about 1 case per million persons per year per rad, in good agreement with the Japanese data.

b) <u>Bone cancer</u>. Most of the human data relates to alpha irradiation from Radium-224 and Radium-226. Whereas the Ra-224 data are consistent with linearity, the Ra-226 data are best fitted with a dose-squared relation, as shown in Figure 14 particularly at the lowest doses[2]. No increase in bone sarcoma has been found in the A-bomb survivors. There is a large amount of animal data, briefly referenced in the BEIR III Report, which demonstrates a strong square-law response (concave upward) for bone cancer following the administration of strontium-90, a pure beta ray emitter (Figure 15).

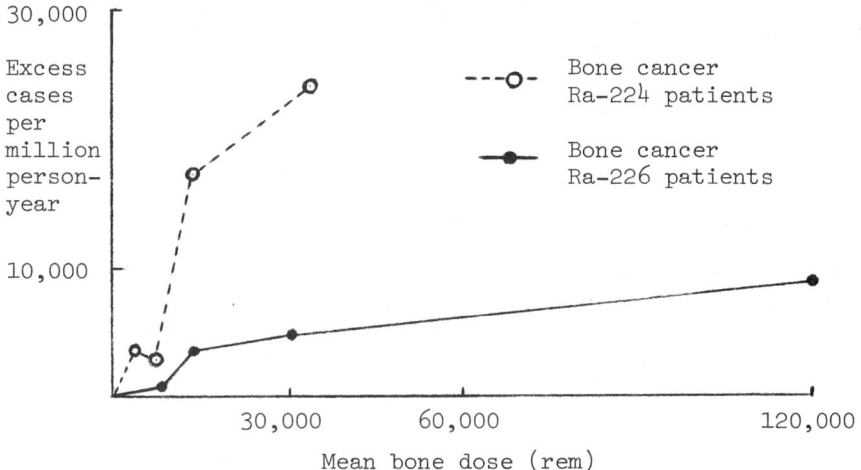

FIGURE 14 Dose response curves for bone cancer produced by alpha emitters (BEIR I 1972)

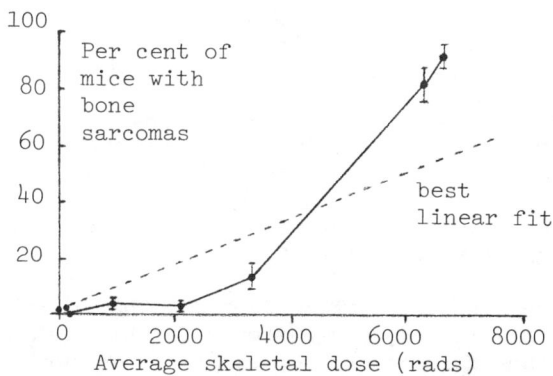

FIGURE 15 Bone sarcomas induced in CF-1 female mice injected with Strontium-90 at 70 days of age. (Data from M. Finkel in Biomedical Implications of Radiostrontium Exposure. Goldman and Bustad: USAEC CONF-710201, 352, 1972)

c) <u>Thyroid cancer</u>. Much of the thyroid cancer data in humans comes from the follow-up of persons irradiated as infants by x rays for enlarged thymus glands[19]. The typical dose was 200 to 600 rads, and of 2650 children treated, 24 have developed thyroid cancer. Incidence per 1000 person-years of follow-up is shown in Figure 16. The number of cases is shown in parentheses at each data point and is very small. Although a linear dose response has been claimed for these data, it is apparent that a linear-quadratic relation would provide a better fit (the dotted line in Figure 16). Indeed a very recent paper[20] which has re-analyzed these data confirms this appearance. The risk on a linear basis is about 3 cases per million per year per rad.

The case for linearity has been strengthened by the 1974 study by Modan of Israeli children who received therapeutic x radiation to the scalp for treatment of ringworm[13]. The thyroid dose was estimated as only 6 rads and the observation of 10 cases of thyroid cancer in 10,000 persons fits well on the linear relation shown in Figure 16. However, this study remains controversial for several reasons:
1. excess thyroid cancer was not found in a smaller study of similar cases in the USA[21];
2. much higher doses were received during the treatment by the pituitary gland and this may be associated with the thyroid cancer incidence which is known to have hormonal dependence;
3. facial and neck structures may not have been well shielded during the treatment of some of these children who were immigrants into the State of Israel in its early years;
4. the thymus gland series [19, 20] shows a special predisposition towards radiogenic thyroid cancer among persons, particularly females, of Jewish extraction.

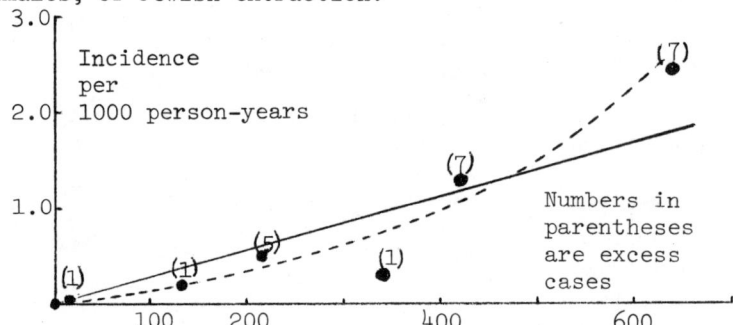

FIGURE 16 Radiation-induced thyroid cancer following x-ray treatment in infancy[19]

d) <u>Lung cancer</u>. There are also some indications that lung cancer while consistent with a linear dose response for high LET radiation, as in the uranium miner population, for example as shown[22] in Figure 17, may not be linear for low doses of low LET radiation (Figure 18). Mortality from lung cancer in Nagasaki[15] shows a significant deficit for doses below 100 rads. However in BEIR III the evidence for non-linearity has not been accepted for partial-body irradiation of the lung and a risk of 3 cases per million-year-rem based mainly on the miners' follow-up is proposed.

e) <u>Breast cancer</u>. As indicated earlier, the human data[12] on radiogenic breast cancer induction is consistent with linearity (Figure 19), but the data at low doses are weak and indeed essentially non-existent except for the Japanese A-bomb survivors. The Japanese data in Figure 19 are for the combined results in Hiroshima and Nagasaki[3]. Figure 20 shows the age-adjusted data separately for the two cities[3] together with the standard errors. There is some apparent curvilinearity in the data for each city but it is more pronounced for Nagasaki. The prudent assumption at present based on all the data is that the relationship is linear although this cannot be regarded as proven, and the absolute risk is about 6 cases per million-year-rad after a latent period of 10 years.

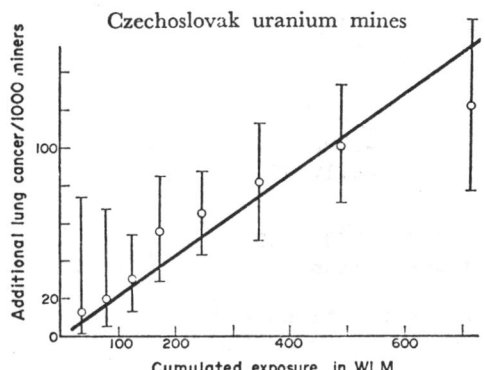

FIGURE 17 Excess lung cancer among Czech uranium miners and the regression line for cumulative radon exposure in working-level-months. (Courtesy of Health Physics)

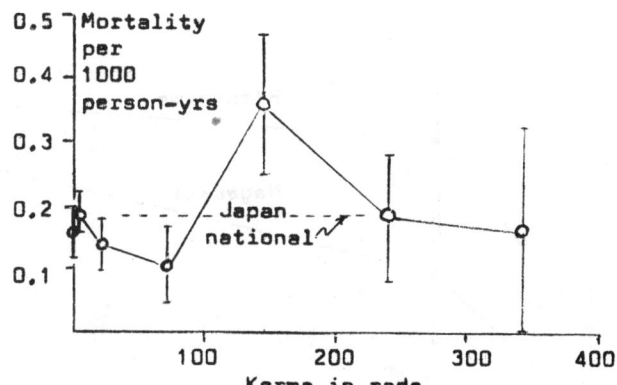

FIGURE 18 Mortality in Nagasaki 1950-74 from cancer of the trachea, bronchus, lung. (Life Span Study[15])

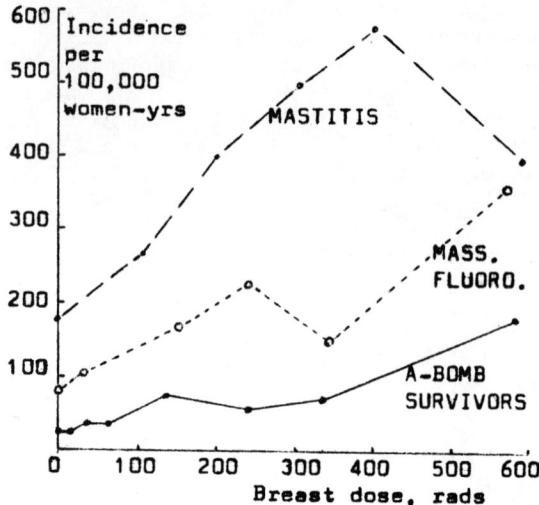

FIGURE 19 Dose response relations for radiation-induced breast cancer (after Boice et al[3])

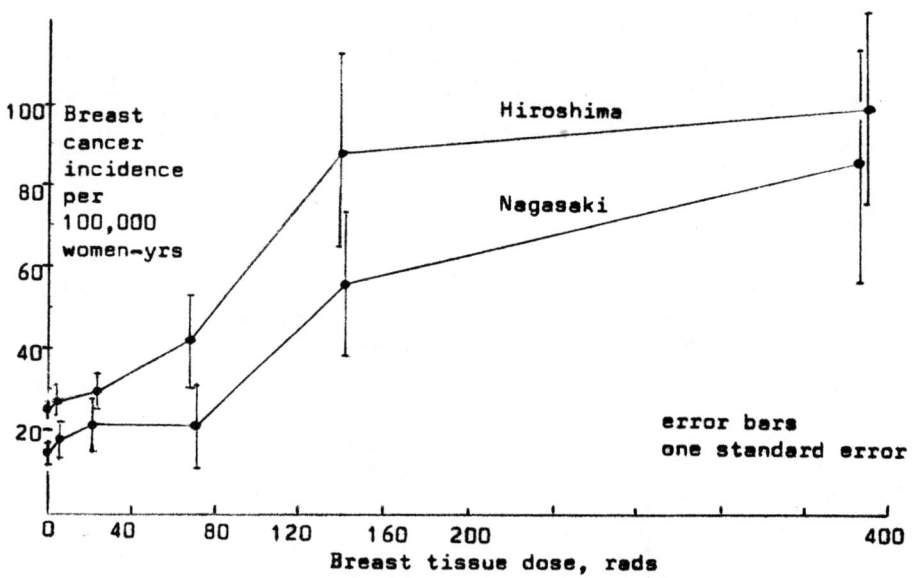

FIGURE 20 Age-adjusted breast cancer incidence rates versus dose for Japanese A-bomb survivors in Hiroshima and Nagasaki (based on data from Tokunaga et al[3])

SUMMARY OF SPECIFIC ORGAN RISKS

The risk estimates in BEIR III for cancer incidence per year per rad of absorbed dose to the thyroid, lung, breast and other internal organs based on the <u>linear</u> hypothesis are set out in Table 3 below.

Table 3 Estimated excess cancer incidence per million persons per year per rad (linear hypothesis)

Site	Males	Females
Thyroid	2.2	5.8
Lung	3.6	3.9
Esophagus	0.3	0.3
Stomach	1.5	1.7
Intestine	1.0	1.1
Liver	0.7	0.7
Pancreas	0.9	1.0
Urinary	0.8	0.9
Lymphoma	0.3	0.3
Breast	---	5.8
Other	1.5	1.6
Total	12.8	23.1
Mean	18	

The sum of the site-specific estimates is used in one of the estimates of cancer incidence following whole-body exposure but this estimate is considered to be overly high and is therefore not "preferred".

CANCER FOLLOWING EXPOSURE IN UTERO

The studies of association of childhood cancer, particularly leukemia, with diagnostic abdominal irradiation of the mother during pregnancy are reviewed in BEIR III. These studies are widely quoted as evidence of a) a carcinogenic effect of radiation at the 1 rad level; and b) considerably greater (5 times) sensitivity to radiation of the fetus compared to the adult. The principal data in studies of this type are those of Stewart and her associates in the Oxford survey of childhood cancer deaths in England[23,24]. Based on these studies which show a greater frequency of <u>in utero</u> exposure in children dying from malignant disease, it has been estimated that between 300 and 800 extra cancer deaths per million children per rad received will occur. These studies are clouded by the possibility that prenatal exposure entails a process of selection which accounts for the increased incidence of malignancy in the exposed population. The most convincing evidence that the irradiation is causal comes from a recent analysis of the Oxford data by Mole[25] which found an excess risk in irradiated twins where the frequency of x-ray examination in twin births was 55%.

Nevertheless, two important negative studies of the cohort

type cast considerable doubt on the reality of the Stewart conclusions. In the prospective study of Court-Brown and Doll[26] follow-up of 39,000 children irradiated in utero showed zero excess cancer whereas at least 11 excess cases would have been expected on the evidence of Stewart et al. Furthermore, in the study of Jablon and Kato[27] of 1292 children born to women who were pregnant at the time of the A-bombing, no excess of cancer was found up to age 10. For the mean fetal dose of 13.5 rads the Stewart risk estimate predicts an excess of 5 cancer cases. Thus the effect of 1 rad and the postulated greater sensitivity of the fetus remains to be substantiated.

RECENT CLAIMS OF INCREASED RADIATION RISKS

The BEIR III Report contains comments on and evaluations of several recent controversial studies which claim carcinogenic effects in occupational or medically exposed groups receiving low LET radiation doses of the order of 1 rad. In each case the allegations are found to be unproven.

a) <u>The Mancuso Report</u>. This is an analysis of 3500 male deaths in the work force of the Hanford Atomic plant, Richland, Washington over the period 1944 to 1972 as related to radiation doses recorded on film badges[28,29]. Excess risk was claimed for cancer of the lung, pancreas, bone marrow and lymph system. A thorough review by Hutchison, MacMahon, Jablon and Land[30] has concluded that there was <u>no</u> association with worker exposure levels for lung cancer, leukemia, lymphoma or all cancer; but there was a significant association for two cancers: multiple myeloma and cancer of the pancreas, even though the mean dose of persons dying with cancer was only 2.1 rad compared with the mean dose for all deceased workers of 1.7 rad. The risk for multiple myeloma was judged to have increased 67% per rad received and for cancer of the pancreas 20% per rad. These risk estimates are extremely high compared with those deduced from other studies; for example, the absolute risk for pancreatic cancer of 10 deaths per million per year per rad derived by Hutchison et al[30] must be compared with 0.44 derived from the ankylosing spondylitis cases and 0.83/M-Y-rad for the Nagasaki survivors (BEIR III). Such high risks may be discounted on the grounds that they imply an improbably large role for background radiation (1 rad in 10 years) in the etiology of these two cancers. Doubt is also cast upon this study by the failure after careful review to find an association of leukemia with dose, which is generally considered the most likely association.

b) <u>The Bross papers</u>. In 1977 and 1979 Bross and his associates presented two papers[31,32] claiming supersensitivity of certain types of subjects to diagnostic x rays. Both of these papers have been subject to critical analyses by Oppenheim[33] and Boice and Land[34] which point to very serious errors, omissions and biasses in the studies. These and other reviewers conclude that the data utilized and the methods of analysis do not lead to the stated conclusions.

c) <u>Portsmouth Naval Shipyard</u>. In 1978 Najarian and Colton published a study of relative cancer deaths in two groups of dockyard workers who were reported as exposed or unexposed to radiation[35]. This classification was established by interviews with next of kin without reference to the radiation exposure records in the possession of the U.S. Navy. The preliminary findings are shown in Table 4. Subsequently the radiation records were released to the National Institute of Occupational Safety and Health and the study was repeated with a reclassification of the deceased workers as exposed or unexposed. Table 4 also includes the results of the second study based on 354 deaths among monitored nuclear workers. Expected deaths are computed from population rates based on the age distribution at death of the nuclear workers.

Table 4 Results of Portsmouth Naval Shipyard Study

Cause of death	Method of classification as nuclear workers					
	Next of kin			Naval Shipyard records		
	Observed	Expected	O/E	Observed	Expected	O/E
Leukemia	6	1.1	5.5	4	2.7	1.5
All hematol. ca.	10	2.9	3.4	9	7.1	1.3
All cancers	56	31.5	1.8	99	74.7	1.3

In the NIOSH study the ratio of observed to expected are similar to those found in employed populations. There was no statistically acceptable evidence of an increasing mortality as a function of dose. The original results are attributed to a bias in reporting workers who died from cancer as nuclear workers.

d) <u>Infant mortality from Chinese A-bomb fallout</u>. Dr. Ernest Sternglass has claimed that fallout from Chinese bomb testing in 1976 led to increased activity in milk in Eastern seaboard states which increased infant mortality in those states. The BEIR Committee concluded that there was no clear evidence of a universally applicable change in infant mortality rates and that the alleged association did not fit the time course for radioisotope movement into the milk food chain.

REFERENCES

1. The effects on populations of exposure to low levels of ionizing radiation. Report of the Committee on the Biological Effects of Ionizing Radiations. National Academy of Sciences-National Research Council, Washington, D.C. (1980).
2. The effects on populations of exposure to low levels of ionizing radiation. Report of the Advisory Committee on the Biological Effects of Ionizing Radiations. National Academy of Sciences - National Research Council, Washington, D.C. (1972).
3. Tokunaga, M., Norman, J. E. et al. Malignant breast tumors among atomic bomb survivors, Hiroshima and Nagasaki, 1950-74. J. Nat. Cancer Inst. $\underline{62}$, 1347 (1979).
4. Sources and Effects of Ionizing Radiation. United Nations Scientific Committee on the Effects of Ionizing Radiation. Report to the General Assembly. United Nations, New York (1977).
5. Purrott, R.J. and Reeder, E. The effects of changes in dose rate on the yield of chromosome aberrations in human lymphocytes exposed to gamma radiation Mutat. Res. $\underline{35}$, 437 (1976).
6. DuFrain, R.J., Littlefield, L.G., et al. Human cytogenetic

dosimetry: a dose-response relationship for alpha particle radiation from ^{241}Am. Health Physics 37, 279 (1979).
7. Ullrich, R. L., Jernigan, M. C. et al. The influence of dose and dose rate on the incidence of neoplastic disease in RFM mice after neutron radiation. Rad. Res. 68, 115 (1976).
8. Ullrich, R. L., Jernigan, M. C. and Adams, L. M. Induction of lung tumors in RFM mice after localized exposures to x rays or neutrons Rad. Res. 80, 464 (1979).
9. Shellabarger, C. J., Bond, V. P. et al. Relationship of dose of total-body ^{60}Co radiation to incidence of mammary neoplasia in female rats. In Radiation-Induced Cancer 161-172 International Atomic Energy Agency, Vienna (1969).
10. Kellerer, A. M. and Rossi, H. H. The theory of dual radiation action. Current Topics in Radiat. Res. Quart. 8, 85 (1972).
11. Rossi, H. H. The effects of small doses of ionizing radiation Rad. Res. 71, 1 (1977).
12. Boice, J. D., Land, C. E. et al. Risk of breast cancer following low dose radiation exposure. Radiology 131, 589 (1979).
13. Modan, B., Baidatz, D. et al. Radiation-induced head and neck tumors. Lancet 1, 277 (1974).
14. Stewart, A. M. and Kneale, G. W. Radiation dose effects in relation to obstetric x-rays and childhood cancers. Lancet 1, 1185 (1970).
15. Beebe, G. W., Kato, H. and Land, C. E. Mortality experience on atomic bomb survivors, 1950-74. Life Span Study Report 8. Technical Report TR1-77. Radiation Effects Research Foundation, Hiroshima (1978). See also Studies of the mortality of A-bomb survivors, 6. Mortality and radiation dose, 1950-74. Rad. Res. 75, 138 (1978).
16. Ishimaru, T., Otake, M. and Ichimaru, M. Dose response relationship of neutrons and gamma rays to leukemia incidence among atomic bomb survivors in Hiroshima and Nagasaki by type of leukemia, 1950-71. Rad. Res. 77, 377 (1979).
17. Land, C. E., Beebe, G. W. and Jablon, S. Role of neutrons in late effects of radiation among A-bomb survivors. Paper at Health Physics Soc. Annual Meeting, Minneapolis, Minn. June 21, 1978.
18. Webster, E. W. in Low-Level Ionizing Radiation. Hearings before the Sub-Committee on Energy Research and Production, Committee on Science and Technology, U. S. House of Representatives, 96th Congress First Session, June 13-15, 1979. No. 41. Figure 1 pg. 554 U. S. Government Printing Office (1979).
19. Hempelmann, L. H. et al. Neoplasms in persons treated with x-rays in infancy: fourth survey in 20 years. J. Nat. Cancer Inst. 55, 519 (1975).
20. Shore, R. E. et al. Radiation and host factors in human thyroid tumors following thyroid irradiation. Health Physics, 38 451 (1980).
21. Shore, R. E., Albert, R. E. and Pasternack, B. S. Follow-up study of patients treated by x-ray epilation for tinea capitis. Arch. Env. Health, 31, 17 (1976).
22. Sevc, J., Kunz, E. and Placek, V. Lung cancer in uranium miners and long term exposure to radon daughter products. Health Physics, 30, 433 (1976).

23. Stewart, A., Webb, J. and Hewitt, D. A survey of childhood malignancies. Brit. Med. J. 1, 1495 (1958).
24. Stewart, A. and Kneale, G. W. Radiation dose effects in relation to obstetric x-rays and childhood cancers. Lancet 1, 1185 (1970).
25. Mole, R. H. Antenatal irradiation and childhood cancer: causation or coincidence. Brit. Jour. Cancer 30, 199 (1974).
26. Court-Brown, W. M., Doll, R. and Hill, A. B. The incidence of leukemia following exposure to diagnostic radiation in utero. Brit. Med. J. 2, 1539 (1960).
27. Jablon, S. and Kato, H. Childhood cancer in relation to prenatal exposure to atomic-bomb radiation. Lancet 2, 1000 (1970).
28. Mancuso, T. F., Stewart, A. and Kneale, G. W. Radiation exposures of Hanford workers dying from cancer and other causes. Health Physics 33, 369 (1977).
29. Kneale, G. W. Stewart, A. and Mancuso, T. F. Re-analysis of data relating to the Hanford study of the cancer risks of radiation workers. In Late Biological Effects of Ionizing Radiation, Vol. 1. p. 386. International Atomic Energy Agency, Vienna (1978).
30. Hutchison, G. B., MacMahon, B., Jablon, S. and Land, C. E. Review of report by Mancuso, Stewart and Kneale of radiation exposure of Hanford workers. Health Physics 37, 207 (1979).
31. Bross, I. D. J. and Natarajan, N. Genetic damage from diagnostic radiation, J. A. M. A. 237, 2399 (1977).
32. Bross, I. D. J., Ball, M. and Falen, S. A dosage response curve for the 1 rad range: adult risks from diagnostic radiation. Am. J. Public Health 69, 130 (1979).
33. Oppenheim, B. E. Genetic damage from diagnostic radiation? A critique of the Bross and Natarajan study. J. A. M. A. 242, 1390 (1979).
34. Boice, J. D. and Land, C. E. Adult leukemia following diagnostic x-rays? Am. J. Public Health 69, 137 (1979).
35. Najarian, T. and Colton, T. Mortality from leukemia and cancer in shipyard nuclear workers. Lancet 1, 1018 (1978).

UPDATE ON THE UNSCEAR* REPORT

Fred A. Mettler, Jr., M.D.
University of New Mexico, Albuquerque, NM 87131

ABSTRACT

The UNSCEAR Committee plans to expand the 1977 report by inclusion of pertinent data generated since the previous report. To date there appears to be little justification for changing genetic risk estimates; the linear-quadratic dose response function appears satisfactory for low-LET radiation; the non-stochastic effects of low dose radiation will be carefully examined. Additionally, the Committee feels that life-shortening in most animal species and in humans is probably the result of induction of malignant neoplasms. Medical radiation will be considered in terms of describing somatic detriment and essentially using the model described by the ICRP.

INTRODUCTION

The information presented here is an update of the 1977 UNSCEAR report. Although many documents will be presented in the forthcoming 1981 report, not all of them have direct reference to the biological risks of medical irradiation. The portion of the report presented here is still in draft form and may change somewhat in content before final approval by the UNSCEAR Committee and the United Nations General Assembly. This material is restricted for purposes of quotation.

GENETIC EFFECTS OF RADIATION

Emphasis in the new UNSCEAR report will be on updating the 1977 report with new data bearing on the evaluation of genetic radiation hazards in man. The relevant human data include naturally occurring hereditary diseases and defects. The results of the British Columbia survey[1] on the frequency of liveborn individuals affected by hereditary or partially hereditary defects and diseases has been reappraised. It was concluded from this and other studies that for the purpose of estimating genetic radiation hazards in man it is appropriate to use the following revised figure: A) 1.0% dominant and X-linked diseases, B) 0.1% recessive diseases, C) 0.4% chromosomal diseases, and D) 9% congenital malformations multifactorial and irregularly inherited diseases (a total of 10.5%).

A compilation of surveys of numerical and structural chromosome abnormalities includes several involving newborn infants. The data available in the 1977 report indicated that of 55,679 babies tested, 336 (0.6%) had abnormal chromosome constitutions. More recent surveys indicate percentages ranging from 0.48% to 0.83%. Thus, with the addition of new data, 0.62% of babies examined appear to be chromosomally abnormal.

*United Nations Scientific Committee on Effects of Atomic Radiation

The frequency of "clinically significant" abnormalities has also been estimated. Included in this category are the non-mosaic XXY and chromosome 45, X instances, XYY and XX (male) genotypes, all autosomal trisomies and all unbalanced structural rearrangements associated with congenital malformations at birth. The estimate arrived at is 2.91 per 1000 (0.29%), i.e. about one-half of the total of all chromosomal abnormalities detected in newborns. There are several reasons why this number may prove to be an underestimate. Firstly, of the chromosomal abnormalities detected in newborns since 1977, only long term studies will answer questions as to the full clinical significance. Second, the frequency of sex-chromosome mosaics detected in many surveys may be low since the number of cells analyzed may not have been adequate, and finally, data is slowly accumulating, indicating even an apparently balanced structural rearrangement in man can have deleterious effects.

In the few studies carried out on the incidence of chromosomal abnormalities detected in perinatal deaths, the frequency of anomalies appears to be approximately 6%. Additional new data regarding chromosome anomalies in spontaneous abortion has supported and extended the conclusions of the Committee in the 1977 report, i.e. that the overall frequency of chromosomal anomalies among spontaneous abortions may be as high as 50%, and that trisomies as a group constitute the most common anomaly.

The detection of aneuploidy was also discussed in the 1977 UNSCEAR report and there was hope that the intensely fluorescent dot in interphase nuclei following staining with quinacrine dichloride might be useful for estimating nondisjunction in the Y chromosome. Recent work indicates that the F bodies may not at present provide a useful means of estimating the Y chromosomal nondisjunction because not all F bodies represent Y chromosomes. A recent technique has been described in which human spermatozoa can be fused with zona-pellucida-free eggs of the golden hamster. With this technique it may be possible to directly study these sperm chromosomes in a manner similar to the analysis used for somatic cells.

Down's Syndrome is one of the better known autosomal aneuploidies in man. Use of the fluorescent banding techniques gives evidence of the paternal origin of the extra chromosome 21, and the search for a paternal age effect has once again begun. Maternal age has long been known to be an important factor in Down's Syndrome. The Committee had earlier reviewed several studies designed to inquire whether parental (particularly maternal) radiation may increase the risk of Down's Syndrome. An additional recent study has been performed, the Baltimore Case Control[2] study, which found no significant effect of maternal irradiation on the incidence of Down's Syndrome.

The introduction of banding techniques has demonstrated that contrary to earlier belief, partial monosomies are not necessarily lethal and are in fact relatively frequent, involving most of the human chromosomes. Banding has also given some insight into the possible role of chromosomal changes in the origin of some human neoplasias. Chromosomal changes are well known, in the association of the Philadelphia chromosome with chronic myelogenous leukemia.

Acute leukemia victims exhibit chromosomal abnormalities in approximately 50% of the cases, and other studies report chromosomal abnormalities in patients with Burkitt's lymphoma, retinoblastoma and meningiomas.

A large amount of new data (too extensive to be presented here) has become available concerning chromosomal abnormalities in translocations in animals. Recent work of interest comparing radiation sensitivity of human lymphocytes to that of various animal species indicate that human lymphocytes are 1.5 to 2 times more sensitive than mouse lymphocytes. Cat lymphocytes appear to have only about one-fifth the sensitivity of human lymphocytes while experiments in primates indicate close similarity to the data obtained in humans. Other relevant data on the incidence of chromosome aberration in workers exposed to mixed neutron and gamma radiation during refueling of nuclear reactors has become available. There is a positive correlation between the incidence of cells containing aberrations and radiation dose when the population is grouped into cumulative dose categories of five rem intervals. Although the population groups were relatively small, it was clear the yield of dicentric aberrations in cells from individuals who prior to occupational exposures scored approximately 1 in 700 cells, rose four fold afer cumulative doses of 20 to 30 rems.

The 1977 report of the Committee present the available human and experimental data concerned with the evaluation of genetic hazards in man, and discussed assumptions and uncertainties involved in making use of this data as well as giving quantitative estimates of hazards using both the "direct" and the "doubling dose" methods. With the "direct" method it was pointed out that with respect to hazards from induction of mutation, what was desired was an assessment of the risk of induction of dominant effects in the progeny with some indication of handicaps and disabilities. For this purpose, the mouse data on gamma ray induction of dominant mutations in the skeleton was used. The reasoning remains unchanged that many of the skeletal abnormalities in the mouse experiments are similar to rare dominant and irregularly inherited dominant conditions in man which constitute a sizeable proportion of human genetic disease. The estimate of risk arrived at was 20×10^{-6} per rad of paternal low-LET, low dose or low dose-rate irradiation. There appears no reason at the present time to alter this estimate.

Newly available date indicating that radiation induction of dominant mutations causes cataracts in mice may also prove useful. Several reasons appear at the present time for revising estimates of the hazards from induction of balanced reciprocal translocations in man. These reasons include data that 1) the rhesus monkey spermatogonia are much less sensitive than human spermatogonia to translocation induction; and 2) spontaneously arising de novo balanced reciprocal translocations in man can have deleterious effects such as mental retardation, obviousl of clinical significance. To date there are no new data which justify revision of the estimate for induction of sex chromosome losses and other chromosome anomalies.

No new data is available pertaining to the "doubling dose" method for hazard evaluation. The discovery of partial deletion and duplications involving almost every chromosome is of clinical interest but at the present time has not been shown to be induced by radiation. One of the main assumptions involved in the use of doubling dose method is that of proportionality between the average spontaneous and induction rates of mutation. Again no new data have accumulated to suggest an inconsistency in this area.

In summary, with regard to the genetic effects of radiation, there does not appear to be any justification for altering any of the estimates presented in the 1977 report of the Committee.

DOSE RESPONSE RELATIONSHIPS FOR RADIATION-INDUCED CANCER

Malignant neoplasms induced by ionizing radiation probably represent the most important late somatic effect on exposed populations. The probablistic nature of the relation between the dose and frequency of malignancy has been given the term "stochastic." Knowledge of the dose/response function is necessary for assessment of risk from environmental and occupational doses received by man. The most controversial and environmentally important area is the relationship at low doses. The 1977 UNSCEAR report indicated that the lack of "threshold" dose had not been proven. Analysis of the data has been complicated by the great variability and sensitivity of various tissues to induction of malignancy as well as the interaction of other agents such as viruses.

In general, since the publication of the 1977 report there has been relatively little new data concerning experimental induction of malignant neoplasm by radiation. In the 1977 report the Committee presented a comprehensive review of all the epidemiological evidence on radiation induced cancer in man and gave the probability of incidence and mortality per 10^{-6} per unit dose. Most of this evidence related to doses above 100 rads. Additionally, a lifetime risk of cancer incidence was estimated. Direct application of these risk factors has involved the procedure of linear extrapolation. Due to uncertainties in the shape of the dose-response function, such extrapolation can lead to over or underestimation of the risk. The uncertainties in the shape of the dose-response function in man derives from four conditions: 1) the narrow range of doses to which populations studied long term have been exposed; 2) questionable accuracy of dosimetric estimates; 3) wide confidence limits due to the small number of excess cases observed; and 4) the relatively short follow-up periods which do not allow for full manifestation of the expected cancer incidence.

In view of these many difficulties, the Committee has elected to take an alternative approach to assessing the character of the dose-response relationship. Other evidence obtained at subcellular and cellular levels, which theoretically has some inference regarding cancer induction is reviewed in the hope it can contribute a better understanding of the dose response relationship. Such understanding is particularly desirable with regard to limiting the margin of uncertainty felt to exist in following the principle of linear extrapolation.

A large amount of data has been reviewed by the Committee since the 1977 report. Most of the reviewed quantitative models involve over simplifications, and none of the models take into account all possible interacting factors. Some models are linear-quadratic while others such as the Marshall and Groer's[3] model of bone cancer induction do not consider such systemic factors as the immune response and possible virus-host interactions. The role of physiological promoting factors has rarely been considered.

In spite of these limitations the reviewed models permit approximate assessment of tumor rate or cumulative incidence particularly with regard to radiation quality and dose rate. They are also the only available methods by which an approximate, although meaningful, extrapolation is possible in the range from one to several hundred rads. The models require several assumptions which include the stochastic nature of the induction, the unicellular (clonal) origin of cancer and the proportionality of the probability of cancer induction by a given dose of radiation to the number of cells at risk.

None of the models allow estimation of the effect of the genetic heterogeneity of the human population. If this has a significant effect it could lead to a biomodal distribution or to different dose response relationships for subgroups.

Initiation of cancer at the cellular level appears to involve nuclear DNA as the target. Examination of dose response relationships for various effects at the cellular level leads to the following conclusions. For high-LET radiations, the dose response relationships are commonly linear. When sparsely ionizing radiation is delivered at high dose rates, both linear and supralinear relationships are seen for some of the end points e.g., point mutations and somatic cells, terminal deletions of chromosomes, and cell inactivation. At low dose rates and small increments of dose of low-LET radiation, linearity is observed for all end points considered, although when the yield is expressed per unit dose, the results are much below those seen at high dose rate. In general, although some experiments demonstrate a linear response for some effects at the cellular level, assumption that this is a general rule appears unwarranted.

The linear-quadratic model of radiation induced cancer was carefully examined. For sparsely ionizing radiation, equal contribution of the linear and quadratic terms to the total effect occurs in mammalarian cells between about 50 and a few hundred rads. For high-LET radiation, the contribution of the dose-squared term remains negligible below 1000 rads. The effects of radiation quality and time of dose delivery can both be explained by the theory of dual radiation action. With dose protraction or fractionation it is the contribution of the dose-squared term which decreases with increasing time of dose delivery. The linear terms remain unaffected. Thus, at low dose rates or doses applied in small fractions, the dose-response relations tend to become linear. To account for decreasing yields of tumors at high dose values, any model of cancer induction requires the introduction of an additional factor which is usually interpreted as the radiation-induced sterilization of the transformed cell at high doses.

Various models indicate that with respect to tissues of relatively high sensitivity to cancer induction by radiation, the dose response relationships with densely ionizing particles display linearity over the initial portion of the curve. For low-LET radiation, curvilinear relations are observed so that linear extrapolation to low doses should overestimate the risk. At low dose rate for both high and low-LET radiation, a linearity of the response would be expected with the high RBE of neutrons and alpha particles.

For tissues of low sensitivity, of which bone and skin may be examples, curvilinear dose response relations would be expected with pronounced fractionation. Gross overestimation of the risk in the low dose/dose-rate domain should apply if estimates are obtained by linear extrapolation of risk factors from the high dose region. For high-LET particles the respective situation can vary with the spacial relationships of the source and target. Both linear and curvilinear relations may describe the situation.

These analyses of the dose-response relationship of cancer induction are limited by the understanding of the process of cancer induction itself. Further studies aimed at the elucidation of carcinogenesis may diminish some of this uncertainty.

RADIATION-INDUCED AGING AND LIFE SPAN SHORTENING AFTER LOW DOSES OF WHOLE BODY IRRADIATION

Multiple experiments in the 1950's indicated life span shortening due to radiation. A link was established between the life shortening action of radiation and natural senescence. In the late 1950's and early 1960's, reviews of the literature criticized the establishment of a close relationship between aging and certain effects of irradiation, since it was difficult to maintain that irradiation simply advanced the onset of senescence unless it could be accepted that the aging of various organs could be advanced by different degrees.

Many of the experiments performed used death as an end point since it can be precisely defined; however, this is biologically unsatisfactory since it is more informative to know the reason why an animal dies. With aging, the cause of death often becomes obscure since there are multiple lesions and the primary one is difficult to discern.

A large amount of data has been reviewed by the Committee since the 1977 report, including the effects of physical variables, biological variables and modifying effects as well as the human experience. When acute single doses are considered and a plot is made of all the data reviewed, it can be concluded that the life shortening data for the mouse may be considered to follow a linear relationship as a function of the x- or gamma ray acute dose, indicating a life shortening efficiency of about 5% per 100 rads down to the smallest doses. The data may equally well be fitted by a linear-quadratic function where the quadratic term is negligible. Since this curve is a combination of multiple experiments, it is also possible that in a highly non-homogenous mammalian population where all ages, sexes, and strains are randomly represented, the use of a linear or quadratic function to describe the dose effect relationship for acute exposures is not an unreasonable proposition. Data obtained with neutron irradiation are best described by a relationship having a convex upward trend with dose. The data on single acute exposures of animals other than the mouse is much more limited; however, no large differences from the mouse data can be traced from the small series available in the literature.

Continuous lifetime irradiation and its effect on life span shortening may be analyzed either as a function of dose rate or of the total dose received. There have been enough experiments in the mouse to examine both types of dependencies. Sigmoid relationships of the type

$$y = 100 (1 - e^{-a A}) \tag{1}$$

where A is the dose rate in rads/day may be reasonably fitted to the data. The solutions were, in the case of low-LET radiation

$$y = 100 (1 - e^{-0.0379A}) \tag{2}$$

and in the case of neutrons

$$y = 100 (1 - e^{-0.4883A\, 2/3}). \tag{3}$$

When life span shortening is plotted as a function of dose accumulated, the low-LET data show that as the dose increases, the life-shortening effect also increases in an apparently linear fashion at low doses and then with a progressively accentuated upper concavity up to doses of about 6,000 rads. It is of interest to examine the change of effectiveness observed in amounts between the single acute dose and the extremely low dose rate data. When the linear term of the acute single exposure (aboug 5% life loss per 100 rads) is divided by the slope of the curve for the duration of life exposure obtained the loss of efficiency is about a factor of 7.

The effect of variation of dose rate upon life shortening is modest in the case of low-LET radiation and doubtful for neutrons (with treatments lasting a few hours to a few days). Only when extremely low dose rates and correspondingly long radiation times are involved, x- and gamma rays (but not neutrons) show consistent reduction of effectiveness by a factor in the range of 10 - 20.

Only a very few experiments have been conducted where the observations on survival have been accompanied by careful pathology of the animals at death, or serial sacrifices done, to investigate the development of the pathology of aging. In general, analysis of the data of these experiments appears to justify the conclusion that life-shortening, which was clearly apparent when all causes of death were considered together disappears when tumors are excluded from analysis of the data.

Thus, the vast majority of the data obtained on different species of rodent and non-rodent mammals irradiated with sparsely and densely ionizing radiation and with acute and chronic doses appears to be consistent with the following conclusions: the long-term life-shortening action observed on animals surviving the acute effects of radiation may be reasonably accounted for by an acceleration or increased incidence of neoplastic conditions taking some of the animals to premature death. Starting at doses around the $LD_{50/30}$ but progressively more so at higher doses, other pathological conditions may also advance or accelerate death, including fibrosis and vascular changes. The notion of nonspecific aging is based only on actuarial analogies between irradiated and aging animal populations, but it cannot be substantiated by accurate pathology.

Concerning biological variables, there appears to be sufficient data available for discussions on genetic constitution as well as the influence of sex and age at the time of irradiation. It does not appear from the data that the differences between various mammalian species tested is very large. Taking the mouse and the dog to be in the middle of an ideal radiosusceptibility scale, all species may fall within a range covered by a factor of two in both directions.

The basic conclusion drawn from the vast majority of data indicate that within a given strain, sex has a constant effect in the sense that the female animals are more sensitive to radiation-induced life-shortening, which effect is mostly manifested by an increased incidence of tumors of the female genital tract. Body weight, as a biological variable, appears to be of rather minor importance.

Regarding age at time of irradiation, most data agree that irradiation in utero of the mouse produces less marked life-shortening than irradiation during post-gestational ages. The observations on life-shortening as a function of extra-uterine age are rather numerous but limited only to the mouse and rat. In both species invariably irradiation late in life produces less life-shortening than treatment at younger ages. The change in sensitivity between young and old animals may be up to a factor of three when life-shortening per unit dose is considered, but if the effect is evaluated in terms of percentage loss of the remaining life span, this is found to be on the order of a few percent. The data concerning the modifying effects was also reviewed. It appears that keeping animals under environmental temperature conditions which are thought to be suboptimal decreases rather than enhances the life-shortening effect of irradiation. Other stresses of a nonspecific nature may have some influence on life span presumably due to some interaction between the effects of stress and of radiation exposure. It appears remarkable that the cases reviewed have yielded an increase rather than a decrease in the life span of such irradiated animals.

Treatment before irradiation with a number of radioprotective chemicals affords a certain amount of reduction of the life-shortening effect. In those cases where numerical estimates of dose reduction factors can be performed, values in the region of 1.4 to 1.8 are derived. Whether the protective effect of the drugs on life span operates through a decreased induction of neoplasia and leukemia or other nonspecific diseases is not clear from the available data.

The only obvious generalization to be obtained from the experiments in which whole and partial body irradiation were compared is that partial body irradiation in the range of medium to low doses is less effective than whole body irradiation for induction of life span shortening. In cases where leukemia represents a large component in the reduction of life, the lower incidence of this disease that may result from shielding of the hematopoietic system may explain the lower efficacy of the partial body irradiation.

The human experience regarding the existence of non-specific life-shortening effects comes from three different sources: groups of persons exposed occupationally, patients who have undergone radiation treatments, and a large number of the A-bomb survivors and those exposed to a large amount of fallout. The studies on humans are subject to limitations related to the absence of control of variables, and the sample size. An additional limitation previously mentioned is insufficient time having elapsed between irradiation and complete manifestation of the possible effect.

Data on radiologists leaves no doubt, particularly when the early radiologists are examined, that leukemia and cancer have indeed been induced in these persons. Life-shortening per unit dose is not possible to determine since the exact doses are unknown. There is unanimity in the conclusion that the effect of induction of neoplastic conditions together with nonspecific life-shortening in this group has disappeared in recent times presumably due to appropriate radiation protection measures.

In spite of the small sample (about 1,200 persons) the data of the radium dial painters are quite clear in demonstrating that the only causes of deaths significantly contributing to the life span shortening are bone sarcomas and carcinoma of the cranial sinuses.

What may be safely concluded from the studies of occupationally exposed persons is that the induction of neoplastic diseases, particularly leukemia and skin cancer, are true effects, particularly in the old radiologists. Some life span reduction may also have been present, but this effect has disappeared.

In principle, radiotherapy patients have not been useful for determination of life span shortening since the size of the epidemiological surveys has been small and since, in general, only a small fraction of the body was irradiated. On the whole, all the evidence coming from the study of radiotherapy patients is negative for the presence of life-shortening effects.

Induction of leukemia and other tumors throughout the years of experience of the Japanese survivors of the A-bombs has given rise to some shortening of life. The magnitude of shortening can be entirely accounted for by the induction of neoplasms. This group has been particularly valuable due to the large size of the sample and the long term of follow-up.

In conclusion, the evidence concerning a non-specific radiation induced life-shortening effect in man has produced essentially negative answers. In the case of the old United States radiologists, the amount of data was small and are in sharp contrast to the much larger and more reliable epidemiological evidence from the A-bomb survivors. Pending further evidence, it should be concluded that radiation induced life-shortening in man is essentially due to the induction of specific neoplastic conditions.

NON-STOCHASTIC EFFECTS OF IRRADIATION

Non-stochastic effects are those for which the severity of an effect varies with the dose, and for which a threshold dose must occur. In contrast, stochastic effects arethose for which the probability of an effect occurring increases as a function of the dose with some probability existing at all dose levels. Throughout the topic covered in this report, difficulties were encountered since the concept of a threshold depends on the sensitivity of the measuring technique. One may, for example, use a clinical threshold, although structural abnormalities may be detected with much smaller doses through the use of an instrument such as an electron microscope. The report discusses the basic cellular response to irradiation, the radiation effects on individual animal tissues, and a review of data obtained in man mostly from radiation therapy results.

Tissue injury by radiation results from sterilization of the cells of that tissue. Processes of repair and repopulation will increase the threshold level of dose when irradiation is given over a long period or fractionated. There have been several attempts to express these parameters in terms of iso-effect formulae.

Review of the data on effects on tissues of experimental animals indicates the following results. Skin has an enormous capacity to repair radiation damage so that very large doses are needed in order to produce threshold changes. On the basis of repair of sublethal damage alone, the single dose may be increased by a factor of five if given over a long period. The other tissue repair process observed is that of repopulation. The esophagus demonstrates considerable ability to recover from sublethal damage with extensive cellular proliferation. From these results and from clinical studies it is clear that the esophagus is unlikely to be a limiting factor in thoracic irradiation. The gastrointestinal tract can withstand very large daily doses of radiation although all studies reviewed have concentrated on early forms of radiation injury. Little information exists on late damage to the intestine.

Growing cartilage is one of the more radiosensitive tissues. The threshold dose for causing stunting of growth is perhaps nonexistent, with doses of 20 to 30 rads producing 1% stunting in growing rodents. Lung tissue is more radiosensitive than the skin, probably because of its less rapid proliferative ability. The lung's large capacity for repair of sublethal damage enables it to tolerate a high level of fractionated irradiation without necrosis, although function is impaired.

Data on the radiosensitivity of the liver is scarce, probably because its size and position make irradiation of the whole liver exceptionally difficult without causing severe damage to other more rapidly proliferating organs. It is well known that the liver has an enormous reserve capacity and the hepatocytes have an extraordinary capacity for regeneration. The kidney is nowadays thought to be one of the more sensitive organs. Under normal circumstances there is little cell proliferation and, except for large radiation doses, the effects of irradiation occur late. The pathological changes are multiple and it is by no means clear whether vascular or parenchymal damage to the kidney is the more important. Irradiation of the spinal cord may result in myelopathy, the probability and time of onset being dose dependent. The effect of increasing the number of fractions was large in comparison with most other tissue; i.e., the spinal cord has a large capacity for accumulation and repair of sublethal damage. Some results indicate that there is no slow repair in the spinal cord, but rather delayed repopulation. The brain is fairly radiation resistant and doses in excess of 2,000 rads are required to produce morphological changes.

The normal thyroid is non-proliferating tissue in which radiation effects occur after many years. Over 1,000 rads of x-rays are required in a single exposure to cause a 50% reduction in epithelial cells, whereas irradiation with radioiodine at a low dose rate requires at least 4,000-10,000 rads to cause a slight reduction in gland weight.

Irradiation of the testes causes temporary sterility and with large doses sterility may be permanent. The testes are unlike other normal tissues in that repair of sublethal damage does not occur. Fractionated or continuous irradiation renders the tissue more, rather than less, sensitive. The ovary is more resistant than the testes, although in fetal animals, the ovaries are severely damaged by much lower doses of irradiation than that required to cause serious changes in the adult ovary.

The eye is generally considered to be one of the more sensitive tissues with damage to any part of the eye being possible. The most sensitive structure is felt to be the lens. A minimum of 300 to 500 rads are required to produce signficant opacities in animals which are not especially prone to cataract development as is the case for man. In animals who are especially prone, very much lower doses increases the incidence. More dose is required when fractionated irradiation is used, but the dose sparing effect is less than seen in some other tissues.

With acute single exposures the most critical tissue is the bone marrow. For animals of similar size to man, the LD_{50} is 200 to 300 rads. The bone marrow is capable of considerable repair between dose fraction or during low dose rate continuous irradiation. Observations on mice indicate that daily treatment with 5% of the LD_{50} dose can be tolerated. Extrapolating this to large animals, a dose of 10 rads per day could be tolerated.

In analysis of radiotherapy results, the Committee has chosen to place emphasis on the effects of fast neutrons. For single treatments sufficiently large to cause nonstochastic injury, neutron RBE values range between one and five compared with photons. Repair from sublethal damage is less with high-LET radiation so that the N factor is small. In some cases there is no further dose sparing by increasing N beyond 2 fractions. Also, the dose rate effect with high-LET radiation is small. This will cause an increase in RBE with decreasing dose per fraction (and thus, with increasing number of fractions). Where cellular repopulation occurs rapidly such as the skin or intestine, there is no reason to think that it will be dependent on the quality of the radiation. For slowly dividing tissues for which radiation damage occurs a long time after irradiation, repair by repopulation will be small for both x-rays and neutrons.

The Committee also chose to review data on the role of vascular damage. After doses of radiation in the radiotherapy range,

progressive changes occur in all elements of the vasculature such
that at late times following exposure vascular function is reduced.
There is a clear suggestion that vascular damage plays an extremely
important role in all late radiation injury. The fact that in a
given species there is a wide variation between the threshold doses
for different tissues suggests that there may be different sensi-
tivities of the vascular system in different tissues and that
the gross response of a tissue will depend on both parenchymal and
vascular components and it may not be possible to separate these.

MEDICAL IRRADIATION

Medical irradiation includes diagnostic x-ray procedures,
diagnostic nuclear medicine, and radiation therapy procedures.
In highly developed coutries medical exposure equals approximately
the contribution from natural radiation sources. The UNSCEAR
Committee has previously presented data on medical irradiation. Most
of this was generally focused on gonadal doses in order to evaluate
genetic risk. A 1977 UNSCEAR report gave more attention to dose to
other organs to identify examinations in which particular organs may
receive high doses.

The wide variation of organ doses received in medical
irradiation and the different radiosensitivity of organs has prompted
the ICRP to seek a method for deriving radiation protection limits.
The Committee has seen fit to develop this concept further and to
formulate a somatic detriment, G, to an individual from medical
exposure.

The somatic detriment to an individual is defined according
to the equation

$$G = \sum_1 s(i) \; \alpha \; (i) \; \overline{D} \; (i) \tag{4}$$

where s (i) is the relative severity of the somatic effect induced
in the small ith organ and is intended to be a qualitative measure
of the observed excess morbidity or mortality. It is assumed
that s (i) is independent of the absorbed dose: α (i) is the
risk factor for the effect in the ith organ per gray (Gy). This
factor is according to the hypothesis of linear response assumed to
be independent of the absorbed dose and the absorbed dose rate. D(i)
is the average absorbed dose in the ith organ given in gray. The
effective dose D_E is the uniform whole body dose which has the same
potential for causing somatic damage as the set of nonuniform doses
D(i) in individual organs. The calculation of the weighting factors
w(i) requires knowledge of the risk factors $\alpha(i)$ for cancer induction
and the relative severity s(i) of the effect for all organs or tissues
of the body.

The aim of this work done by the Committee is to use the concept of
effective whole body dose, D_E, for all kinds of medical irradiation.
This means that the absorbed dose is estimated not only for the target
organ but also for the tissue of the gondas, breasts, red bone marrow,
lungs, thyroid, and boen surfaces. The total weighting factors

used in this document are those recommended by the ICRP. Calculation of the effective dose is extremely difficult since there are very little experimental data on the actual absorbed dose. One reason for this is the large variation in the performance of examinations including the number of films, types of screens, and other technical factors. The frequency of diagnostic x-ray examinations in different countries is important particularly in calculating the total collective dose.

The estimates of the somatic effective dose for various typical x-ray examinations is also called the "somatic dose index, ID," and the average of male and female differs only slightly from the effective dose calculated from the ICRP recommended weights. To arrive at the somatic dose index for the whole population the individual somatic dose index has to be multiplied by the estimated number of examinations for each sex. An analysis of the formula indicates that when an adult male and an adult female receive the same uniform dose in organs, the potential for somatic detriment to the individual under the selected typical conditions are mammography, thoracic spine and ribs of the female. In the remainder of the report the Committee expects to examine special interest diagnostic radiology procedures such as mammography, and organ doses in computerized tomogarphy. Other areas in which effective dose will be examined in terms of trend and weighting factors is the diagnostic as well as therapeutic use of radiopharmaceuticals, radioisotope, implants and external beam radiotherapy.

In summary, the UNSCEAR Committee plans to extend the 1977 report by reviewing pertinent data derived since the previous report. To date there appears to be little reason to change genetic risk estimates; the linear-quadratic dose response function appears to be satisfactory for low-LET radiation, the non-stochastic effects of low dose radiation will be carefully examined. Additionally, the Committee feels that life-shortening in most animal species and in humans is probably the result of induction of malignant neoplasms. Medical radiation will be considered in terms of describing somatic detriment and essentially using the model described by the ICRP.

REFERENCES

1. B. K. Trimble, J. H. Doughty, The Amount of Hereditary Disease in Human Populations. Ann. Hum. Genet. 38:199-233 (1974).
2. B. H. Cohen, A. M. Lilienfeld, S. Kramer, et al., Parental Factors in Down's Syndrome. pp. 301-352, Population Cytogenetics: Studies in Humans (Academic Press, New York, 1977).
3. J. M. Marshall, P. G. Groer, A Theory of Bone Cancer Induction by Alpha Radiation, Radiat. Res. 71:51-74 (1977).

DISCUSSION - BIOLOGICAL BASIS

W. Kendall: Is there enough confidence in the data to reach the risk estimate conclusions or would the statistical uncertainty impugn the etimates?

P. Selby: I think that I've made it clear that the risk estimates should only be treated as rough estimates. The BEIR III estimates make this very clear because they are presented only as wide ranges. While it is true that there are no statistical measures of uncertainty incorporated into them, this should not alter their validity as rough estimates. For example, the direct estimate is based on the mutation frequency of 37/2646 and not on the 95 percent confidence limits of this frequency. However, it seems unlikely that the factor of about two of uncertainty between the upper and lower 95 percent confidence limits of this frequency is of much consequence in view of the wide range of uncertainty built into the estimate by other terms used in the risk calculation.

K. Banerjee: In one of your earlier slides you showed that the slope for high-dose rate effect was three times that for the low-dose rate effect. The data for high-dose rate was not available for total dose of about 250 rads or less. Why do you expect the slope of both the lines to be same at low doses?

P. Selby: I expect this because Mary Lyon and some of her colleagues found that 626 R given as 60 equal daily acute fractions gave the same mutation frequency expected for such a total exposure administered chronically.

K. Banerjee: You calculated the risks for populations which receive 22 mrem for 30 years. How does your risk estimate compare to the genetic effects on a population in an area like costal regions of Brazil (500 mR/yr) or in Kerala in India (1300 mR/yr)? These background radiations are much higher than the man-made radiation of 22 mrem/yr.

P. Selby: There are no estimates of overall genetic effects induced in humans by living in such high background radiation areas. Not only would very detailed epidemiological studies be needed on such people and on valid control population, but results could easily be confounded by many other variables. Migrations into and out of the area would add to the complexity of such a study.

A. Boyer: What is the increased incidence rate of genetic damage for those individuals exposed to medical irradiations vis a vis to the average over the whole population? What data and estimation procedure should one use when answering the concerns of individuals considering procedures about to be performed on them?

P. Selby: The last application to medical irradiation that I gave illustrated the general type of approach that could be used in estimating risk to an individual. Perhaps you have in mind the need for explaining the genetic risk to someone receiving a very small diagnostic exposure of, for example, if risk from 100 R of acute exposure is only increased from about 13.5 percent to 13.66-14.95 percent, then the genetic risk to one individual from 15 mR would be very slight. In actual calculations for such an exposure, you could assume a dose-rate effect and you would have to take into account the germ-cell stage. Also, only the exposure of the gonads would be of importance for this risk estimate.

E. Gregg: Do you believe that a human female will resemble a mouse female in having no radiation-induced mutations in oocytes ovulated more than six weeks after irradation?

P. Selby: It's possible that both species might be the same in this regard, but this is not known. I suppose that it is quite unlikely that a shift in oocytes from being mutable to being essentially immutable would occur precisely after six weeks in both species; however, if such a shift does occur in women, it might occur at roughly the same time.

S. Jayaraman: Can't we explain the 44 percent value you quoted for abnormalities in oocyte response based on the repair capabilities of the eggs compared to sperms? This has been demonstrated in literature, for example, with Ascaris eggs.

P. Selby: The 44 percent value is based on the highest of four estimates for mature and maturing oocytes, the other three estimates being considerably lower. The explanation suggested by W.L. Russell for the pronounced dose-rate effect in oocytes was that the primary oocytes were exceedingly capable of repairing premutational damage induced by low-dose rate or low-dose irradiation. Examples of repair in oocytes or eggs reported in the literature are, of course, not inconsistent with Russell's hypothesis. They are also consistent with other hypotheses.

S. Jayaraman: In the split-dose technic, why did you choose a small conditioning dose of 100 R followed by a test dose of 500 R, knowing one effect of the magnitude of conditioning dose on the overall effects?

P. Selby: We chose the split dose for our first experiment because this was the exposure that gave the highest mutation frequency in Ehling's earlier studies, and we wanted to be sure of having many presumed mutations to test.

S. Jayaraman: Won't there be an effect of the differences in radiosensitivity of the sperm cells as they progress through the Type A, Type B Spermatocytes, Spermatid stages with progressive differentiations?

P. Selby: Yes, there are differences in radiosensitivity, both for genetic effects and for cell killing. Genetic effects would be transitory, however, for all germ cells in the male except for the A_s spermatogonia. By this, I mean that only in A_s spermatogonia would mutations be induced that would continue to occur in sperm for the rest of the lifetime of the irradiated man.

J. Kereiakes: I have the impression, from your presentation, that you are using the term "threshold" in terms of total dose and also using the term "threshold" in terms of dose-rate; could you clarify the terminology?

P. Selby: Yes, I am thinking both in terms of a threshold dose rate and a threshold dose. Perhaps your confusion stems from the fact that the lower mutational response (referred to as the dose-rate effect) occurs with chronic exposures and with acute exposures if the total dose is small (about 10 R or less). There thus appears to be both a threshold dose-rate and a threshold dose in the female mouse (for mature and maturing oocytes in young females) because in large experiments no clear-cut induction of mutations has been seen at low dose rates or at low doses administered at a high dose rate. In contrast, in the male there appears to be no threshold dose or threshold dose rate in the stem cells because it seems that any dose or any dose rate will induce some mutations.

J. Kim: Are there any efforts for biochemical characterizations of damage lesions in chromosomes now or in the future? This would be useful for finer studies.

P. Selby: Yes, attempts are being made to define radiation-induced mutations in mammals at a molecular level, but this has not yet been accomplished.

M. Meltz: Concerning the table you just showed, the valve of 22 mrem per year of medical radiation is averaged over the entire population. Shouldn't the value, before being used in risk estimating, be separated in components: i.e., those people who receive radiation each year vs those who don't; and further, how many receive radiotherapy vs diagnostic exposure, etc.: For each of those groups, will not the risk be higher?

P. Selby: Certainly, genetic risk is higher for those individuals who are actually exposed. However, it would be expected that if the much more complex task were undertaken of attempting to estimate risk for each of these subgroups individually, the summation of all the individual estimates would be reasonably in accord with the population estimates given here, which are based on the BEIR III report.

S. Jayaraman: What is the estimated magnitude of the components of irreparable radiation damage? This irreparable component may have a bearing on the long-term effects, such as aging, carcinogenesis, leukaemogenesis, etc., particularly under chronic exposures to low levels of radiation.

V. Bond: The concept of "irreparable radiation damage" was based on relatively high doses in which actual (harmful) effects were observed in each of the animals studied. With "low-level radiation", it is widely considered that only carcinogenesis and mutagenesis represent serious types of harm. With these endpoints, there is only risk to the overwhelming majority of individuals with actual harm appearing only in an extremely small fraction. Therefore, there is no "damage" to be irreparable and the concept does not apply to "low-level" radiation effects. There is, of course, the small probability of the all-or-none stochastic (i.e., cancer) effect in the individual (maximum incidence of 1 in 10,000 per rem). This is conceptually different from "irreparable damage" in each individual exposed.

E. Gregg: Were your data for curvilinear dose response curves with dose in rems or rads?

V. Bond: Rads.

T. Fields: Slope of incidence of deaths vs distance is dependent upon speed of the vehicle. Actually slope may be negative instead of positive at low speed. This may or may not be similar to low gamma radiation exposures.

V. Bond: You are of course right in a sense, but let me make the following observations. The curve I showed represents the mean for a very large population. This large popultaion can be regarded, of course, as being composed of a number of subpopulations, with differing risks due to various factors such as age, sex, driving habits (including speed), condition of roads traveled, state of sobriety, etc. For each subgroup, the curve would have a different slope, even though all of the curves would be linear. My curve is a "weighted average" for all. The similarity with radiation comes in that involved in both are processes that are all or nothing, occur by chance (or are "stochastic"), and are produced with single hit kinetics.

M. Meltz: Caution should be observed in relating mutagenesis to carcinogenesis; the evidence is still based on observations that carcinogens (and very few are proven human carcinogens) cause mutations and even then not all suspected carcinogens are demonstrated mutagens, either in bacteria or mammalian cells. The relationship may prove fortuitous; carcinogenesis may be related, as you suggested, to DNA damage, rather than to inheritable mutagenic events. Secondly, it is important that both inheritable mutagenic hazards and somatic carcinogenic hazards be of concern in their own right.

V. Bond: With respect to your first point, I agree and certainly
I didn't mean to imply that carcinogenesis depends on a mutation,
in the usual sense of the word. What was meant is that both processes involve broadly similar changes in the cell that alter pro-
foundly the subsequent behavior of the cell, at least operationally speaking. With respect to the second point, I certainly
agree.

E. Banerjee: Sometimes we calculate the incidence of an effect
from a group of people who might be predisposed to an effect. For
example, the incidence of cancer predosed in patients who were repeatedly fluoroscoped for having TB. How valid is our extrapolation to the general population from a group of predisposed persons? How does one separate the predisposed factor from the effect of radiation plus predisposed factors?

V. Bond: the question you raised does come up often and although
one tries to control for it, this is not always possible. There
are some clear-cut situations (e.g., the British spondylitis patients) in which one might expect that the previous drug therapy
could have contributed to the tumor incidence which might be confounded with the contribution from radiation. Careful studies of
control populations using the same drug spectrum, however, showed
no evidence of an effect of the drugs. One must also note that
there are relatively few well-identified "added" carcinogens to
which large groups are exposed. If one has in mind carcinogens in
general that may may be in the diet, etc., then presumably the
control population used would have had the same exposure as would
the irradiated group.

J. Kim: My question concerns the ovarian tumor incidence vs dose
graph. What is the minimum dose used to obtain the graph? Down
to 10 rads? Lower than 10 rads? Some of us are interested in
effects of doses as low as one rad or even less.

V. Bond: The lowest dose on the ovarian tumor incidence vs dose
graph was 10 rads. With respect to lower doses, one could presumably obtain meaningful data and still use animal populations of
manageable size. With low-LET radiation, however, this would
probably be impossible. For this reason, I showed data in "sim-
pler" systems in which one can use large populations and therefore
work at lower doses. As I indicated, the data from a number of
species and endpoints indicate that, in principle, the relationships we see in lower systems, with respect to dose and dose rate,
appear to describe adequately, or even well, what we see in
"higher" systems. Hence, it is probably that a slope generated by
using the smallest "reliable" data points will not underestimate
the true effect at still lower doses.

J.Kim: Since ther is no quantitative model for carcinogenesis at
the biomolecular level, one cannot really say the dose-incidence
curve will be linear, say, below one rad (1 rad) for example.

However, many of us are interested in this low, low dose level. This requires research at a fundamental level, using biochemical and recombinant DNA technologies beyond the traditional approach to characterize cancer incident. What is your view on the value of some new approachs? For example, "error-prone" repair may, if accumulated or evoked, give rise to eventual carcinogens.

V. Bond: I would say that all of us are interestd in the low-dose levels and I believe that a number of approaches are relevant to investigating this area. I believe none should be excluded. My personal view is that while biochemical and molecular studies are important, actual observations with the endpoint of interest are necessary in order to establish the overall shape of the dose response curve. With respect to "error-prone" repair, I would look at this as another possible mechanism in the overall picture of carcinogenesis that would help determine the shape of the curves obtained.

D. Plewes: You made the comment that the biological response to various fractionation schedules indicated that the time constant for repair was on the order of two hours. Is there any biochemical data on the kinetics of repair enzymes that would support this two-hour value?

V. Bond: I do not know of any studies on repair enzymes with respect to ionizing radiation, although I believe there are such studies with respect to UV radiation damage. It is generally accepted, however, that one can observe the state of the cell's repair capability for ionizing of UV radiation by doing fractionation and dose-rate studies. It is from this kind of study that the repair constant on the order of 10's of minutes to hours is deduced. A great deal more work will have to be done, however, before we have data on repair kinetics that are adequate to predict, with reasonable precision, what one might expect with different patterns of dose size, of dose rate, and dose fractionation.

P. Steward: You stated that supralinear incidence vs dose curves do not hold up under close scrutiny of the data. Can you expand on this statement, since these curves continually arise in the literature recently, for example, as incidence as a function of dose for cell transformation in vitro?

V. Bond: A lengthy presentation would be required to respond fully to your qustion. In short, on close examination the findings reported rarely, if ever, permit such a conclusion ("supralinear" curve at low doses, low-LET radiation), either because of poor dosimetry, inadequate "experimental" and/or control population, methodology, statistical analysis approach, or some combination. Some additional comments can be found in a recent NCRP publication of mine, "Quantitative Risk in Radiation Protection Standards", Radiat. Environ. Biophys. 17:1-28 (1979), and elsewhere.

As to the data on cell transformation in vitro, the findings there are unusual and have not been observed in other systems. It remains to be seen exactly what they mean. At any rate, the observations are at relatively high doses and I suspect that they may not turn out to have major importance, with respect to the low-dose region.

P. Steward: In one of your slides, it appeared that the transit time in the hematopoietic system from stem-cell to functional blood cell was about seven days. Yet, the nadir in the peripheral blood count was about 30 days. Why wouldn't the nadir be closer to seven days than to 30?

V. Bond: Your question is good and the answer is widely assumed to involve injured rather than killed cells. Large doses of radiation stop completely the reproductive capacity of some cells, impair that of others such that they can reproduce only for a limited number of generations, and leave others pristine. The second rise in the peripheral blood cells and the later nadir is known as the "abortive rise" and is assumed to be due to those cells that can proliferate for some period of time, following which they and all of their progeny disappear and thus produce the "second nadir". The final recovery is from the relatively small pool of remaining cells that are intact, at least with respect to proliferative capacity.

V. Collins: Please comment on the usefulness and validity of the "10-day rule". (Clarify from onset of menses.)

L. Russell: the "10-day rule" and the "14-day rule" were committee recommendations growing out of a suggestion my husband and I published in 1952 (Radiology 58(3):369-376). Our suggestion was made at a time when diagnostic doses could still be quite high and was based on the experimental finding that the period of major organogenesis was the most sensitive for the induction of gross malformation, and that at least the early portion of this period could take place before a woman might realize she was pregnant. We stated our proposal as follows (p. 373): "Prior to pelvic irradiation of women of childbearing age, the radiologist should always inquire whether there is even the remotest possibility of a very early pregnancy. The safest procedure is to restrict pelvic irradiation, whenever possible, to the two weeks following (onset of) menstruation, as there is almost no chance of an unsuspected pregnancy during that time (ovulation probably occurring half-way between menstrual periods)."

Some medical groups have argued aginst the rule, mainly for practical reasons, citing scheduling difficulties for hospital facilities, and the inconvenience of requiring repeated communication between the radiologist and the referring physician. These groups have stated that the low-dose levels most commonly employed would not present an undue risk to the embryo, in any case. It has also been argued that if the mother really required the radiation, she needs it right then; that if radiation can be postponed, she doesn't need it at all.

If I were to propose the rule today, I should make it not a 14 but a 23-day rule, since irradiation during the (roughly) 9-day preimplantaion period is virtually without risk of abnormality in a surviving child. This means that no re-scheduling would be necessary in 82% (= 23/28) of women of childbearing age who might have conceived and, of course, the question of re-scheduling does not arise at all for any other women.

S. Bushong: We need a fuller discussion of the bomb survivor data that was on chalkboard. Percent effect values seem very high and not consistent with major organogenesis stage.

Russell: Microcephaly was diagnosed when head circumference was more than two standard deviations less than normal. Using this criterion, the control frequency for Hiroshima was 4% (relatively high) and this should be taken into account when looking at the following Hiroshima frequencies for children who were exposed as embryos during the most sensitive period for induction of microcephaly, namely between weeks 6-11 post-conception.

Kerma (Air Dose)	Incidence	Percent	
1-9 Rad	2/19	11	Not significantly higher than the 4% frequency for controls or the 6% frequency for other stages irradiated at this dose.
10-19	4/24	17	Significantly higher than control.
20-29	3/10	30	Significantly higher than control.
30-49	4/10	40	Significantly higher than control.
50-99	7/10	70	Significantly higher than control.
100 +	7/7	100	Significantly higher than control

At Nagasaki, for all doses combined, there were only less than 20 embryos at risk during the sensitive period. Had the frequency of induced microcephaly been the same as at Hiroshima, one would have expected seven cases; only one occurred. The difference between the cities could be the result of the considerable neutron component at Hiroshima. If so, one must assume a high RBE for induction of microcephaly.

J. Kim: There was an interesting article by Canadians recently in their support of the 14-day rule on theoreticl grounds alone: There is a higher probability of transmitting "damaged" components of chromosomes during mitosis than during meiosis. And since formation of a fetus or an embryo is a process of mitosis, there is a higher probablity of transmitting the damaged chromosome. Therefore, given a choice, choose the period before the fetus is formed or 10 to 14 days after menstruation to avoid the period of rapid mitosis.

L. Russell: the 10 or 14-day rules are designed to avoid irradiation post-conception (see my response to Dr. Collins). Irradiation pre-conception, while avoiding teratogenic effects, does not, of course, avoid genetic risks. For a discussion of these, see the talk by Dr. Selby.

E. Gregg: Of what significance is the high sensitivity of the oocytes in teratogenesis? Particularly the LD_{50} of 5 rads.

L. Russell: I probably failed to make it clear that the oocytes I was talking about were those of a female fetus, not those of the mother. Therefore, the radiation-induced death of these oocytes is merely another example of teratogenic damage--in principle, no different from the damage (probably cell killing) that eventually results in skeletal malformations.

R. Gould: Would you comment on whether or not to recommend abortion following medical irraditaion to the fetus in a critical time period? Is there any credence to the "Hammer-Jacobsen" rule?

L. Russell: I feel that the total dose to the embryo or fetus should be carefully determined and the probability of a measurable effect be presented to the mother. For most radiological procedures, this probability will be exceedingly low. My estimate is that if the dose to the embryo was < 2 R, radiation-induced effects would less than double the "spontaneous" incidence of birth defects.

S. Jayaraman: Keeping the developmental stage constant for irradiation, have you looked at the influence of the age of the mother at conception on the teratological effects observed in the offspring?

L. Russell: The age effect in the case of Down's Syndrome has nothing to do with teratogenesis; it is an effect on a genetic (pre-conception) phenomenon, namely the frequency of non-disjunction in the maternal reproductive cells. With respect to impacts occurring post-conception, it is not inconceivable that advanced age of the mother could produce a poorer intrauterine environment and thus make the embryo slightly less viable--even in the absence of radiation. This type of environmental effect would be difficult to distinguish from genetic changes brought on by age, except by experimental procedures such as embryo transfer. To my knowledge, this has not been done for the study of age effects.

S. Jayaraman: If irradiation were done at or before the preimplantation period, at what dose levels will there be intrauterine absorption of the fetus itself? What is your dose guesstimate for humans?

L. Russell: If irradiation were given <u>before</u> the preimplantation period, it would be pre-conception and thus fall outside the sphere of teratogenesis. If irradiation is given during the preimplantation period, the magnitude of the embryo toxic effect varies with the stage attained during that period. At the most sensitive stages, the probability of killing the conceptus is 90-100% for 200 R, and 50-60% for 100 R. Some investigators have noted slightly increased mortality also, following low doses (5 to 25 R) administered on days 0.5 or 1.5 post-conception.

P. Steward: Dr. Russell has pointed out that the incidence of abnormalities in children due to their irradition <u>in utero</u> varies drastically from day to day, in mice at least. Wouldn't this make any data on the incidence of cancer in children who had been irradiated <u>in utero</u> difficult to interpret?

E. Webster: I believe Dr. Russell was discussing developmental abnormalities and not cancer. There do appear to be many other variables affecting the former--such as smoking status. For cancer, the primary problems at low doses are statistical (population size needed for a positive finding) and the proper choice of control populations. The reality of <u>in utero</u> radiation induction of cancer at low doses is not yet settled, but the Stewart findings are often accepted on the grounds of "prudence".

S. Bushong: Jablon's leukemia data (<u>Lancet</u> 1972) is so much lower than teratogenetic findings reported today by Russell. Why?

E. Webster: In Nagasaki, the Jablon data on childhood cancer developing in children irradiated <u>in utero</u> is reasonably consistent with the teratogenic findings (e.g., microcephaly) reported by Dr. Russell--in one case, zero excess cancer and in the other case, no microcephaly below 150 rads. The difference may well be due to differences in mechanisms between two widely different effects, but there is also the suggestion of a threshold for gamma-ray induced teratogenesis. In Hiroshima, there does appear to be a discrepancy insofar as microcephaly was observed with kerma (neutron plus gamma) in the 10 rad range and above, whereas no leukemia excess was observed. The failure to observe leukemia or any other form of childhood cancer suggests that the fetus may be no more sensitive than the adult regarding induction of malignancies. The lower doses for microcephaly in Hiroshima are consistent with the adult leukemia data which show a larger effect for fast neutrons than for gamma rays. Overall, it would seem that microcephaly, a developmental anomaly, does carry a higher risk than childhood cancer, on the basis of the Japanese results.

K. Banerjee: Children who were treated for ringworm or thymus had a certain risk of cancer of the thyroid. The present data indicate that the people treated with I-131 (with high doses) for hyperthyroidism usually become hypothyroid and very small number, if any, become cancerous. Would you comment on this? Also, what theory, "linear or quadratic", fits this data?

E. Webster: It is well-known that because of the "cell-killing" effect at high doses, leaving fewer cells at risk, the probability of cancer induction falls at the higher doses; e.g., 500-1000 rads. Treatment for hyperthyroidism involves gland doses of this magnitude or greater. It is also believed that there is a large dose-rate effect in thyroid cancer production, particularly evident in contrasting the effects of radioiodine with those of external x-ray beams. The thyroid cancer risk from ringworm treatment is not well-established--the Modan study is in disagreement with the study by Shore and Albert (1976). I don't believe there is adequate data to test a dose-effect model for radioiodine treatments.

M. Bank: Please comment on the Stewart data on irradiation of the fetus in utero and the development of cancer (leukemia) in the first eight years of life.

E. Webster: A number of epidemiolgoists (e.g., Professor Brian MacMahon of the Harvard School of Public Health) have pointed out that the methodology of the Stewart-type study leads to an association between abdominal irradiation during pregnancy and the subsequent development of childhood cancer, and that the association does not prove causation. There might be a selection process in the administration of abdominal x-rays which leads to a greater predilection for childhood cancer. The Stewart data on leukemia in twins (Mole, Brit. J. Cancer, 1974) does strengthen the Stewart risk estimates. But, as my paper notes, there are two cohort studies in disagreement with the Stewart conclusions.

S. Jayaraman: Knowing that irradiation of the pituitary can lead to abscopal effects, why can't the incidence of thyroid cancer be just an abscopal effect? The fact that radiation could be carcinogenic is also borne out by the observation that pneumothorax cases develop cancer of the breast corresponding to which lung was collapsed under fluoroscopy. The other breast did not develop breast cancer.

E. Webster: This possibility has been suggested by others (e.g., R.D. Evans) and is appealing insofar as the pituitary doses in the ringworm treatments is much higher than the thyroid case. However, there is some animal evidence that thyroid cancer might be inhibited by pituitary irradiation (Doniach). I agree with your comment that there appears to be such an association, although there are evident exceptions. The fluoroscopy was sometimes given bilaterally.

Kendall: In the data for which the models were evaluated, were all cancers (or deaths) assumed to be caused by radiation or were other etiological agents excluded?

E. Webster: It is desirable (but not always possible) in epidemiologic studies to compare the irradiated population with a control population identical in all respects except for the irradiation. This ideal is seldom completely realized in human studies and therefore confounding factors (e.g., smoking habits, ethnic differences) may be present and not evaluated.

J. Kim: On lung cancer data, was the effect of smoking taken into account at all? There could have been synergistic effects giving rise to a more complicated curve.

E. Webster: Those involved in lung cancer epidemiology are well aware of the confounding effects of smoking. Attempts have been made to evaluate this (e.g., in Appendix A of the 1980 BEIR Report and in the Archer study of lung cancer in uranium miners (Annals NY Acad. Sci., 1976). The BEIR report suggests an additive rather than a synergistic effect.

V. Collins: Carcinogens are more effective on regenerating liver in rats after partial resection of liver. Comparably, could functioning breast tissue in young women be more susceptible to carcinogenesis?

E. Webster: I am not sure whether this is a statement of fact or a question. There is clear evidence that radiation-induced breast cancer is more likely in young women in the 10-19 age group than in older women and this is attributed to hormonal influences at puberty.

T. Fields: Is there greater evidence of breast Ca among Catholic nuns?

E. Webster: My mammographer friends tell me that the childbearing history (e.g., multipara) of women is one of the factors bearing on the breast cancer risk.

J. Kim: Do you know of any effort to really arrive at a "unified picture" of basic process of carcinogenesis taking into account DNA damage, repair mechanism, membrane alterations (possibly due to alteration in regulatory mechanism), etc., so that whether the cause is radiation, carcinogens, or virus we get to understand the nature of the low-dose effect? This should explain the truer character of linear, linear-quadratic, or quadratic nature and probably many other sundries which appear puzzling at the present.

E. Webster: Such complete understanding is highly desirable, but we are far from it. There are many current theories of carcinogenesis, including the factors you mention, and probably as many relating to radiation carcinogenesis (see book by P.R.J. Burch; also, article in <u>Radiation Research</u> Vol. 71, 1977, by J. Martin Brown).

II. Risk Evaluation and Reduction

DOSE EVALUATION IN DIAGNOSTIC RADIOLOGY

Stewart C. Bushong
Baylor College of Medicine, Houston, Texas 77030

INTRODUCTION

The evaluation of radiation doses received in diagnostic x-ray procedures required consideration of a number of modifying conditions. It should be kept in mind that all dose evaluation is prompted by our desire to predict the effect of any given dose of radiation administered diagnostically. To this end, radiation dose-response relationships are developed, and these are much of the basis for activity in radiation biology.

There are four principal characteristics of radiation dose-response relationships. They are either linear or nonlinear and they are either threshold or nonthreshold. All of the suspected effects that are possible following diagnostic levels of x-radiation are presumed to follow a linear, nonthreshold dose-response relationship. There is currently some consideration that this relationship overestimates the response at low dose levels, however, nearly all would agree that there is not sufficient evidence at this time for absolute conclusions.

QUANTITIES AND UNITS

There are a number of units in medical health physics that are used to express various quantities of radiation, radioactivity and other intensities. Three basic units are applied to radiation intensity and one unit is applied to radioactivity. Various other units principally associated with one of the three areas of medical radiation applications - diagnostic roentgenology, radiotherapy and nuclear medicine - are also in routine use.

SI Units

Unfortunately, the situation regarding units in medical health physics is clouded because of the current change from classical units with origins in history to units of the International System (Le Systeme International d'Unités of SI)[1,2] which are principally based on the meter, kilogram, second (MKS) system. In 1960 the 11th General Conference of Weights and Measures adopted SI Units and today SI has been officially adopted by most of the world and is gradually being introduced into regular use. A notable laggard in this adoption is the United States. SI units are founded on seven base units, the meter (m), the kilogram (kg), the second (s), the ampere (A), the kelvin (K), the candela (cd) and the mole (mol)[3]. Other units that can be formed as products of these base units are called derived units. The SI units for radiation are derived units and therefore are more slowly being integrated into routine use. Table 1 lists the derived SI units for radiological application. Quantities as expressed in conventional units and the equivalent SI units are summarized in Table 2.

Considerable debate[4-8] has raged over the advisability of adopting SI units for routine radiation specification. The debate has continued with increasing intensity in the U.S. since the ICRU has suggested the <u>special</u> SI radiation units, the gray, the becquerel and seivert[9].

Table 1. Derived Radiologic Units of the SI and Their Present Equivalent.

Quantity	Derived SI Unit	Symbol	Present Equivalent
Activity	reciprocal second	s^{-1}	$\sim 2.703 \times 10^{-11}$ Ci
Absorbed dose	joule per kilogram	$J\ kg^{-1}$	100 rad
Absorbed dose rate	watt per kilogram	$W\ kg^{-1} = J\ kg^{-1}s^{-1}$	100 rad s^{-1}
Exposure	coulomb per kilogram	$C\ kg^{-1}$	$\sim 3.876 \times 10^3$ R
Exposure rate	ampere per kilogram	$A\ kg^{-1} = C\ kg^{-1}s^{-1}$	$\sim 3.876 \times 10^3$ R s^{-1}

Table 2. Conventional and SI Units and Conversion Factors

	Conventional Unit		SI Unit	
Quantity	Name	Symbol	Name	Symbol
electric charge	coulomb	C = A s	coulomb	C = A s
energy	electron volt	eV	joule	J
exposure	roentgen	R	coulomb per kilogram	C/kg
absorbed dose	rad	rad or rd	gray	Gy = J/kg
dose equivalent	rem	rem	seivert	Sv
activity	curie	Ci	becquerel	Bq = s^{-1}
Multiply # of to obtain # of	→ by ← by		→ to obtain # of Divide # of	
eV	1.6021×10^{-19}		J	
R	2.58×10^{-4}		C/kg	
rad	0.01		Gy	
rem	1		Sv	
Ci	3.7×10^{10}		Bq	

Radiation Intensity

For the first thirty years or so after the discovery of x-rays, their use in medicine was without the aid of a precise unit of measure. The earliest attempt at quantitating x-ray intensity was based on the radiation dose that the practitioner reckoned would produce an erythema or sunburn-like reddening of the skin. The quantity was the skin erythema dose (SED) and fractional SEDs were specified for both patient treatments and maximum permissible occupational exposures.

<u>The Roentgen (R)</u>: The first precise definition of radiation intensity was not official until 1928 when the Roentgen was adopted by the International Congress of Radiology in Stockholm[10,11]. At this time the principal emphasis was on the measurement of x-rays and radium gamma

rays and such measurements were then possible by determining the magnitude of ionization in air exposed to such beams. As originally defined,

> "The roentgen is the quantity of x-radiation which, when the secondary electrons are fully unilized and the wall effect of the chamber is avoided produces in 1 cm^3 of atmospheric air at 0°C and 76 cm of mercury pressure such a degree of conductivity that 1 esu of charge is measured at saturation current."

Following discussion of the International Committee for Radiological Units in Zurich in 1934[12] and the same committee in Chicago in 1937[13] the definition of the roentgen was refined to,

> "the roentgen shall be the quantity of x or gamma radiation such that the associated corpuscular emission per 0.001293 gram of air produces, in air, ions carrying one electrostatic unit of quantity of electricity of either sign."

These definitions of the roentgen held until the 1962 report of the International Commission on Radiation Units and Measurements (ICRU)[14]. The ICRU defines the roentgen as the unit of exposure specifically as follows:

> "the exposure (x) is a quotient ΔQ by Δm, where ΔQ is the sum of the electrical charges on all the ions of one sign produced in air when all of the electrons (negatrons and positrons), liberated by photons in a volume element of air whose mass is Δm, are completely stopped in air:
> $$X = \frac{\Delta Q}{\Delta m}$$

The special unit of exposure is the roentgen (R). 1 R = 2.58×10^{-4} C/kg (exactly).

This expression for the roentgen is numerically identical with the older definition of 1 e.s.u. of charge per 0.001293 gm of air.

Currently the transition from this classical Roentgen unit to the SI equivalent is taking place slowly and with some resistance. The unit of exposure in the SI system is the coulomb per kilogram, and therefore, the conversion factors are 1 R = 2.58×10^{-4} C/kg and 1 C/kg = 3.88×10^3 R.

The roentgen, therefore, is the unit of radiation exposure or simply exposure. It is a measure of the ionization produced in air by x and gamma ray photons having energy from a few keV to 3 MeV. It is also the unit measured by most portable survey instruments in the course of an area radiation survey. In such a situation, one usually records total exposure in R or mR (C/kg) and exposure rate in mR/hr (C/kg-hr).

Absorbed Dose (rad): It was recognized very early in medical health physics that the roentgen was not a very satisfactory unit for predicting the biological effect of radiation. Such effects are dependent upon the type of radiation, its energy and the rate and manner in which its energy is transferred to the biological target. It has been shown by numerous radiobiological experiments that equal radiation exposures produced widely different biological responses. What was needed was a unit that could usefully be used to accurately predict the biological result.

The first attempt at such a unit was suggested by Gray and Read[15] in 1939. They defined the energy unit to be that dose of ionizing radiation, either photon or particulate, that would deliver to tissue the same energy per gram as that delivered to water by exposure to 1 R of x or γ radiation. Numerically the energy unit was 93 ergs per gram. This unit never enjoyed widespread adoption and therefore at the time of the postwar activity in nuclear development we were still without a suitable unit of dose.

Since the roentgen was applicable only with photon radiation, a unit was needed to accommodate particulate radiation. Parker[16] in 1948 defined the Roentgen Equivalent Physical (rep) as "that dose of ionizing radiation which produces an energy absorption of 84 ergms/cm^3 in tissue." This value also approximates the energy absorbed by 1 gm of air exposed to 1 R x or γ radiation. What was needed, however, was a unit associated with energy absorption in soft tissue. Consequently, the value of the rep was later changed to 93 ergs/cm^3 and still later to 93 ergs/gm. Understandably, there was confusion in the use of the unit rep.

At the 1953 Copenhagen meeting of the International Congress of Radiology, the ICRU introduced the concept of absorbed dose and its unit the rad[17]. In its 1956[18] and 1962[14] reports, the ICRU attempted to explicitly define the unit of absorbed dose as the rad.

"The absorbed dose (D) is the quotient of ΔE_D by Δm, where ΔE_D is the energy imparted by ionizing radiation to the matter in a volume element, Δm is the mass of the matter in that volume element...
$$D = \Delta E_D / \Delta m$$
The special unit of absorbed dose is the rad.
1 rad - 100 erg/g = 0.01 J/kg"

The rad is applicable to all ionizing radiation, both directly ionizing particles (electrons, protons, alpha particles, etc.) and indirectly ionizing particles (neutrons, photons, etc.). It is also applicable to all different types of absorbing material. Consequently, the rad is a more useful and universal quantity than the roentgen. The rad applies to all radiation and all target materials, not just x and gamma rays in air.

The precise application of the rad (gray) seems to be confusing to some. If one gram of tissue is irradiated to a dose of 5 rads the energy absorbed in that gram will be 500 ergs. If three grams of tissue receive 5 rads, then each individual gram would absorb 500 ergs, but the total energy absorbed would be 1500 ergs. In both cases, however, the dose is 5 rads.

The SI equivalent of the rad is the gray (Gy) and one gray is equal to one joule per kilogram.

Therefore:
$$1 \text{ Gy} = 1 \text{ J/kg} \times \frac{10^7 \text{ ergs}}{J} \times \frac{10^{-3} \text{ ergs}}{gm} \times \frac{10^{-2} \text{ rad}}{erg/gm} = 100 \text{ rads}$$
and 1 rad = 0.01 Gy

<u>Radiation Equivalent Man (rem)</u>: The rem is a unit specifically reserved for use in radiation protection. It is an attempt to normalize all occupational radiation exposure according to the type and energy to which the worker is exposed. For instance, a one rad dose of fast neutrons will produce two to five times the biological damage that a one rad dose of x rays would. A worker receiving a low dose of neutrons, therefore, might consider himself only moderately exposed if his dose were reported in rads. In fact, the biological damage could be severe, but his monitoring report, in rads, would convey a false sense of safety.

The dose equivalent (H) is the quantity applied to this measure of occupational radiation intensity and its unit is the rem. The dose equivalent attempts to take into account the biological effectiveness of the occupational exposure by modifying factors (N), most important to which is the quality factor (Q). The ICRU[19,20] defines these quantites as follows,

> "The dose equivalent, H, is the product of D, Q, and N, at the point of interest in tissue, where D is the absorbed dose, Q is the quality factor and N is the product of any other modifying factors.
> $$H = DQN$$
> The special unit of dose equivalent is the rem or its SI equivalent, the seivert. When D is expressed in rads, H is in rem."

A further restriction is placed on the quantity dose equivalent and its unit, the rem (Sv). It is to be used only for <u>normal</u> radiation protection activities--those activities that result in exposures near or below the maximum permissible dose equivalent. Accidental exposures to high radiation intensities that are life threatening, or otherwise serious, are to be expressed in rads.

Diagnostic Radiology

There are a number of quantities and units that have special application to diagnostic radiology. Undoubtedly, there are some complimentary applications to some of these quantities and units to the health physics of other medical specialties.

<u>Kilovolt Peak (kVp)</u>: The potential difference impressed across an x-ray tube is measured in <u>kilovolts peak</u> (kVp). The electrons so accelerated will arrive at the anode with energies, expressed in kiloelectron volts (keV), that are equal to or less than the kVp of operation.

In conventional full wave rectified generators, electrical potential impressed across the tube is pulsed from zero to a maximum value 120 times per second. It can be shown that 120 instances per second the electrical potential is zero, and therefore, electron flow ceases. Also, 120 instances per second electrons will arrive at the anode with a maximum accelerating voltage. Should that voltage happen to be, say 90 kVp, these electrons would arrive with 90 keV of kinetic energy and it is this energy which is available for conversion into electromagnetic energy -- x-rays. At all other times, the voltage potential will be somewhere between zero and maximum, and consequently, the kinetic energy of the projectile electrons arriving at the anode will have kinetic energy from zero to the maximum keV. This electrical potential is expressed in kVp rather than kV since it is pulsating in nature.

Diagnostically useful x-rays are produced at or near the peak kV. At low kV, the number and energy of the emitted x-rays are too low. The x-ray emission spectrum is considerably influenced by this pulsating electrical potential.

Milliamperes (mA): The smallest indivisible unit of electric charge is that charge contained in one electron. This is called the basic electronic charge. The unit of basic electronic charge is the coulomb (C) and one coulomb is equal to 6.25×10^{18} electronic charges. When electronic charges are set in motion, as in a conductor by an electrical potential difference, expressed in volts, then an electrical current is set to flow. This is electricity and it is measured in amperes (A). One ampere is the movement of one coulomb of charge per second in a conductor. Therefore, an x-ray machine operated at the 100 mA station will cause 6.25×10^{17} electrons to flow through the x-ray tube from cathode to anode each second. An exposure of 10 mAs would represent total electron flow of 6.25×10^{16} electrons. Conventional diagnostic x-ray machines have discretely selectable mA operating stations from 50 mA to 600 mA or 800 mA in five to eight steps. Special, high capacity machines are capable of up to 1200 mA.

Milliampere Seconds (mAs): During fluoroscopy, the undertable x-ray tube is energized by a "dead-man" type switch for many seconds or even minutes, depending upon the nature of the examination. The important operating characteristic is the tube current, mA. Image intensified fluoroscopy is usually accomplished at a tube current of 0.5-2.0 mA.

For radiographic exposures, the important operating characteristic is somewhat different. A tube current is selected, and a timer station is also selected so that the current is terminated after a predetermined exposure length at that tube current. The product of the tube current and the exposure time is expressed in milliampere seconds (mAs). The unit mAs is, in fact, a unit of charge ($Q/t \times t = Q$) which is appropriate since the total number of x-rays produced is directly related to the total number of electrons that interact with the target.

DOSE MODIFYING FACTORS

Whole vs. Partial Body Irradiation
Nearly all of our available dose-response relationships are derived either experimentally with laboratory animals or from observations on irradiated humans and they are generally based on whole

body irradiation. Diagnostic x-ray procedures constitute partial body irradiation and only a small portion of the body at that. Consequently, there is considerable inprecision when one attempts to project dose-response relationships following whole body irradiation to the situation present in diagnostic radiology.

When a patient receives a diagnostic x-ray examination, the radiation is incident on a relatively small portion of the body and with penetration, is readily absorbed, attenuated and reduced in intensity. In general, less than 5% of the radiation incident on a patient will exit the patient to interact with the image receptor. The radiation that exits the patient includes both primary x-rays and scattered x-rays that are collectively identified as remnant radiation.
The patient is exposed to the useful beam and those tissues and organs in that useful beam will absorb energy from this primary radiation. Tissues and organs outside of the useful beam will receive a dose of radiation due to scattered x-rays, and this dose will be necessarily much smaller.

Fractionation and Protraction

If a dose of radiation is delivered over a long period of time rather than quickly, the effect of that dose will be less. Stated differently, if the time of irradiation is lengthened, a higher dose will be required to produce the same effect. This lengthening of time can be accomplished in two ways.

If the dose is delivered continuously but at a lower dose rate, it is said to be protracted. Six hundred rad (6 Gy) delivered in 3 min (200 rad/min, 2 Gy/min) is lethal for a mouse. However, when 600 rad (6 Gy) are delivered at the rate of 1 rad/hr (10 m Gy/hr), the mouse will survive. Dose protraction is less effective because of the lower dose rate and the longer irradiation time.

If the 600-rad (6 Gy) dose is delivered at the same dose rate, 200 rad/min (2 Gy/min), but in twelve equal fractions of 50 rad (500m Gy), each separated by 24 hr, the mouse will survive. In this situation the dose is said to be fractionated. Dose fractionation occurs when the total dose is delivered at a high dose rate but intermittently.

Dose protraction or fractionation is less effective because, during the lengthened time interval of irradiation, the body has an opportunity to recover and repair some of the radiation damage. Dose fractionation is the irradiation scheme experienced in diagnostic radiology.

SPECIFICATION OF PATIENT DOSE

Entrance Exposure

Undoubtedly the easiest specification of radiation dose in x-ray procedures is entrance exposure or skin exposure. This quality is usually expressed as a radiation exposure in mR (C/kg). Entrance exposure is easy to measure. Ionization chambers or thermoluminescent dosimeters find particular application in this measurement. They would normally be placed on the patient's skin but the measurement of exposure at any distance from the x-ray tube target can be used with some accuracy to measure skin exposure.

The measurement technique most often employed is TLD. The size, sensitivity and accuracy of TLDs makes them very satisfactory patien radiation monitors. A small grouping or pack of 3 to 10 TLDs can be easily taped to the patient's skin in the center of the x-ray field. Since the response of the TLD is proportionate to dose they can be used to measure all levels experienced in diagnostic radiology. With proper laboratory technique, the results of such measurements will be confident to within 5%.

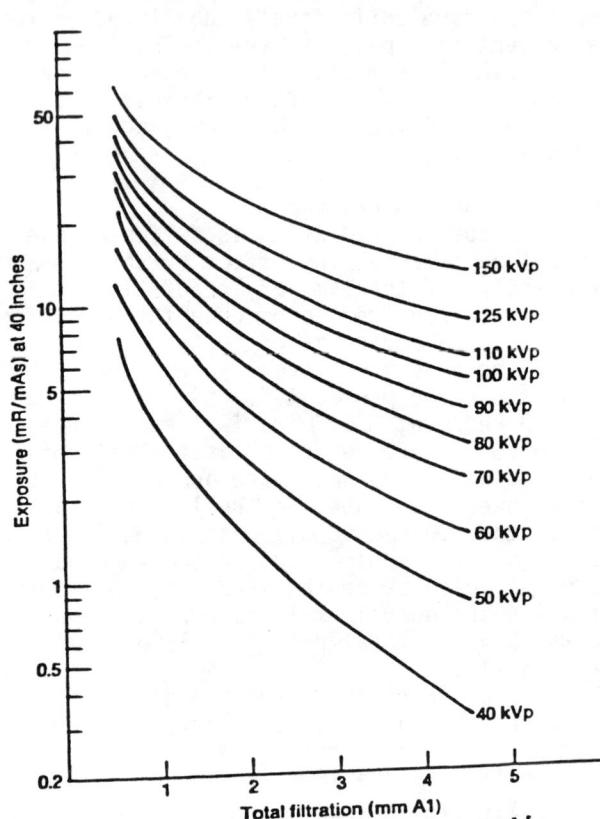

Figure 1. This nomogram is for estimating x-ray intensity from a single-phase radiographic unit. (Courtesy J.R. Cameron, Univ. of Wisconsin.)

There are two rather straight forward methods for estimating sk dose in the absence of patient measurements. This requires the use a nomogram such as that shown in Figure 1[21]. This figure contains a family of curves from which one can estimate the output intensity of a radiographic unit if you know or assume the technique. The output intensity varies widely so that use of this nomogram methods is only good to perhaps ± 50%.

The second method for estimating patient skin dose requires that one know the output intensity for at least one operating condition. During the annual or special radiation control survey and calibration of an x-ray facility, the physicist will indicate this output intensity usually in units of mR/mAs or mR/100 mAs at 32 in (80 cm), the approximate source to skin distance (SSD) or at 40 in (100 cm) the SID. At 70 kVp radiographic output intensity varies from about 2 mR/mAs to 10 mR/mAs at 32 in (80 cm) SSD. With this calibration value available one would alter by inverse square law to another SSD if necessary and adjust the value linearly for both kVp and mAs.

The assumption that the output varies linearly with kVp is not precisely correct but is satisfactory for such an estimate. In actual fact it varies from near linear at 50 kVp to almost kVp^2 at 120 kVp.

Skin dose in fluoroscopy is much more difficult to estimate because the radiation field moves and sometimes varies in size. If the field were of one size and stationary, skin dose would be directly related to exposure time. It is usually satisfactory, in the absence of measurements, to estimate maximum fluoroscopic skin dose at 2.0 rads/mAmin. Stated differently, <u>for every mA of fluoroscopic technique one can assume tabletop intensity of 2.0 rads/m</u>.

Organ Dose

Although entrance radiation exposure is that which is routinely measured or estimated, it is not the radiation quantity which is particularly useful in estimating radiation risk or predicting a biological effect.

Since our experimental radiation dose-response relationships are based on radiation doses uniformly distributed over the whole body, they are of limited value in diagnostic radiology. Consequently, our principal interests should be aimed at radiation dose to certain organs considered to be somewhat at risk.

We know that if sufficient radiation dose is imparted to any organ or tissue of the body as a localized exposure, a radiation response will follow. Following high levels of radiation acutely delivered, the response is generally atrophy and dysfunction. Following low level, long term exposure, such as that experienced in diagnostic radiology, the responses may not be so identifiable or relatable to the previous radiation exposure.

There are three organ doses of particular significance in diagnostic radiology. These relate to exposure of the eyes, the bone marrow and the gonads. An additional specific area exposure that is not strictly an organ dose but that is extremely important, is that of the unborn. Consequently, fetal dose will also be treated here.

<u>Lens Dose</u>: The radiation dose delivered to the lens of the eyes is easily measured with thermoluminescent dosimeters. As a patient, such exposure becomes of concern during multidirectional tomographic procedures and computed tomography. Several investigators have measured lens dose during multidirectional tomography[22-26] and taken, collectively suggest that the lens dose during a conventional inner ear study is in the range of 0.5 to 2 rads per view. Our early in-

vestigation[27] of lens dose in computed tomography resulted in an average of 400 mrads unless the lens was in the primary beam in which case a dose of several rads was possible with different types of CT scanners. These estimates have subsequently been verified by others[28-37].

The lens dose is of importance because of suspected radiation induced cataracts following a latent period of perhaps 20 years. Radiation induced cataracts are considered to follow a non-linear, threshold type dose response relationship and the threshold for low LET radiation such as diagnostic x-rays is approximately 200 rads[38]. Lens dose can be reduced significantly with the use of lead eye shields but too often such use interferes significantly with the image production.

Mean Marrow Dose: Another of the suspected human responses to low level radiation exposure is leukemia. Radiation leukemogenesis is apparently a consequence of exposure of the hematologic stem cells particularly those residing in the bone marrow. Therefore, the average radiation dose to the active bone marrow is an important index of exposure relating to a latent somatic effect. Such an index is known as the mean marrow dose, and it refers not only to an average over the body but also to a population average.

In the U.S., the mean marrow dose has an estimated value of 103 mrad/hr from medical and dental applications of x-rays, with 77% of the dose attributed to radiography[39]. This value is obtained by first estimating the mean marrow dose for specific x-ray examinations and averaging that value to the entire population with regard to the frequency of various types of x-ray examinations that are conducted each year. Table 3 summarizes estimates of mean marrow dose made by different types of examinations. Recent reports[49-54] on mean marrow dose in chest radiography review the procedures involved in estimating mean marrow dose from a given examination from a measurement of entrance exposure.

EXAMINATION	Mean Marrow Dose
skull	35
chest	12
cervical spine	55
lumbar spine	275
IVP	550
abdomen	125
pelvis	135
pelvimetry (to fetus)	1000
extremity	<5
full mouth dental	20

These values are averages and should be used only as an indication. They have been obtained from many sources[40-48], but it should be clear that the dose delivered in any radiological procedure is very dependent upon the technical factors of application.

Table 3. Approximate mean marrow dose for various radiographic examinations.

Gonad Dose: Following high doses to both the male and female gonads, infertility and even permanent sterility can occur.

Evidence following human testicular radiation[38] suggests that sterility occurs at approximately 500 rads, transient infertility at perhaps 100 rads and a minimal spermatocyte depression at as low as 5 rads. There is, of course, considerable animal evidence to support these findings. The risk following diagnostic x-ray exposure is none of the above, but rather the possibility of genetic consequences.

In males, the gonad dose is easily measured since the male gonads lie superficially and are not shielded by overlying layers of tissue. Gonad dose in the male has been measured by a number of investigators[40-42, 55-56] and these findings are summarized in Table 4.

Examination	Gonad dose (mrads)
skull	<5
chest	<5
cervical spine	<5
lumbar spine	275
IVP	850
abdomen	350
pelvis	350
pelvimetry (to fetus)	900
extremity	<1
full mouth dental	<1

Table 4. Approximate gonad dose for various radiographic examinations.

These reports stress that during each examination for which the gonads are in the useful beam, the dose to the male gonad is considerably higher than that of the female gonad as is expected.

Fetal Dose: The fetal dose is a unique radiation index for diagnostic radiology in that it is, depending upon the time of gestation, essentially equal to the ovarian dose. However, the risk estimate is considerably more important. Not only is the fetus known to be more sensitive to radiation exposure than the postnatal individual, but also the fetal dose represents a whole body dose. A determination of fetal dose will equal all organ doses and the gonad dose for the fetus. Consequently, the suspected late somatic effects and genetic effects may be amplified.

In as much as the fetal dose is essentially equivalent to the ovarian dose, one could refer to Table 4 for such information if a crude estimate is sufficient. Better still, one could employ the summary data developed by the BRH using the procedures described above and published in several documents[63-65]. Essentially, this analysis allows one to estimate fetal dose from a knowledge of entrance exposure. Table 5 is reproduced from NCRP Report No. 54[65] and shows the fetal dose in millirads as a function of entrance exposure in roentgens.

This approach to dose determination for nearly all anatomical organs has been estimated using computer assisted methodology and Monte Carlo techniques[63]. This methodology has been developed by the Bureau of Radiological Health and is presently being extended conceptually into an organ dose index - an index of population dose averages for both somatic and genetic organs.

Projection	View	SID (inches)	Image Receptor Size (inches)[c]	Beam Quality (HVL, mm Al) 1.5	2.0	2.5	3.0	3.5	4.0
Pelvis, lumbopelvic	AP	40	17" × 14"	142	212	283	353	421	486
	LAT	40	14" × 17"	13	25	39	56	75	97
Abdominal[d]	AP	40	14" × 17"	133	199	265	330	392	451
	PA	40	14" × 17"	56	90	130	174	222	273
	LAT	40	14" × 17"	13	23	37	53	71	91
Lumbar Spine	AP	40	14" × 17"	128	189	250	309	366	419
	LAT	40	14" × 17"	9	17	27	39	53	68
Hip	AP (one)	40	10" × 12"	105	153	200	244	285	324
	AP (both)	40	17" × 14"	136	203	269	333	395	454
Full Spine (Chiropractic)	AP	40	14" × 36"	154	231	308	384	457	527
Urethrogram Cystography	AP	40	10" × 12"	135	200	265	327	386	441
Upper G.I.	AP	40	14" × 17"	9.5	16	25	34	45	56
Femur (one side)	AP	40	7" × 17"	1.6	3.0	4.8	6.9	9.4	12
Cholecystography	PA	40	10" × 12"	0.7	1.5	2.6	4.1	6.0	8.3
Chest	AP	72	14" × 17"	0.3	0.7	1.3	2.0	3.1	4.3
	PA	72	14" × 17"	0.3	0.6	1.2	2.0	3.0	4.5
	LAT	72	14" × 17"	0.1	0.3	0.5	0.8	1.2	1.8
Ribs, Barium Swallow	AP	40	14" × 17"	0.1	0.3	0.5	0.9	1.4	2.0
	PA	40	14" × 17"	0.1	0.3	0.5	0.9	1.5	2.2
	LAT	40	14" × 17"	0.03	0.08	0.2	0.3	0.4	0.6
Thoracic Spine	AP	40	14" × 17"	0.2	0.4	0.8	1.4	4.1	3.0
	LAT	40	14" × 17"	0.04	0.1	0.2	0.4	0.5	0.8
Skull, Cervical Spine, Scapula, Shoulder, Humerus	—	40	—	<.01	<.01	<.01	<.01	<.01	<.01

[a]Average dose to the uterus (mrad) for 1 roentgen entrance skin exposure (free-in-air).
[b]From Rosenstein (1976).
[c]Field size is collimated to the image receptor size.
[d]Includes: Retrograde Pyelogram, KUB, Barium Enema, Lumbosacral Spine, IVP, Renal Arteriogram.

Table 5. Fetal dose for selected radiographic examinations.

Genetically Significant Dose

Just as the mean marrow dose is a dose index for a suspected somatic effect - leukemia, so the genetically significant dose (GSD) is a dose index for suspected genetic effects. It must be emphasized that both are dose indices. They are our current best estimate of the population dose of these organs. Neither dose in any way is used to predict an effect

The genetically significant dose is the gonad dose which, if received by every member of the population, would be expected to produce the sum total effect on the population as the sum of the individual doses actually received. The general formulation is:

$$GSD = \frac{\Sigma \; D\bar{N}P}{\Sigma \; NP}$$

where D = the average gonad dose per examination
$\bar{N}$ = the number of persons receiving x-ray examination
N = the total number of persons in the population
P = the expected number of children per person

For computational purposes we consider age, sex and type of examination for each patient. The general formulation becomes:

$$GSD = \frac{\Sigma_i \Sigma_j \; (\bar{N}_{ij} P_i D_{ij})_{male} + (\bar{N}_{ij} P_i D_{ij})_{female} + (\bar{N}_{ij} P_i D_{ij})_{fetus}}{\Sigma_i \; (N_i P_i)_{male} + (N_i P_i)_{female} + (N_i P_i)_{fetus}}$$

where i indexes age
j indexes the type of examination performed

Inspection of the above equation would reveal that the GSD is determined by consideration of estimates of gonad dose for each type of examination, the age and sex of each individual so irradiated (including those not irradiated) and the expected progeny of each. The GSD, therefore, relies on measurements of gonadal radiation dose coupled with estimates of various statistics of medical x-ray examinations.

In the U.S. the most recent estimate of GSD was 20 mR/yr. Table 6 presents the results of reports from several countries summarizing the respective GSD for each. The estimates shown for the United States were later revised downward because of errors in the earlier computer assisted analyses.

Table 6. Estimated GSD due to diagnostic x-ray examination.

Population	Time of Study	GSD (mrads)
New Zealand	1963	12
Great Britain	1957-58	14
Denmark	1956	22
United States	1970	36 (20)*
Japan	1960	39
United States	1964	55 (16)*
Sweden	1955	72
Australia	1950-55	159

* Corrected values

CURRENT CLINICAL SITUATIONS

The exposure of patients to medical x-rays is assuming increasing importance in our society for two reasons. First, the frequency of x-ray examination is increasing every year among all age groups at a rate of between 6% and 10% per year in the United States, a rate of increase exceeded in many other countries. This indicates that physicians are relying more and more on x-ray diagnosis to assist them in patient care. Second, there is increasing concern among public health officials and radiation scientists that the risk associated with medical x-ray exposure may be increasing more rapidly than the benefits derived therefrom. It attention is given to good radiation-control practices, the same level of diagnostic information can be obtained with reduced risk of latent injury.

Patient Dose in Mammography

Because of the very considerable application of x-rays for examination of the female breast and the concern for the induction of breast cancer by radiation, it is imperative that we have some understanding of the radiation doses involved in such examinations.

There are three principal methods for mammography, only two of which are generally acceptable. The direct exposure method is not acceptable because of high patient dose. In direct exposure mammography, the patient dose will vary from perhaps 6 to 15 rads/view, and this is unacceptable because the other two methods result in equal if not better images at considerably less patient dose.

When xeromammography was first introduced, it required patient doses ranging from one to five rads/view. More recently, these average doses have been reduced to the range of 0.5 to 1.5 rads/view[66-74].

Screen/film mammography is the lowest dose procedure. Patient doses in the range of 0.2 to 1 rad per view are experienced with screen/films[75-82]. Faster films and screens may make even lower dose screen/film mammography possible.

The values just cited for patient dose in mammography can be misleading. Because of the low x-ray energies employed in mammography, the dose falls off very rapidly as the beam penetrates the breast. If the entrance dose for a craniocaudad view mammogram is for example, 1 rad, the dose to the midline of the breast may be only 250 mrad and that at the image receptor perhaps 20 mrads. The biological effect of such an examination is presumed to be more closely associated with the total energy absorbed by the breast or the average dose rather than the skin dose. Consequently, when using such dose estimates to predict response, it is the midline dose that should be employed.

Specification of a skin dose can also be misleading when one considers a multi-view examination. Figure 2 illustrates this dilemma. Consider a three view mammogram consisting of a craniocaudad, mediolateral and axillary view. The cranio-caudad and the mediolateral views produced a skin dose of 1 rad each and the axillary view a dose of 2 rads. It would be incorrect to describe this total examination procedure as resulting in a patient dose of 4 rads. Skin doses from different projections cannot be added. We must either specify the skin dose for each view or attempt to estimate the total midline dose or integral dose.

To estimate the total midline dose we can make the approximation that the contribution from each view will be 25% of the skin dose. Consequently, the total midline dose would be the sum of a 250 mrad contribution from each of the cranio-caudad and mediolateral views and a 500 mrad contribution from the axillary view. The total midline dose, therefore, would be 1000 mrad.

From this discussion it would seem that patient dose in mammography can be considerably reduced if the number of views is restricted. The axillary view should not be done routinely. For screening programs perhaps only a single view would be advisable.

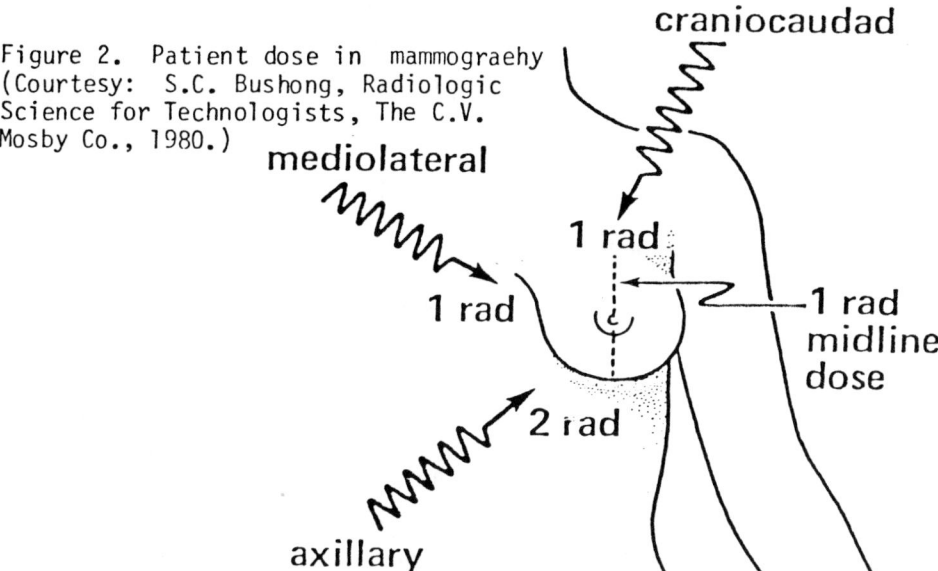

Figure 2. Patient dose in mammograehy (Courtesy: S.C. Bushong, Radiologic Science for Technologists, The C.V. Mosby Co., 1980.)

Patient Dose in CT Scanning

An important consideration in CT scanning, as with any diagnostic procedure is patient dose. The skin dose delivered to a patient by a series of contiguous CT scans is roughly equivalent to that delivered by a single conventional skull or abdominal radiographic view. However, a typical conventional head or body procedure often involves several views. Thus, the dose from CT is frequently less than the cumulative dose produced by a series of conventional radiographic views. Furthermore, for most CT examinations considerably less tissue volume is irradiated than in conventional radiography. The CT dose is significantly less than most fluoroscopic procedures.

Part of the dose efficiency of CT is due to the precise collimation of the x-ray beam. The precise collimation used in CT means that only a very well defined volume of tissue is irradiated during each scan. The ideal x-ray beam for CT would have sharp boundaries. There would be no overlap between adjacent scans. Thus, aside from a minimal contribution due to scatter, the dose delivered to a patient from a series of ideal adjacent CT scans would be the same as from a single scan. Figure 3 illustrates how this ideal situation, however, cannot be attained in practice. The finite focal spot size of the x-ray tube produces some penumbra and blurs the sharp boundaries of the slice. Also the beam is not precisely parallel and some spreading occurs as the beam traverses the scan field. If series of adjacent scans are performed with an automatically indexing patient couch, the couch movement must be precise. Finally and perhaps most importantly, if the pre-patient collimators are open too wide, tissues near the interface of each scan will receive higher dose than they otherwise should. It is essential that CT collimators be periodically monitored for proper adjustment. Thus, in practice, a series of adjacent scans deliver a higher dose than a single scan because of the overlap of beam peripheries.

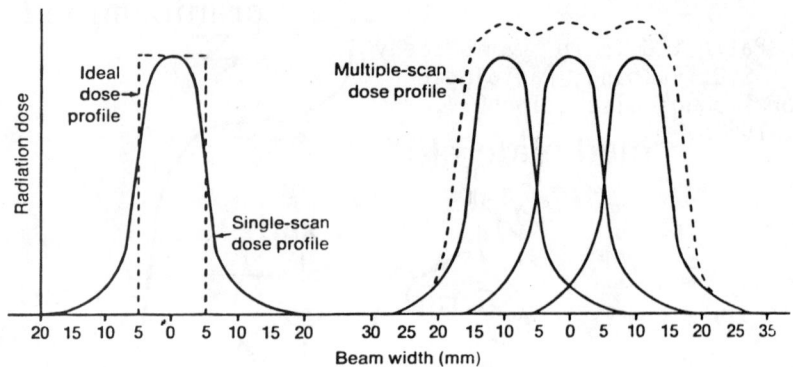

Figure 3. Patient dose distribution in CT is somewhat complicated when contiguous scanning is employed. (Courtesy: S.C. Bushong, Radiologic Science for Technologists, The C.V. Mosby Co., 1980.)

Dose is more uniformly distributed in CT than in conventional radiography. This is because the x-ray source rotates about the patient through at least 180 degrees.

Typical skin doses range from 0.5 to 4 rad during head scans and 1 to 10 rad during body scans. Midline doses are somewhat less than the skin doses. These values are only approximate and vary widely depending on the machine and the radiation technique. Because the CT beam is well collimated, the area of irradiation can be precisely controlled. Thus radiosensitive areas such as the lenses of the eye can be selectively avoided. Shields as protection from the primary x-ray beam in CT are of little use. Not only does the metal from these shields produce terrible artifacts in the image, but also the rotational scheme of the x-ray source greatly reduces their effectiveness.

As with any radiographic procedure, many factors influence patient dose. For CT the following general proportionality holds true:

$$\text{Dose} \, \alpha \, \frac{I \, E}{\alpha^2 w^3 h}$$

where   means "is proportional to"
  I = beam intensity in mAs
  E = average beam energy in keV
  α = system noise
  w = pixel size
  h = slice thickness

All other things being equal, a CT scanner that produces a low noise - high resolution image does so at the sacrifice of higher patient dose. The challenge in CT, as indeed with all radiographic imaging procedures, is not so much to deliver fantastically good resolution and low noise for this could be achieved at the cost of very high patient dose, but to use the x-ray beam efficiently, producing the best possible image at a reasonable dose to the patient.

OCCUPATIONAL EXPOSURE

Although the maximum permissible dose for radiologic personnel is 5000 mrem/year, experience has shown that considerably lower exposures than this should be routine. The occupational exposure of radiologic personnel engaged in general x-ray activity should not normally exceed about 1000 mrem/year. Table 6 is a summary of the personnel-monitoring experience of four large general hospitals in Houston, Texas. Each hospital conducts over 100,000 x-ray examinations per year and has a reasonably proficient radiation-control program. Note that there is little difference between the exposures of radiologists and x-ray technologists, although the radiologists generally receive slightly higher exposures.

Table 6. Average occupational exposure (mrem/year) of radiology personnel in four general hospitals in Houston, Texas.

	1967-68	1969-70	1971-72	1973-74	1975-76	1977-78	Average
Hospital A							
Radiologists	407	380	590	1138	1143	657	688
Technicians	315	389	334	207	103	965	255
Hospital B							
Radiologists	295	631	864	367	302	282	447
Technicians	170	311	285	361	176	427	280
Hospital C							
Radiologists	790	520	416	457	829	448	.553
Technicians	337	603	259	260	266	305	357
Hospital D							
Radiologists	894	2219	1895	616	214	106	954
Technicians	667	957	472	241	57	32	412

Unquestionably, the highest occupational exposure of diagnostic x-ray personnel occurs during fluoroscopy and portable radiography. During radiographic exposures, the radiologist is rarely present, and the technologist should be positioned behind a protective barrier. When protective barriers are not available, such as during portable examinations, the portable x-ray machine should be equipped with an exposure cord long enough to allow the technologist to leave the examination area and the technologist should be provided with a protective apron.

During fluoroscopy, both radiologist and x-ray technologist are exposed to relatively high levels of radiation. However, personnel exposure is directly related to the x-ray beam - on time so that, with care personnel exposures are acceptably low. Image-intensified fluoroscopy generally results in lower personnel exposures because smaller field sizes and lower mA are used.

Personnel engaged in special procedures often receive higher exposures than those in general radiologic practice because of the longer fluoroscopic times experienced, the frequent absence of an intensifier tower protective curtain and the extensice use of cineradiography.

Personnel exposures associated with mammography are low because the low kVp of operation results in reduced scatter radiation. Frequently a long exposure cord and a conventional wall are sufficient to provide adequate protection.

CT scanning is another new activity in radiology contributing to personnel exposure. Since the CT x-ray beam is finely collimated and only scatter radiation is present in the scan room, personnel can be permitted to remain in the room during scanning. Protective apparel should be used in such situations.

It should NEVER be necessary for diagnostic x-ray personnel to exceed 5000 mrem/yr. In smaller hospitals, emergency centers and private clinics, occupational exposures will rarely exceed 500 mrem/yr. Average exposures in such facilities arecloser to 100 mrem/yr.

REFERENCES

1. W.A. Jennings, Brit. J. Radiol. 45:784, 1972.
2. K. Liden, H.O. Wycoff and A. Allisy, Brit. J. Radiol. 46:561, 1973.
3. The International System of Units, N.B.S., Special Publication 330, 1972.
4. N.W. Ramsey, Brit. J. Radiol. 47:269, 1974.
5. A.R. Reddy and A. Nagaratnom, Brit. J. Radiol. 47:295, 1974.
6. M.J. Day, Brit. J. Radiol. 47:821, 1974.
7. N. Goodwin, Brit. J. Radiol. 49:898, 1976.
8. A. Feldman, Brit. J. Radiol. 50:296, 1977.
9. H.O. Wyckorr, A. Allisy, K., Liden, Brit. J. Radiol. 49:476,1976.
10. International Congress of Radiology Recommendations, X-ray and Radium Protection. Radiol. 12:519, 1929.
11. National Bureau of Standards Circular No. 374, 1929.
12. Recommendations of the International Committee for Radiological Units, Radiology 23:580-581, 1934.
13. Recommendations of the International Committee for Radiological Units, Radiology 29:634-636, 1937.
14. Radiation Quantities and Units, Report 10a of the ICRU, NBS Handbook 84, 1962.
15. L.H. Gray and J. Read, Nature 144:439-440, 1939.
16. H.M. Parker, Health Physics, Instrumentation and Radiation Protection, Advances in Biol. and Med. Phys. 1:223-285, 1948.
17. International Commission on Radiological Units, 1953, Brit. J. Radiol. 27:243, 1954.
18. Report of the International Commision on Radiological Units and Measurements (ICRU) 1956, NBS Handbook 62, 1957.
19. ICRU Report No. 19s, Dose Equivalent (Supplement to ICRU Report 19), 1973.
20. ICRU Report No. 25, Conceptual Basis for the Determination of Dose Equivalent, 1976.
21. E.C. McCullough and J.R. Cameron, Brit. J. Radiol. 43: 448, 1970.
22. J. Robert Cassady and R.N. Pierce, BRH/DEP 70-27, 1970.
23. F.K. Chin, W.B. Anderson and J.D. Gilbertson, Radiology 94:623-627, 1970.
24. J.S. Krohmer, Radiology 103:447-450, 1972.
25. H. Dahlin, Acta Rad. 14:353-367, 1973.
26. J.T. Littleton, Radiology 129:3, 1978
27. R.C. Whitmore, Radiologic Technology, Vol 51, No. 1, 1979.
28. O. Krauss, Der Radiologe 16:7, 1976.
29. S. Balter, Medicamundi, Vol. 22, No. 3, 1977
30. D.G. Bhave, Radiology, Vol. 124, No. 2, 1977.
31. D.G. Bhave, Radiology, 124:379-380, 1977.
32. T. Villafana, Health Physics 34:71-82, 1978.
33. D.E. Raeside, Radiology 129:814-815, 1978.
34. B. Alexxson, Acta Radiol., Vol. 17(4), 1978.
35. E.C. McCullough, Radiology, Vol. 129, No. 2, 1978.
36. B. Skalnik, Applied, Radiology, Jan-Feb, 1979.
37. B.F. Wall, Br. Jr. of Radiol., Vol. 52, No1. 615, 1979.

38. The Effects of Populations of Exposure to Low Levels of Ionizing Radiation, NAS-NRC Report, 1972.
39. B. Shlein, Health Physics, 34:587-601, 1978.
40. E.R. Epp, Br. Jr. of Radiol., April, 1963.
41. S. Antoku, Radiology, 101:669-678, 1971.
42. S. Antoku, Radiology, 101:669-678, 1971
43. J.G. Kereiakes, Radiology 103:651-656, 1972.
44. T. Hashizume, Health Physics, Vol. 23, 1972
45. B. Shleien, "A review of determinations of radiation dose to the active bone marrow from diagnostic x-ray examinations", FDA publication, No. 74-8007, 1973.
46. L. Seidlitz, Investigative Radiol., 9:419-424, 1974.
47. Y. Takaku, Nippon Acta Radiol, Vol. 35, 1975.
48. B. Shleien, HEW Publication (FDA) 77-8013, 1973.
49. E.R. Epp, Measure. of Bone Marrow and Gonad Dose, 2/61.
50. L. Koblinger, Health Physics, 1972.
51. T. Kitabatake, Radiology 109:37-40, 1973.
52. R.E. Ellis, DHEW Publication (FDA) 76-8015, 1975.
53. S.C. Bushong, Health Physics 35:886, 1978.
54. B.R. Archer, Radiology 133:211-216, 1979.
55. S.C. Bushong, Am. J. Ob-Gyn. 117:933-938, 1973.
56. G.M. Ardran, Gonad Rad. Dose from Diag. Proce., 30:295, 1975.
57. H.A. Bishop, California Medicine 90:20-25, 1959.
58. W.D. Norwood, Am. J. Roentg. 82: #6, 1959.
59. B.S. Pasternack, Radiology 90:217, 1968.
60. M. Gileadi, Health Physics, 25:43-49, 1973
61. Gonad Doses and Genetically Significant Dose from Diagnostic Radiology, HEW Publication (FDA) 76-8034, 1976.
62. K.E. Kivinitty, Health Physics, 34:387-389, 1978.
63. M. Rosenstein, HEW Publication (FDA) 76-8030, 1976.
64. M. Rosenstein, HEW Publication (FDA) 76-8031, 1976.
65. Medical Radiation Exposure of Pregnant and Potentially Pregnant Women, NCRP Report No. 54, p. 18, 1977.
66. S.C. Bushong, Health Physics 27:625, 1974.
67. J.H. Baxt, Health Physics, 30:91-94, 1976.
68. R.C. Palmer, Radiology 101:697-699, 1975
69. R.L.A. Kirch, Radiology 117:701, 1975.
70. F. Willgeroth, Strahlentherapie 152:533, 1976.
71. W.G. Van De Riet, Am. J. Roent, 128:821-823, 1977.
72. W.G. Van De Reit, Am. J. Roent, 128:821, 1977.
73. J.B. Buchanan, Radiology 123:63, 1977.
74. E.P. Muntz, Radiology 127:517, 1978.
75. R.C. Palmer, Radiology 95:395-397, 1970.
76. J.L. Price, Brit. J. Radiol. 43:251-255, 1975.
77. B.J. Ostrum, Radiology 109:323-326, 1973.
78. J. Stillman, Br. J. Radiol., Vol 48:228, 1975.
79. J.P. Weiss, Jr. Appl. Photo. Engineer., Vol. 2(1), 1976.
80. M. Karlsson, Acta Radiologica, 15:252, 1976.
81. R.A. Mintzer, Invest. Radiol., 12:465-466, 1977.
82. I. Andersson, Acta Radiologica, 18:264, 1977.

DOSE EVALUATION IN NUCLEAR MEDICINE

James G. Kereiakes, Ph.D., Stephen R. Thomas, Ph.D., Michael J. Gelfand, M.D., Harry R. Maxon, M.D. and Eugene L. Saenger, M.D., Eugene L. Saenger Radioisotope Laboratory, University of Cincinnati, Cincinnati, Ohio 45267

INTRODUCTION

The increasing use of radionuclides in medical diagnosis and research demands accurate knowledge of the radiation exposure sustained during these procedures. Estimates of absorbed radiation dose can be made when information on radionuclide properties and decay scheme, amount injected, and biological fate and distribution of the radionuclide are available. Today's knowledge of radionuclide properties is adequate but physiological data are often very limited. Factors that can influence the physiological distribution of radioactive materials within the patient are alterations of organ size, uptake, and excretion in the disease state. Most current approaches to radiation dose estimates assume the following: (a) that the tissue in question is homogeneous throughout the region of interest and (b) that the radionuclide is uniformly distributed. These assumptions usually result in a dose value which is considered to be an average value for the tissue.

Of special interest to this symposium is the estimation of absorbed doses to several pediatric age groups and to the embryo and fetus. The spatial and temporal distribution of radiopharmaceuticals may differ greatly in children from that accepted for adults.

This presentation will provide available information on the various parameters involved in estimating the radiation doses in clinical nuclear medicine. We have attempted to include the most commonly employed radionuclides.

DOSIMETRY MODEL

The mean absorbed dose $\bar{D}(r_k \leftarrow r_h)$ expressed in rad to a target organ r_k from a radionuclide distributed uniformly in a source organ r_h has been formulated by the MIRD Committee[1,2] as

$$\bar{D}(r_k \leftarrow r_h) = \frac{\tilde{A}_h}{m_k} \Sigma_i \Delta_i \phi_i (r_k \leftarrow r_h)$$

$$= \tilde{A}_h \Sigma_i \Delta_i \Phi_i (r_k \leftarrow r_h)$$

where $\tilde{A}_h$ (µCi·h) is the cumulated activity in source organ r_h; m_k (g) is the mass of the target organ r_k; Δ_i (g-rad/µCi·h) is the mean energy emitted per unit cumulated activity for radiation of a particular type and energy, here indicated by i; and $\phi(r_k \leftarrow r_h)$ and $\Phi_i(r_k \leftarrow r_h)$ represent, respectively, the absorbed fraction and the specific absorbed fraction (g^{-1}) of energy for target organ r_k for particles i emitted in source organ r_h.

PHYSIOLOGICAL CONSIDERATIONS

Most of the biologic data needed for the estimation of dose are embodied in the cumulated activity $\tilde{A}_h$. The biologic data in estimating dose relate only to the anthropomorphic model used (size, shape, density, and composition) and to the distribution and retention of the radionuclide in source organ r_h.

The cumulated activity is related to the activity function $A_h(t)$ by the expression

$$\tilde{A}_h = \int_{t_1}^{t_2} A_h(t) dt$$

where $t_2 - t_1$ is the exposure time interval for which the dose is computed. The activity $A_h(t)$ in an organ or tissue, at any time t_1, is in general governed by the following factors: the amount of administered activity, the site and rate of radiopharmaceutical uptake and removal, and the physical characteristics of the radionuclide.

Administered Activity, A_o

The initial activity in the area of interest will depend on the uptake and the administered activity. Table 1 shows recommended administered activity schedules based on body weight. These schedules are intended only as guidelines. Considerations of individual patient conditions, pathological processes and physiology must be taken into account in determining the administered activity to be used in performing nuclear medicine procedures.

Table 1. ADMINISTERED ACTIVITY

Radioisotope & Chemical Form	Study	Activity	Adult Activity	Pediatric Activity Maximum	Pediatric Activity Minimum
^{67}Ga-citrate	gallium scan	50 µCi/kg	5 mCi	3 mCi	--
^{99m}TcEHDP disphosphonate	bone scan	165 µCi/kg for benign disease; 220 µCi/kg for known malignancy	15-20 mCi	15 mCi	1 mCi
^{99m}Tc-Sn-DTPA	renal imaging	150 µCi/kg	10 mCi	7 mCi	500 µCi
^{99m}Tc glucoheptonate	renal imaging	60 µCi/kg	15 mCi	3 mCi	400 µCi
^{99m}Tc-glucoheptonate	brain imaging	280 µCi/kg	15 mCi	15 mCi	1.5 mCi
^{99m}Tc-HIDA	hepatobiliary imaging	90 µCi/kg	3-8 mCi	3 mCi	400 µCi
^{99m}Tc-human serum albumin	cardiovascular imaging	150 µCi/kg	15-20 mCi	12 mCi	1 mCi
^{99m}TcMAA	lung scan	80 µCi/kg	3 mCi	2 mCi	400 µCi
^{99m}TcO$_4$ pertechnetate	brain scan	280 µCi/kg	15 mCi	15 mCi	1.5 mCi
^{99m}TcO$_4$ pertechnetate	cardiovascular imaging	150 µCi/kg	15-20 mCi	10 mCi	1 mCi
^{99m}TcO$_4$ pertechnetate	ectopic gastric tissue (e.g. Meckel's diverticulum)	50 µCi/kg	5 mCi	4 mCi	500 µCi

Table 1. ADMINISTERED ACTIVITY (cont.)

Radioisotope & Chemical Form	Study	Activity	Adult Activity	Pediatric Activity Maximum	Pediatric Activity Minimum
$^{99m}TcO_4$ pertechnetate	testicular scan	200 µCi/kg	10 mCi	10 mCi	1 mCi
$^{99m}TcO_4$ pertechnetate	thyroid scan	80 µCi/kg	5 mCi	4 mCi	300 µCi
^{99m}Tc-red cells	cardiovascular imaging	150 µCi/kg	15-20 mCi	12 mCi	1 mCi
^{99m}Tc sulfur colloid	liver scan	80 µCi/kg	3 mCi	2 mCi	400 µCi
^{111}In-DTPA	cisternogram or rhinorrhea study	17 µCi/kg	500 µCi	250 µCi	80 µCi
^{111}In-DTPA	cerebrospinal fluid shunt imaging			150 µCi	150 µCi
^{123}I-sodium iodide	thyroid scan	2.6 µCi/kg	200 µCi	100 µCi	15 µCi
^{131}I-sodium iodide	thyroid uptake		10 µCi	10 µCi	5 µCi
^{131}I-hippuran	renogram	7.7 µCi/kg if under 14 kg; 5.5 µCi/kg if greater than 14 kg	300 µCi	300 µCi	50 µCi
^{133}Xe-gas	ventilation study	0.5 mCi/liter			
^{169}Yb-DTPA	cerebrospinal fluid imaging		1 mCi	1 mCi	200 µCi
^{201}Tl-chloride	myocardial scan		1.5 mCi	1.5 mCi	200 µCi

Quantitation of Radioactivity

Quantitative methods for in vivo measurements of radioactivity are receiving increased attention. Quantitation using conjugate counting views has been proposed by Budinger[3], Sorenson[4] and Thomas et al.[5] The approach provides corrections for source thickness, inhomogeneity, and attenuation.

Effective Half-Life, T_e

In practice, measurements are made for a period of time over the area or organ of interest and the effective half-life (T_e) is determined.

Cumulated Activity, $\tilde{A}_h$

Having determined T_e and having quantified the initial activity, A_o, in the organ of interest the cumulated activity can then be calculated from

$$\tilde{A}_h \ (\mu Ci \cdot h) = A_o(\mu Ci) \cdot 1.44 \ T_e(h)$$

The above assumes single exponential time dependency and usually can be used as a first approximation. More accurate determination of the activity-versus-time function may require more exponential terms or in some cases a different type of function. Numerical integration of the activity-versus-time curve using the trapezoidal rule is another alternative. In this case, it is unnecessary to assume a particular form for the function $A_h(t)$.

Table 2 presents published values for cumulated activities (whole body and investigated or critical organ) for the radiopharmaceuticals.[20] The cumulated activity values are based on distributions obtained mostly from animal studies but also from human clinical studies.

PHYSICAL CONSIDERATIONS

The terms $\Sigma_i \Delta_i \phi_i (r_k \leftarrow r_h)/m_k$ involves physical and anatomical data. Values for these terms can all be tabulated for specific radionuclides and for specific source-target configurations commonly used in nuclear medicine. It is assumed that the activity is distributed uniformly in the source organ, and the phantom used in estimating the specific absorbed fractions is essentially that of MIRD pamphlet No. 5 with some modifications.[7]

Mean Energy Emitted per Unit cumulated Activity, Δ_i

The nuclear parameters for many radionuclides appear in the work of Dillman[8,9]. The mean energy emitted per unit cumulated activity, in units of $g \cdot rad/\mu Ci \cdot h$, is defined as:

$$\Delta_i = 2.13 \cdot n_i \cdot E_i$$

Table 2. CUMULATED ACTIVITIES FOR VARIOUS RADIOPHARMACEUTICALS

Radiopharma-ceutical	Study	Cumulated Activity μCi·hr per μCi administered		
		Total Body	Organ	Remaining Body
^{67}Ga-citrate	tumor and abscess imaging	88.4	11.5-bone (.13) 4.5-liver (.05) 4.8-red marrow (.05) 0.63-spleen (.007)	58.4
^{75}Se-selenomethionine	pancreas imaging	1650.0	188.0-liver (.24) 40.8-lungs (.036) 26.3-renal corgex (.022) 12.4-spleen (.015)	1370.0
^{99m}Tc-DTPA	renal imaging	8.9	0.43 -kidneys (.05) 5.0 -bladder	2.8
^{99m}Tc-glucoheptonate	renal, brain imaging	3.9	1.6-kidneys (.25)	2.16
^{99m}Tc-human serum albumin	cardiovascular imaging	4.3		
^{99m}Tc-iron complex	renal imaging	3.7	1.7-renal cortex	
^{99m}Tc-macroaggregates, microspheres	lung imaging	8.0	5.6-lungs 0.56-liver	
^{99m}Tc-pertechnetate	brain, thyroid imaging	7.8	0.15 -thyroid (.03) 0.35 -stomach (.06)	7.17
^{99m}Tc-polyphosphate, pyrophosphate	bone imaging	8.7	4.3 -bone (.50)	4.33

Table 2. CUMULATED ACTIVITIES FOR VARIOUS RADIOPHARMACEUTICALS (cont.)

Radiopharmaceutical	Study	Cumulated Activity µCi·hr per µCi administered		
		Total Body	Organ	Remaining Body
^{99m}Tc-sulfur colloid	liver, spleen imaging	8.7	7.36-liver (.85) 0.43 -red marrow (.05) 0.61 -spleen (.07)	0.26
^{111}In-colloid	liver imaging	97.0	84.0 - liver	
^{111}In-DTPA	cerebrospinal fluid imaging	3.3	3.3 - bladder	
^{111}In-iron hydroxide	lung imaging	7.8	5.1 - lungs	
^{123}I-iodide	thyroid	17.8 15.9 14.0	0.94-thyroid (.05) 2.81-thyroid (.15) 4.68-thyroid (.25)	16.9 13.1 9.3
^{123}I-iodohippurate	renal imaging	0.6	0.2 -kidneys	
^{123}I-rose bengal	liver imaging	12.0	1.9 -liver	
^{131}I-iodide	thyroid imaging	46.0 72.0 100.0	12.1-thyroid (.05) 36.3-thyroid (.15) 60.5-thyroid (.25)	20.9 19.5 17.0
^{131}I-iodohippurate	renal imaging	0.7	0.157-kidneys (.30)	0.743
^{131}I-macroaggregates	lung imaging	35.0	9.0 (.82)-lungs 4.1 -liver (.20) 21.7 -thyroid (.08)	
^{131}I-rose bengal	liver imaging	30.0	2.2 -liver	

Table 2. CUMULATED ACTIVITIES FOR VARIOUS RADIOPHARMACEUTICALS (cont.)

Radiopharma-ceutical	Study	Cumulated Activity μCi·hr per μCi administered		
		Total Body	Organ	Remaining Body
^{133}Xe-gas	lung perfusion and ventilation	5870.0	170 - blood	(1 mCi/liter)
^{169}Yb-DTPA	cerebrospinal fluid imaging	8.5	7.7 -kidney	
^{201}Tl-chloride	cardiac imaging	96.4	1.03 -liver 0.14 -heart 0.74 -kidneys	

*number in parentheses indicate percent uptake

where n_i is the mean number of particles or photons per nuclear transformation, E_i is the mean energy of this radiation in MeV, and 2.13 is a unit conversion constant. Each type of emission may be classified as either penetrating (that is electromagnetic radiation having energy greater than 10 keV) or nonpenetrating (that is electromagnetic radiation of energy less or equal to 10 keV, and all particulate radiation). Table 3 provides values for nonpenetrating, penetrating, and total mean energy emitted per cumulated activity.

Mass of Target Organ, m_k

Kereiakes, et al.[10] have provided information for a series of standard children - newborn, 1, 5, 10, and 15 years old - derived by supplementing values of the 50 percentile for heights and weights of certain ages with pertinent information on organ weights and physiology. Body weights and weights of most organs of interest are listed in Table 4. The weights used for the Φ calculation (Poston[11]) are given in this table and agree closely with the previously reported values.

Absorbed Fraction, ϕ

The absorbed fraction as a function of photon energy is available from MIRD[13,7]. Ellett and Humes[14] have calculated tables of absorbed fractions for small unit-density-absorbing volumes of 1-100g containing a uniformity distributed photon source. The data for small volumes are specifically helpful for absorbed dose calculations involving sizes of organs in children. The data for small volumes differ in one important aspect from absorbed fractions published earlier; it is assumed that the volume containing the activity is imbedded within a large scattering medium of the same composition. Backscatter radiation from these surroundings is included in the tabulated absorbed fractions. These tables are useful only when source organ and target organ are the same.

Specific Absorbed Fraction, Φ

Dividing the absorbed fraction, ϕ, by the mass of the target organ, m_k, provides the specific absorbed fraction, Φ. Values have been developed for the specific absorbed fraction to several target organs from activity located in certain source organs. These values of Φ for reference man, for several gamma energies, are given by Snyder, et al.[15]

Mean Dose Per Unit Cumulated Activity, S

It is convenient to introduce the term

$$S(r_k \leftarrow r_h) = \sum_i \Delta_i \Phi_i (r_k \leftarrow r_h)$$

where $S(r_k \leftarrow r_h)$ is defined as the mean dose (rad/μCi·h) to target

Table 3. Δ, MEAN ENERGY EMITTED PER UNIT CUMULATED ACTIVITY[8,9]

Radionuclide	Mean Energy Emitted per Unit Cumulated Activity Δ_i (g·rad/μCi·hr)		
	nonpenetrating	penetrating	total
^{51}Cr	0.0101	0.0694	0.0795
^{67}Ga	0.0862	0.3307	0.4169
^{75}Se	0.0401	0.7828	0.8229
^{99m}Tc	0.0369	0.2660	0.3029
^{111}In	0.0773	0.8648	0.9421
^{123}I	0.0610	0.3592	0.4202
^{125}I	0.0434	0.0884	0.1318
^{131}I	0.4084	0.8047	1.2121
^{133}Xe	0.2928	0.0950	0.3878
^{169}Yb	0.4142	0.5311	0.9453
^{201}Tl	0.0874	0.1931	0.2805

Table 4. SUMMARY OF ORGAN WEIGHTS FOR PEDIATRIC PHANTOMS

Organ	Newborn		1-year		5-years		10-years		15-years	
	Wellman et al. (12)	ORNL(11)	Wellman et al.	ORNL	Wellman et al.	ORNL	Wellman et al.	ORNL	Wellman et al.	ORNL
Brain	350	372	945	1005	1214	1180	1313	1651	1350	1367
Bladder Wall	---	3	---	7	---	14	---	23	---	34
Intestines	146	32†	398	140†	550	301†	820	339	1350	1265
Kidneys	23	19	72	68	112	116	187	177	247	230
Liver	136	110	333	300	591	608	918	896	1289	1267
Lungs	52	40	172	130	291	260	523	430	701	650
Red Marrow	---	40	---	150	---	400	---	---	---	950
Yellow Marrow	---	0	---	0	---	50	---	---	---	1500
Ovaries	0.29	0.3	1.0	0.7	2.0	2	3.5	3.1	6.5	5
Pancreas	2.8	2.6	14	9	23	19	30	27	68	57
Skeleton	---	500	---	1600	---	2800	---	3162	---	8700
Spleen	9.4	8.8	31	27	54	50	101	80	138	145
Stomach	6.5	5.9	27	27	57	52	90	88	120	118
Testes	0.67	0.8	1.5	1.5	1.7	1.6	2.0	1.9	18	16
Thyroid	1.5	1	2.2	2	4.7	5	8.0	9.0	11.2	13
Total Body	3540	3990	12100	10400	20000	20000	33500	32170	55000	56980
Total Height (cm)	50	52	75	76	108	112	---	140	166	167

† Not complete, does not include mass of contents for lower large intestine.

organ r_k per unit accumulated activity in source organs r_h. $S(r_k \leftarrow r_h)$ can also be expressed as

$$S(r_k \leftarrow r_h) = \frac{\sum_n \Delta_n \phi_n (r_k \leftarrow r_h)}{m_k} + \frac{\sum_p \Delta_p \Phi_p (r_k \leftarrow r_h)}{m_k}$$

where n and p denote nonpenetrating and penetrating emissions, respectively. If the source and target organs do not coincide ($r_h \neq r_k$), it is usually assumed that $\phi_n (r_k \leftarrow r_h) = 0$. Thus, the first term in the above equation has a non-zero value only when $r_h = r_k$, in which case all of the energy emitted in r_h is assumed to be absorbed in r_h.

Values for S (due to both nonpenetrating and penetrating emissions) for several target organs and for uniform distribution of the radionuclide in source organs are given in Tables by Snyder, et. al.[16] S factors for pediatric age groups (for specific source-target organ configurations) have been developed recently by the Health Physics Division, Oak Ridge National Laboratory[17,18]. It is not possible to present all the S factor tables in this manuscript, but representative values for S factor for ^{99m}Tc for an adult and for a 5 year old are given in Tables 5 and 6. Symbols used in these tables have the following meaning: * - includes nonpenetrating component $\Sigma\Delta_n/2m$ contents; + - includes nonpenetrating components $\Sigma\Delta_n/m$ target; and $\pm$ - includes nonpenetrating components $\Sigma\Delta_n/m$ total body. Table 7 has S values for several radionuclides and various organs with embryo as the target organ.[19]

RADIATION DOSES

Table 8 gives a tabulation of published whole body or organ doses (express in mrad/µCi administered) for the different radiopharmaceuticals and different age groups.

Table 9 includes dose estimates to the embryo for certain radiopharmaceuticals. Table 10 gives an estimate of the dose to the thyroid of the fetus from maternally administered radiodine.

PEDIATRIC MEASUREMENTS

At a time when the use of radionuclides in diagnostic procedures is increasing in infants and children, accurate and detailed information concerning the radiation dose during these procedures is frequently not available. Differences between the temporal and spatial distribution of radiopharmaceuticals in children and in adults indicate the need for specific pediatric data. These type of data are being accummulated at the Eugene L. Saenger Radioisotope Laboratory. Activity in the area of interest is quantified by a conjugate view counting technique, developed by Thomas, et.al.[5], using a gamma camera interfaced to a computer system. The effective half-life is determined by serial

TABLE 5. S, ABSORBED DOSE PER UNIT CUMULATED ACTIVITY, (RAD/UCI-H)
TECHNETIUM-99M   HALF-LIFE 6.03 HOURS

SOURCE ORGANS

TARGET ORGANS	ADRENALS	BLADDER CONTENTS	STOMACH CONTENTS	SI CONTENTS	ULI CONTENTS	LLI CONTENTS	KIDNEYS	LIVER	LUNGS	OTHER TISSUE (MUSCLE)
ADRENALS	3.1E-03	1.1E-07	2.7E-06	1.0E-06	9.1E-07	3.6E-07	1.1E-05	4.5E-06	2.7E-06	1.4E-06
BLADDER WALL	1.3E-07	1.6E-04	2.7E-07	2.2E-06	6.9E-06	2.6E-06	2.8E-07	1.6E-07	3.6E-08	1.8E-06
BONE (TOTAL)	2.0E-06	9.2E-07	9.0E-07	1.3E-06	1.6E-06	1.8E-06	1.6E-06	1.1E-06	1.5E-06	9.8E-07
GI (STOM WALL)	2.9E-06	1.6E-07	1.3E-04	3.7E-06	3.8E-06	1.8E-06	3.6E-06	1.9E-06	1.8E-06	1.3E-06
GI (SI)	8.3E-07	3.0E-06	2.7E-06	7.8E-05	1.7E-05	9.4E-06	2.9E-06	1.6E-06	1.9E-07	1.5E-06
GI (ULI WALL)	9.3E-07	2.2E-06	3.5E-06	2.4E-05	1.3E-04	4.2E-06	2.9E-06	2.5E-06	2.2E-07	1.6E-06
GI (LLI WALL)	2.2E-07	7.6E-06	1.2E-06	7.3E-06	3.2E-06	1.9E-04	7.2E-07	2.2E-08	7.1E-08	1.7E-06
KIDNEYS	1.1E-05	2.6E-07	3.5E-06	3.2E-06	2.8E-06	8.6E-07	1.9E-04	3.9E-06	8.4E-07	1.3E-06
LIVER	4.9E-06	1.7E-07	2.0E-06	1.8E-06	2.6E-06	2.5E-07	3.9E-06	4.6E-05	2.5E-06	1.1E-06
LUNGS	2.4E-06	2.4E-08	1.7E-06	2.2E-07	2.6E-07	7.9E-08	8.5E-07	2.5E-06	5.2E-05	1.3E-06
MARROW (RED)	3.6E-06	2.2E-06	1.5E-06	4.3E-06	3.7E-06	5.1E-06	3.8E-06	1.6E-06	1.9E-06	2.0E-06
OTH TISS (MUSC)	1.4E-06	1.8E-06	1.4E-06	1.5E-06	1.7E-06	1.7E-06	1.3E-06	1.1E-06	1.3E-06	2.7E-06
OVARIES	6.1E-07	7.3E-06	5.0E-07	1.5E-06	1.2E-06	1.8E-05	1.1E-06	4.2E-07	9.4E-08	2.0E-06
PANCREAS	9.0E-06	2.3E-07	1.8E-05	2.1E-06	2.3E-06	7.4E-07	6.5E-06	4.2E-06	2.6E-06	1.8E-06
SKIN	5.1E-07	5.5E-07	4.4E-07	4.1E-07	1.1E-07	4.8E-07	5.3E-07	4.9E-07	5.3E-07	7.2E-07
SPLEEN	6.3E-06	6.6E-07	1.0E-05	1.5E-06	1.4E-06	8.0E-07	8.6E-06	9.2E-07	2.3E-06	1.4E-06
TESTES	3.2E-08	4.7E-06	5.1E-08	3.1E-08	2.7E-07	1.8E-06	8.8E-08	6.2E-08	7.9E-09	1.1E-06
THYROID	1.3E-07	2.1E-09	8.7E-08	1.5E-08	1.6E-08	5.4E-09	4.8E-08	1.5E-07	9.2E-07	1.3E-06
UTERUS (NONGRVD)	1.1E-06	1.6E-05	7.2E-07	4.6E-06	5.4E-06	7.1E-06	9.4E-07	3.9E-07	8.2E-08	2.3E-06
TOTAL BODY	2.2E-06	1.9E-06	1.9E-06	2.4E-06	2.6E-07	2.3E-06	2.2E-06	2.2E-06	2.0E-06	1.9E-06

SOURCE ORGANS

TARGET ORGANS	OVARIES	PANCREAS	R MARROW	SKELETON CORT BONE	TRA BONE	SKIN	SPLEEN	TESTES	THYROID	TOTAL BODY
ADRENALS	3.3E-07	9.1E-06	2.3E-06	1.1E-06	1.1E-06	6.8E-07	6.3E-06	3.2E-08	1.3E-07	2.3E-06
BLADDER WALL	7.2E-06	4.4E-07	9.2E-07	1.5E-07	5.1E-07	4.9E-07	1.2E-07	4.8E-06	2.1E-09	2.3E-06
BONE (TOTAL)	1.5E-06	1.5E-06	4.0E-06	1.25E-05	1.0E-05	9.9E-07	1.1E-06	9.2E-07	1.0E-06	2.5E-06
GI (STOM WALL)	8.1E-07	1.8E-05	9.2E-07	5.5E-07	5.5E-07	5.4E-07	1.0E-05	3.2E-08	4.5E-08	2.2E-06
GI (SI)	1.2E-05	1.8E-07	2.6E-06	7.3E-07	7.3E-07	4.5E-07	1.9E-06	3.6E-07	9.3E-09	2.5E-06
GI (ULI WALL)	1.1E-05	2.1E-06	2.1E-06	6.9E-07	1.0E-06	4.7E-07	1.4E-06	3.1E-07	1.1E-08	2.4E-06
GI (LLI WALL)	1.5E-05	5.7E-07	1.2E-06	1.0E-06	4.2E-07	4.8E-07	6.1E-07	2.7E-06	4.3E-09	2.3E-06
KIDNEYS	9.2E-07	6.6E-06	2.2E-06	8.2E-07	8.2E-07	5.7E-07	9.1E-06	4.0E-08	3.4E-08	2.2E-06
LIVER	5.4E-07	4.4E-06	1.6E-06	6.6E-07	6.6E-07	5.3E-07	9.8E-07	3.1E-08	9.3E-08	2.2E-06
LUNGS	6.0E-08	2.5E-06	1.2E-06	9.4E-07	9.4E-07	5.8E-07	2.3E-06	6.6E-09	9.4E-07	2.0E-05
MARROW (RED)	5.5E-06	2.8E-06	3.1E-06	4.1E-06	9.1E-06	9.5E-07	1.7E-06	7.3E-07	1.1E-06	2.9E-06
OTH TISS (MUSC)	2.0E-06	1.8E-06	1.2E-06	9.8E-07	7.2E-07	1.4E-05	1.4E-06	1.1E-06	1.3E-06	1.9E-06
OVARIES	4.2E-03	4.1E-07	2.3E-06	7.1E-07	7.1E-07	3.8E-07	4.0E-07	0.0	4.9E-09	2.4E-06
PANCREAS	5.0E-07	5.8E-04	1.7E-06	8.5E-07	8.5E-07	4.4E-07	1.9E-05	5.5E-08	7.2E-08	2.4E-06
SKIN	4.1E-07	4.0E-07	5.9E-07	6.5E-07	6.5E-07	1.6E-05	4.7E-07	1.4E-05	7.3E-07	1.3E-06
SPLEEN	4.9E-07	1.9E-05	2.2E-07	5.8E-07	5.8E-07	5.4E-07	3.3E-04	1.7E-08	1.1E-07	2.2E-06
TESTES	0.0	5.2E-08	4.5E-08	6.4E-07	6.4E-07	9.1E-07	4.8E-08	1.4E-03	5.0E-10	1.7E-06
THYROID	4.9E-09	6.8E-07	7.9E-06	7.9E-07	7.9E-07	6.9E-07	8.7E-08	5.0E-10	2.3E-03	1.5E-06
UTERUS (NONGRVD)	2.1E-05	5.3E-07	2.2E-06	5.7E-07	5.7E-07	4.0E-07	4.0E-07	5.0E-08	0.0	2.6E-06
TOTAL BODY	2.6E-06	2.6E-06	2.2E-06	2.0E-06	2.0E-06	1.3E-06	2.2E-06	1.9E-06	1.8E-06	2.0E-06

137

Table 6. S, MEAN DOSE PER UNIT CUMULATED ACTIVITY (rad/µCi·h)
TECHNETIUM-99m   5 YEAR OLD

TARGET ORGANS	SOURCE ORGANS					
	BLADDER CONTENTS	STOMACH CONTENTS	STOMACH WALL	SMALL INTESTINE	ULI CONTENTS	LLI CONTENTS
ADRENALS	7.02E-07*	6.04E-06	4.36E-06	2.87E-06	2.74E-06	5.77E-07
BLADDER WALL	1.19E-03	1.84E-06*	1.80E-06+	1.19E-05	9.58E-06	1.99E-05
GI(STOMACH WALL)	2.23E-06	4.89E-04	8.45E-04+	8.01E-06	9.74E-06*	4.92E-06
GI(ULI WALL)	1.00E-05	8.06E-06	9.63E-06	5.53E-05	5.38E-04	1.65E-05*
GI(LLI WALL)	2.23E-05	4.02E-06	3.51E-06	2.04E-05+	1.20E-05	5.40E-04
GI(SI + CONTENTS)	1.14E-05	7.85E-06	8.70E-06	3.19E-04+	5.60E-05	2.74E-05
HEART	3.86E-07	7.71E-06	8.27E-06	1.33E-06	1.33E-06	5.59E-07
KIDNEYS	1.39E-06	6.22E-06	6.44E-06	7.98E-06	6.30E-06	3.22E-06
LIVER	1.38E-06	8.65E-06	9.10E-06	5.32E-06	7.10E-06	1.60E-06
LUNGS	2.74E-07	4.02E-06	4.42E-06	7.98E-07	9.31E-07	3.88E-07
MARROW (RED)	5.69E-06	4.52E-06	4.55E-06	1.18E-05	9.39E-06	1.13E-05
OVARIES	1.73E-05	4.39E-06	2.71E-06	3.86E-05	3.64E-05	4.28E-05
PANCREAS	1.21E-06	2.64E-05	2.71E-05	4.87E-06	5.43E-06	2.38E-06
SALIVARY GLANDS	3.83E-08	2.61E-07	2.05E-07	1.67E-07	9.60E-08	3.96E-08
SKELETON	2.38E-06	2.33E-06	2.36E-06	3.72E-06	3.11E-06	3.88E-06
SKIN	1.32E-06	3.06E-06	3.06E-06	2.62E-06	2.66E-06	2.46E-06
SPLEEN	1.07E-06	1.79E-05	1.76E-05	4.12E-06	4.04E-06	2.50E-06
TESTES	1.69E-05	5.08E-07	8.01E-07	1.39E-06	2.69E-06	7.93E-06
THYMUS	4.02E-08	1.24E-06	1.34E-06	3.25E-07	2.85E-07	1.15E-07
THYROID	2.09E-08	6.06E-07	6.65E-07	--	1.08E-07	--
TOTAL TISSUE	5.03E-06	3.86E-06	6.30E-06	4.76E-06	4.52E-06	4.81E-06
UTERUS	3.40E-05+	2.60E-06+	2.74E-06+	5.11E-05+	2.59E-05+	2.32E-05+
TOTAL BODY	6.77E-06+	6.56E-06+	6.43E-06+	7.17E-06+	7.01E-06+	6.82E-06+

TARGET ORGANS	KIDNEYS	LIVER	LUNGS	RED MARROW	OVARIES	SALIVARY GLANDS
ADRENALS	2.21E-05	6.92E-06	6.17E-06	9.26E-06	2.383E-06	--
BLADDER WALL	1.68E-06	1.27E-06	4.23E-07	3.96E-06	2.58E-05	3.06E-08
GI(STOMACH WALL)	5.99E-06	9.34E-06	4.42E-06	2.69E-06	3.03E-06	2.20E-07
GI(ULI WALL)	6.60E-06	7.29E-06	1.03E-06	6.22E-06	4.81E-05	8.78E-08
GI(LLI WALL)	2.61E-06	1.19E-06	4.04E-07	7.08E-06	9.95E-06	6.17E-08
GI(SI + CONTENTS)	8.88E-06	5.88E-06	1.03E-06	8.09E-06	4.60E-05	4.36E-08
HEART	2.82E-06+	1.23E-05	1.77E-05	2.79E-06	7.77E-07	9.10E-07
KIDNEYS	4.48E-04+	6.46E-06+	2.21E-06	7.05E-06	4.34E-06	1.58E-07
LIVER	6.49E-06	1.12E-04+	5.75E-06+	2.87E-06	3.56E-06	2.93E-07
LUNGS	2.41E-06	6.20E-06	1.83E-04+	3.56E-06+	5.35E-07	1.88E-06
MARROW (RED)	1.04E-05	4.63E-06	5.16E-06	1.10E-04+	1.09E-05+	1.97E-06
OVARIES	4.07E-06	2.59E-06	5.56E-08	8.11E-06	2.05E-02+	--
PANCREAS	1.25E-05	1.56E-06	6.14E-06	3.83E-06	2.22E-06	1.71E-07
SALIVARY GLANDS	7.45E-08	2.18E-07	1.63E-06	1.43E-06	4.31E-08	2.24E-04
SKELETON	3.78E-06	2.58E-06	3.94E-06	7.47E-06	3.48E-06	6.01E-06
SKIN	1.39E-06	1.28E-06	2.93E-06	1.26E-06	1.14E-06	6.62E-06
SPLEEN	2.19E-05	4.68E-06	5.75E-06	4.07E-06	1.90E-06	2.58E-07
TESTES	1.23E-08	8.17E-07	--	6.14E-07	6.33E-06	--
THYMUS	6.94E-07	2.23E-06	1.06E-05	2.21E-06	2.57E-07	3.37E-06
THYROID	5.96E-08	2.28E-07	3.11E-06	9.63E-07		2.65E-05
TOTAL TISSUE	3.88E-06	3.35E-06	3.96E-06	3.40E-06	5.91E-06	2.58E-06
UTERUS	2.30E-06+	2.11E-06+	2.10E-07+	4.42E-06+	9.95E-05+	--
TOTAL BODY	6.24E-06+	6.43E-06+	5.92E-06+	5.65E-06+	7.25E-06+	5.25E-06+

Table 6. S, MEAN DOSE PER UNIT CUMULATED ACTIVITY (rad/μCi·hr)
TECHNETIUM-99m   5 YEAR OLD

TARGET ORGANS	SOURCE ORGANS				TOTAL ± BODY
	SKELETON	SPLEEN	TESTES	THYROID	
ADRENALS	5.53E-06	2.18E-05	1.54E-07	--	5.71E-06
BLADDER WALL	1.64E-06	1.10E-06	2.06E-05	--	4.96E-06
GI(STOMACH WALL)	1.38E-06	1.69E-05	5.85E-07	3.88E-07	4.03E-06
GI(ULI WALL)	1.95E-06	4.12E-06	1.92E-08	9.34E-08	5.12E-06
GI(LLI WALL)	2.09E-06	1.82E-06	1.29E-05	1.73E-08	5.31E-06
GI(SI + CONTENTS)	2.47E-06	4.55E-06	2.79E-06	9.63E-08	5.68E-06
HEART	2.55E-06	6.86E-06	9.84E-08	1.80E-06	5.39E-06
KIDNEYS	2.61E-06	2.19E-05	6.46E-07	1.78E-07	5.28E-06
LIVER	1.75E-06	4.76E-06	4.26E-07	4.39E-07	4.40E-06
LUNGS	2.63E-06	6.36E-06	6.30E-08	3.59E-06	5.79E-06
MARROW (RED)	9.10E-06	6.25E-06	2.82E-06	2.63E-06	1.20E-05
OVARIES	1.79E-06	1.93E-06	3.40E-06	--	2.95E-06
PANCREAS	2.74E-06	4.04E-05	3.14E-07	6.04E-07	4.80E-06
SALIVARY GLANDS	5.40E-06	1.57E-07		3.30E-05	4.25E-06
SKELETON	2.24E-05+	3.30E-06	2.20E-06	4.73E-06	1.01E-05
SKIN	1.52E-06	1.28E-06	2.03E-06	2.45E-06	3.46E-06
SPLEEN	2.28E-06	1.04E-03+	2.63E-07	3.35E-07	5.12E-06
TESTES	2.47E-06	1.40E-07	2.60E-02+	--	3.79E-06
THYMUS	1.95E-06	1.59E-06	3.86E-08	1.29E-05	4.16E-06
THYROID	2.79E-06	2.65E-07		8.45E-03+	4.32E-06
TOTAL TISSUE	2.69E-06	4.28E-06	3.54E-06	4.73E-06	4.91E-06
UTERUS	1.04E-06	3.14E-06	6.14E-06	--	5.76E-06
TOTAL BODY	5.41E-06+	6.53E-06+	5.49E-06+	6.24E-06+	5.55E-06

Table 7. S(embryo←r_h), ABSORBED DOSE PER UNIT CUMULATED ACTIVITY (rad/μCi·hr), FOR SEVERAL RADIONUCLIDES AND VARIOUS SOURCE ORGANS r_h WITH THE EMBRYO AS THE TARGET ORGAN.[19]

Source organs	Radionuclides					
	^{99m}Tc	^{111}In	^{113m}In	^{123}I	^{131}I	^{133}Xe
Adrenals	4.0E-07	1.4E-06	8.6E-07	4.9E-07	1.3E-06	7.0E-08
Bladder contents	1.9E-05	5.7E-05	3.2E-05	2.7E-07	4.9E-05	9.8E-06
Bone (total)	7.6E-07	2.3E-06	1.3E-06	9.0E-07	2.0E-06	2.1E-07
GI tract (stom.cont.)	9.7E-07	3.0E-06	1.8E-06	1.1E-06	2.8E-06	2.1E-07
GI tract (SI & cont.)	1.1E-05	3.1E-05	1.8E-05	1.4E-05	2.7E-05	4.8E-06
GI tract (ULI cont.)	6.1E-06	1.8E-05	9.9E-06	7.4E-06	1.5E-05	2.1E-06
GI tract (LLI cont.)	7.6E-06	2.2E-05	1.2E-05	9.2E-06	1.9E-05	2.7E-06
Kidneys	1.2E-06	3.6E-06	2.1E-06	1.4E-06	3.3E-06	2.5E-07
Liver	6.5E-07	2.1E-06	1.3E-06	7.7E-07	2.0E-06	1.3E-07
Lungs	8.4E-08	3.2E-07	2.4E-07	1.1E-07	3.6E-07	1.2E-08
Marrow (red)	2.3E-06	6.6E-06	3.7E-06	2.7E-06	5.8E-06	7.0E-07
Other tissue (muscle)	2.6E-06	8.0E-06	4.6E-06	3.8E-06	6.9E-06	1.3E-06
Ovaries	2.0E-05	5.8E-05	3.3E-05	2.7E-05	5.0E-05	9.9E-06
Pancreas	6.8E-07	2.2E-06	1.3E-06	8.0E-07	2.1E-06	1.3E-07
Salivary glands	4.5E-09	2.4E-08	2.5E-08	7.3E-09	3.9E-08	4.2E-10
Skin	7.0E-07	2.1E-06	1.2E-07	8.3E-07	1.9E-06	1.9E-07
Spleen	5.4E-07	1.8E-06	1.1E-06	6.5E-07	1.7E-06	1.0E-07
Thyroid	4.5E-09	2.4E-08	2.5E-08	7.3E-09	3.9E-08	4.2E-10
Total body	2.8E-06	8.2E-06	8.4E-06	4.1E-06	1.2E-05	5.3E-06

* The digits following the symbol E indicate the proper of 10 by which the initial number is to be multiplied, e.g., 4.0E-07 = 4.0 x 10^{-7}.

Table 8. RADIATION DOSES FROM RADIOPHARMACEUTICALS[20,21]

Radiopharmaceutical	Study	Age yr	testes	ovaries	Kidneys	Liver	Lungs	Marrow (red)	Spleen	Thyroid	Total Body	Other
^{67}Ga-citrate	tumor and abscess imaging	a	0.26		0.41	0.45		0.58	0.60		0.16	0.44-bone
		15	0.31						0.71		0.20	0.36(SI)[22]
		10	0.44						1.00		0.28	0.56(ULI)[22]
		5	0.60						1.60		0.38	0.90(LLI)[22]
		1	0.93						2.60		0.57	
		0	2.60						8.00		1.40	
^{75}Se-seleno methionine	pancreas, parathyroid	a	8.6	9.9	22.0[23]	25.0		9.7	16.0[23]	16.0[23]	8.0[23]	9-blood
		15				31.0						14-pancreas
		10				39.0						
		5				53.0						
		1				83.0						
		0				190.0						
^{99m}TcDPTA	brain imaging (static or dynamic)	a	0.020	0.027	0.040			0.0095			0.016	0.45-bladder wall
		15	0.024	0.032	0.051						0.021	
		10	0.110	0.049	0.068						0.029	
		5	0.122	0.068	0.100						0.043	
		1	0.132	0.110	0.150						0.062	
		0	0.170	0.330	0.390						0.170	
	renal imaging (dynamic)		(see above)									

Table 8. RADIATION DOSES FROM RADIOPHARMACEUTICALS[20,21]

Absorbed Dose (mrad per microcurie administered)

Radiopharma-ceutical	Study	Age yr	Gonads testes	Gonads ovaries	Kidneys	Liver	Lungs	Marrow (red)	Spleen	Thyroid	Total Body	Other
99mTc-gluco-heptonate	renal imaging		0.004	0.007	0.30			0.012			0.01	
	brain imaging		(see above)									
99mTc-human serum albumin	cardio-vascular imaging	a	.015	0.013				0.02			0.015	0.05-blood
		15	.018								0.018	0.06
		10	.026								0.026	0.094
		5	.040								0.040	0.150
		1	.061								0.061	0.240
		0	.180								0.180	0.810
												0.033-blad-der
99mTc-HIDA	hepato-biliary imaging	a	0.025	0.05		0.09		0.02				0.55(ULI)
99mTc-macro-aggregates, microspheres	lung perfusion imaging	a	0.007	0.009	0.16	0.017	0.20	0.015	0.017	0.008	0.015	0.38-blad-der
		15	0.017	0.010			0.25				0.019	
		10	0.038	0.016			0.35				0.028	
		5	0.043	0.022			0.59				0.042	
		1	0.046	0.038			1.00				0.064	
		0	0.060	0.110			3.10				0.180	

Table 8. RADIATION DOSES FROM RADIOPHARMACEUTICALS[20,21]

Radiopharma-ceutical	Study	Age yr	Gonads testes	Gonads ovaries	Kidneys	Liver	Lungs	Marrow (red)	Spleen	Thyroid	Total Body	Other
^{99m}Tc-pertechnetate	brain imaging (static & dynamic)	a	0.012	0.017		0.015		0.022			0.013	0.053–bladder (resting) 0.085–bladder (active) 0.013–brain 0.25(ST) 0.21(ULI) 0.20(LLI) 0.23(LLI) 0.33 0.46 0.67 1.90
		15	0.014	0.022						0.35	0.016	
		10	0.066	0.032						0.48	0.024	
		5	0.073	0.045						0.77	0.037	
		1	0.079	0.076						1.30	0.055	
		0	1.100	0.220						3.40	0.150	
	thyroid imaging									(see above)		

Table 8. RADIATION DOSES FROM RADIOPHARMACEUTICALS[20,21]

Radiopharmaceutical	Study	Age yr	Gonads testes	Gonads ovaries	Kidneys	Liver	Lungs	Marrow (red)	Spleen	Thyroid	Total Body	Other
99mTc-polyphosphate,pyrophosphate, methylene diphosphnate	bone imaging	a	0.034	0.046	0.030	0.010		0.035			0.013	0.050-bone
		15	0.041	0.055							0.015	0.060
		10	0.190	0.083							0.025	0.089
		5	0.210	0.120							0.040	0.140
		1	0.230	0.190							0.057	0.200
		0	0.290	0.560							0.150	0.640
												0.13-bladder(2 hr)
												0.34-bladder(8 hr)
99mTc-red cells	cardiovascular imaging	a							1.3		0.015	
		15							1.6			
		10							2.3			
		5							3.5			
		1							6.0			
		0							20.0			
99mTc-sulfur colloid	liver, spleen bone marrow imaging	a	0.019	0.023		0.34-n*		0.027-n*	0.21-n*		0.019	
						0.21-e,i		0.045-e,i	0.28-e,i		0.018	
						0.16-i,d		0.079-i,d	0.42-i,d		0.016	
		15	0.023	0.028		0.40			0.40		0.020	
		10	0.100	0.041		0.56			0.60		0.027	
		5	0.120	0.058		0.92			0.80		0.038	
		1	0.130	0.097		1.30			1.20		0.056	
		0	0.160	0.280		4.30			3.70		0.140	

* - n is normal liver; e, i is early to intermediate diffuse parenchymal disease; i, d is intermediate to advanced diffuse parenchymal disease.

Table 8. RADIATION DOSES FROM RADIOPHARMACEUTICALS[20,21]

Radiopharma-ceutical	Study	Age yr	Gonads testes	Gonads ovaries	Kidneys	Liver	Lungs	Marrow (red)	Spleen	Thyroid	Total Body	Other
^{111}In-DTPA	cerebro-spinal fluid imaging, cisterno-gram	a	0.06	0.07	0.6(surface)			0.10			0.10	14-brain (surface)
		15	0.08	0.09							0.12	15
		10	0.13	0.14							0.20	16
		5	0.22	0.25							0.32	17
		1	0.34	0.38							0.52	20
		0	1.10	1.30							1.80	47
												12-spinal cord (normal)
												20-spinal cord (hydro-cephalus)
^{123}I-iodine	thyroid imaging	a	0.025	0.034		0.030		0.044		2.4(5%)	0.030	0.23(ST)
			0.021	0.029				0.040		7.5(15%)		
			0.017	0.024				0.035		13.0(25%)		
		15		0.035						21.0	0.045	
		10		0.051						30.0	0.051	
		5		0.120						51.0	0.079	
		0		0.350						110.0	0.130	
										160.0	0.350	
		a	0.025							55.0 (administered 24 hr after production)		3.0 bladder wall

Table 8. RADIATION DOSES FROM RADIOPHARMACEUTICALS[20,21]

Radiopharmaceutical	Study	Age yr	Gonads testes	Gonads ovaries	Kidneys	Liver	Lungs	Marrow (red)	Spleen	Thyroid	Total Body	Other
^{131}I-iodide	thyroid uptake	a	0.028	0.25		0.20		0.31		260(5%)	0.21	
						0.35		0.41		800(15%)	0.34	
						0.48		0.68		1300(25%)	0.45	
		15	0.53	0.53						2500	0.53	
		10	0.81	0.81						3000	0.81	
		5	1.3	1.3						5200	1.3	
		1	2.0	2.0						11000	2.0	
		0	10.0	10.0						16000	10.0	
^{131}I-iodohippurate	renal imaging	a	0.3	0.3	1.0			0.0094		48	0.30	12.0-bladder wall
		15	0.4	0.4	1.2						0.40	
		10	0.56	0.56	2.2						0.56	
		5	0.77	0.77	3.1						0.77	
		1	1.1	1.1	4.4						1.10	
		0	2.4	2.4	9.5						2.40	
^{133}Xe-gas	regional brain perfusion imaging	a			0.0062							0.017-brain
	lung ventilation imaging-administered activity	a	0.26	0.26			6.0				0.001	0.26-blood 52.2-mucosa single breath (1 mCi/ℓ)
	concentration (mc/ℓ) in inspired gas		3.7	3.7			39.0					3.7-blood 642.0-mucosa rebreath 3 min closed system (1 mCi/ℓ)

Table 8. RADIATION DOSES FROM RADIOPHARMACEUTICALS[20,21]

Radiopharma-ceutical	Study	Age yr	Gonads testes	Gonads ovaries	Kidneys	Liver	Lungs	Marrow (red)	Spleen	Thyroid	Total Body	Other
^{169}Yb-DTPA	cerebro-spinal fluid imaging	a									0.2	3.2-brain
		15										3.4
		10										3.7
		5										3.9
		1										4.6
		0										10.8
												0.78-bladder
												15.0-spinal cord (normal)
												25.0-spinal cord (hydro-cephalus)
^{201}Tl-chloride	myocardial imaging	a	0.30	0.39							0.5	0.17-heart

Table 9. DOSE ESTIMATED TO EMBRYO FROM RADIOPHARMACEUTICALS[a]

Radiopharmaceutical	Embryo Dose (rad/mCi administered)
^{99m}Tc-human serum albumin	0.018*
^{99m}Tc-lungaggregate	0.035*
^{99m}Tc-polyphosphate	0.036*
^{99m}Tc-sodium pertechnetate	0.037
^{99m}Tc-stannous glucoheptonate	0.040*
^{99m}Tc-sulfur colloid	0.032*
^{123}I-sodium iodide (15% uptake)	0.032
^{131}I-sodium iodide (15% uptake)	0.100
^{123}I-rose bengal	0.130
^{131}I-rose bengal	0.680

a-adapted from Smith and Warner.[19]

*-these values were calculated using cumulated activity ($\tilde{A}$) values from company product data and absorbed dose per cumulated activity (S) values from reference.[16]

Table 10. THYROIDAL RADIOIODINE EXPOSURE OF THE FETUS[24]

Gestation Period	Fetal/Maternal Ratio (thyroid gland)	Dose to Thyroid (Fetus) rad/µCi*
10-12 weeks	--	.001 (precursors)
12-13 weeks	1.2	0.7
2nd trimester	1.8	6.0
3rd trimester	7.5	--
birth imminent	--	8.0

* rad/µCi of ^{131}I ingested by mother

measurements over approximately 24 hours. As indicated previously, pediatric S factors (for specific source organ-target organ configurations) were developed by the Health Physics Division, Oak Ridge National Laboratory.[17,18]

The mean dose to specific organs was then calculated according to the basic MIRD schema and are given in Tables 11-12.

For a series of children aged 2 to 18 years undergoing ^{99m}Tc-sulfur colloid scans the absorbed radiation dose, adjusted to 70 µCi/kg administered activity, ranged from 0.59 - 1.17 rad (mean 0.78 rad) for the liver and from 0.78 - 3.34 rad (mean 1.69 rad) for the spleen. Thus the spleen would appear to be the critical organ for pediatric patients undergoing ^{99m}Tc-SC scans.

For five children aged 4 - 16 years, undergoing bone scans, doses to the metaphyseal growth plate were 1.6 to 4.7 rads (mean 2.5 rads) when adjusted for an administered activity of ^{99}Tc-EHDP of 200 µCi/kg. This dose range compares to approximately 0.6 rad to the adult skeleton for a corresponding study.

In recent data involving the administration of ^{67}Ga-citrate for tumor and/or abscess studies in 9 children aged 1.8 to 17.5 years, the absorbed radiation dose to the liver, spleen and metaphyseal growth complex is 0.29 - 5.41 rad (mean 3.16 rad), 0.50 - 9.45 rad (mean 4.95 rad) and 6.0 - 21.7 rad (mean 9.1 rad), respectively, for an adjusted administered activity of 50 µCi/kg.[27] The importance of specific pediatric measurements is evident here because of the high degree of nonspecificity of this radiopharmaceutical.

Table 11. ^{99m}Tc SULFUR COLLOID

DOSIMETRY RESULTS

Patient Age/yr.	Liver		Spleen	
	$\frac{rad}{mCi}$	70 $\frac{rad}{\mu Ci/kg}$	$\frac{rad}{mCi}$	70 $\frac{rad}{\mu Ci/kg}$
2.2	0.54	0.72	1.34	1.79
2.6	0.63	0.59	1.56	1.48
5.5	0.56	0.69	0.63	0.78
10.1	0.40	0.68	1.96	3.34
10.6	0.36	1.17	--	--
10.8	0.40	0.83	0.51	1.05

adapted from:
Thomas S.R., Purdom, R.C., Kereiakes, J.G., et al.[25]

Table 12. DOSE TO THE METAPHYSES FROM ^{99m}Tc-EHDP BONE SCANS[26]

	Dose (rads) Adjusted to 200 µCi/kg Administered Activity	
	Plate Thickness	
	3 mm	4 mm
Patient 1, a 4-year-old boy; administered activity 2.66 mCi; weight 15.4 kg		
Right distal femur	2.7	2.1
Right proximal tibia	2.1	1.6
Left distal femur	2.8	2.1
Left proximal tibia	2.4	1.9
Patient 2, a 6-year-old boy; administered activity 4.47 mCi; weight 20.4 kg		
Right distal femur	2.4	1.8
Right proximal tibia	2.1	1.6
Left distal femur	2.3	1.7
Left proximal tibia	1.9	1.5
Patient 3, a 6-5-year-old boy administered activity 6.33 mCi; weight 25.9 kg		
Right distal femur	4.7	3.7
Right proximal tibia	4.7	3.7
Left distal femur	4.5	3.4
Left proximal tibia	4.5	3.4
Patient 4, an 11-year-old boy; administered activity 6.86 mCi; weight 29.5 kg		
Right distal femur	2.1	1.5
Right proximal tibia	1.9	1.5
Left distal femur	2.2	1.6
Left Proximal tibia	2.2	1.6
Patient 5, a 13-year-old boy; administered activity 10.96 mCi; weight 36.0 kg		
Right distal femur	2.2	2.2
Right proximal tibia	2.8	2.1
Left distal femur	2.8	2.1
Left proximal tibia	2.5	1.9

REFERENCES

1. Loevinger, R. and Berman, M. A Schema for Absorbed-Dose Calculations in Biologically Distributed Radionuclides. MIRD Pamphlet No. 1, J. Nucl. Med. 9, Suppl. No. 1, 7-14 (1968)
2. Loevinger, R., and Berman, M. A Revised Scheme for Calculating the Absorbed Dose from Biologically Distributed Radionuclides. MIRD Pamphlet No. 1, Soc. of Nucl. Med., New York, March (1976).
3. Budinger, T.F. Progress in Atomic Medicine: Recent Advances in Nuclear Medicine. Edited by J.H. Lawrence. (Grune and Stratton, N.Y., 1974), 4, 41.
4. Sorenson, J.A. Quantitative Measurement of Radioactivity in Vivo by Whole Body Counting in Instrumentation in Nuclear Medicine, edited by G. Hine and J. Sorenson (Academic Press, N.Y., 1974).
5. Thomas, S.R., Maxon, H.R. and Kereiakes, J.G. In Vivo Quantitation of Lesion Radioactivity Using External Counting Methods. Med. Phys., 3, 252-255 (1976)
6. Kereiakes, J.G. and Feller, P. In Vivo Dosimetry of Beta and Gamma-Emitting Radiopharmaceuticals. Handbook of Medical Physics, edited by R. Waggener, R. Shalek, and J.G. Kereiakes. (CRC Press, West Palm Beach, Fla., to be published 1980).
7. Snyder, W.S., Ford, M.R. and Warner, G.G. et al. Estimates of Absorbed Fraction for Monoenergetic Photon Sources Uniformly Distributed in Various Organs of Heterogeneous Phantoms. MIRD Pamphlet No. 5. J. Nucl. Med., 10, Suppl. No. 3, 5-12, (1969).
8. Dillman, L.T. Radionuclide Decay Schemes and Nuclear Parameters for Use in Radiation-Dose Estimation. MIRD Suppl. No. 4, Pamphlet No. 6, Soc. of Nucl. Med., New York, March (1970).
9. Dillman, L.T. and Von der Lage, F.C. Radionuclide Decay Schemes and Nuclear Parameters for Use in Radiation Dose Estimation. MIRD Pamphlet No. 10, Soc. of Nucl. Med., New York, (1975).
10. Kereiakes, J.G., Seltzer, R., Blackburn, B. and Saenger, E.L. Radionuclide Doses to Infants and Children: A Plea for a Standard Child. Health Phys. 11, 999 (1965).
11. Poston, J. The Effects of Body and Organ Size on Absorbed Dose: There is No Standard Patient. Radiopharmaceutical Dosimetry Symposium, Oak Ridge, Tennessee, HEW Publication (FDWA) 76-8044, June (1976).
12. Wellman, H., Kereiakes, J.G. and Branson, B. Total and Partial Body Counting of Children for Radiopharmaceutical Dosimetry Data. In Medical Radionuclides: Irradiation Dose and Effects. USAEC Symposium, Series 20, Division of Technical Information (1970).
13. Brownell, G., Ellett, W. and Reddy, A. Absorbed Fractions for Photon Dosimetry. MIRD Suppl. No. 1., Pamphlet No. 3, Soc. of Nucl. Med., New York, February (1968).

14. Ellett, W. and Humes, R. Absorbed Fractions for Small Volumes Containing Photon-Emitting Radioactivity. MIRD Suppl. No. 5, Pamphlet No. 8, Soc. of Nucl. Med, New York, March (1971).
15. Snyder, W.S., Ford, M.R., Warner, G.G. and Watson, S.B. A Tabulation of Dose Equivalent per Microcurie-day for Source and Target Organs of an Adult for Various Radionuclides. ORNL-5000, Oak Ridge National Laboratory, Oak Ridge, Tennessee, November (1974).
16. Snyder, W.S., Ford, M.R., Warner, G.G. and Watson, S.B. "S", Absorbed Dose per Cumulated Activity for Selected Radionuclides and Organs. MIRD Pamphlet No. 11, Soc. of Nucl. Med., New York, (1975).
17. Warner, G.G., Poston, J.W. Health Physics Division, Oak Ridge National Laboratory, Oak Ridge, Tennessee (1978).
18. Kereiakes, J.G. Contribution in "Radiation Protection in Nuclear Medicine and Ultrasound Applied to Children",(draft) NCRP SC-51 B, Washington, D.C.
19. Smith, E.M. and Warner, G.G. Estimates of Radiation Dose to the Embyro from Nucl. Med. Proced. J. Nucl. Med., 17, 836-839 (1976).
20. Kereiakes, J.G., Feller, P.A., Ascoli, F.A., Thomas, S.R., Gelfand, M.J. and Saenger, E.L. Pediatric Radiopharmaceutical Dosimetry Symposium, HEW Publication (FDA) 76-8044, Bureau of Radiological Health, FDA, Rockville, MD, June (1976).
21. Roedler, H.D., Kaul, A., and Hine, G.J. Internal Radiation Dose in Diagnostic Nuclear Medicine. Verlage H. Hoffman, Berlin, (1978).
22. Product Data. Gallium Citrate Ga-67. New England Nuclear, North Billerica, Mass. (1976).
23. Product Data. Selenomethionine Se-75 Injection Code SC.10P. Amersham (Searle), Arlington Heights, IL, (1975).
24. Book, S. and Goldman, M. Thyroidal Radioiodine Exposure of the Fetus. Health Phys., 29, 874 (1975).
25. Thomas, S.R., Purdom, R.C. and Kereiakes, J.G. Dose to Liver and Spleen in Pediatric Patients Undergoing Technetium-99m Sulfur Colloid Scans. Radiol. 133, 465-467 (1979).
26. Thomas, S.R., Gelfand, M.J. and J.G. Kereiakes. Dose to the Metaphyseal Growth Complexes in Children Undergoing ^{99m}Tc-EHDP Bone Scans. Radiol. 126, 193-195 (1978).
27. Thomas, S.R., Gelfand, M.J., Kereiakes, J.G. Burns, G.S.. Purdom, R.C. and H.R. Maxon. Dosimetry Considerations for the Liver, Spleen, and Metaphyseal Growth Complexes in Children Undergoing Gallium-67 Citrate Scanning Procedures. Presented at Soc. of Nucl. Med., Atlanta, GA, June 26-29 (1979).

DOSE EVALUATION IN RADIATION THERAPY

Robert J. Shalek
The University of Texas System Cancer Center
M. D. Anderson Hospital and Tumor Institute
Houston, Texas

INTRODUCTION

In radiation treatment of cancer the question of risk is somewhat different than in radiation protection, diagnostic radiology or nuclear medicine. A patient who has a life threatening disease is willing to take greater risks to regain health than one who has a minor illness or who is exposed to radiation in the course of his employment. A further consideration is the age of the patients. About 93% of cancer patients are 40 years of age or older at the time of diagnosis (1). Thus for the older patients pregnancy at the time of treatment is rare and there is small concern for genetic damage from the radiation treatment. Nonetheless, pregnant patients do appear for radiation treatment and the discussion by Brent in this monograph applies to fetuses irradiated in therapy as well as in diagnosis. Also, there are a growing number of children treated for cancer who survive to adulthood and childbearing. For these young patients concern for the genetic burden which they might transmit is much greater than that resulting from diagnostic radiology or nuclear medicine since the radiation doses are larger and the radiation effects may have been enhanced by adjuvant chemotherapy.

Of more direct concern in radiation treatment are the collateral risks to healthy tissue and organs which are unavoidably irradiated in treatment. Therapeutic doses are measured in terms of thousands of rads and radiation inactivation of an organ function in the short term is a real possibility. Radiation therapists are very concerned about adverse clinical reactions, particularly those occurring within the first 2 or 3 years.

Combined radiation and chemotherapy is becoming increasingly popular. This therapy brings with it new uncertainties in the radiation dose which will be tolerated by normal tissues. Different drugs and different treatment protocols have different effects upon the enhancement of radiation damage in the tumor and in surrounding normal tissue. Thus the hard-won understanding of the clinical boundaries established by the tolerance of normal tissue must be reassessed in very complex circumstances. The adverse effects of radiation and drugs upon normal tissue may not appear until months or years after treatment; so the establishment of tolerable radiadoses will be slow. Necessarily the amount of drugs and radiation will be conservative until the limitations are understood.

ORGAN DAMAGE

A general listing of radiation tolerance for various organs has been given by Rubin and Casarett (2); some of the radiation tolerance doses are contained in Table I. Under the headings 5% and 50% are listed doses which if administered to the organ in question under a standard set of treatment conditions would result in no more than a 5% severe complication rate at 5 years after treatment or in 50% for the higher doses. The standard treatment conditions require photon beams of 1-6 MeV, five 200-rad fractions per week, with the treatment completed in 2-8 weeks depending upon total dose.

TABLE I

Radiation tolerance doses-rad. (Abstracted from Rubin and Casarett (2)

Organ	Injury at 5 years	5%	50%	Volume or lengths
Colon	Ulcer, stricture	4,500	6,500	100cm^3
Rectum	Ulcer, stricture	5,500	8,000	100cm^3
Liver	Liver failure, ascites	3,500	4,500	whole
Kidney	Nephrosclerosis	2,300	2,800	whole
Testes	Permanent sterilization	500-1,500	2,000	whole
Ovary	Permanent sterilization	200-300	625-1,200	whole
Lung	Pneumonities, fibrosis	4,000	6,000	lobe
Heart	Pericarditis, pancardities	4,000	<10,000	whole
Bone, child	Arrested growth	2,000	3,000	10cm^3
CNS (brain)	Necrosis	5,000	6,000	whole
Spinal cord	Necrosis, transection	5,000	<6,000	5cm^3
Eye	Panophthalmitis, hemorrhage	5,500	10,000	whole
Lens	Cataract	500	1,200	whole
Fetus	Death	200	450	

The radiation tolerance of healthy tissues may be reduced because of previous radiation treatment or the administration of chemotherapeutic drugs. The reirradiation of previously irradiated volumes is seldom attempted, but when it is, there are no clear guidelines. When combined with chemical treatment the doses of radiation well tolerated alone may be excessive in combination (3). Reductions of radiation dose by 10 to 80% may be indicated (4).

Judging by the number of publications, organ damage as a result of radiation therapy appears to be receiving increased attention. Perhaps increasing effectiveness of therapy allows longer survival time for the development of complications or perhaps the readiness of patients to seek legal remedies for perceived over treatment has sharpened interest. Some recent publications are noted for bowel (5), kidney (6), lung (7), heart (8), brain (9), eye (10) (11).

Permanent radiation myelitis resulting in paralysis or death is a rare, but potentially serious complication from therapy. Gradations of neuropathy are observed and the progression of disability from numbness to paralysis can sometimes be arrested with steroid or hyperbaric oxygen treatment. Phillips and Buske (12) reported an incidence of 1% of severe complications amongst 350 patients treated with thoracic irradiation or about 8% of long term survivors. Wara et al (13) recommend that the dose to the spinal cord be limited to 2,000 rads in 5 fractions, 3,000 rads in 10 fractions, 4,000 rads in 15 fractions and 5,000 rads in 25 fractions in agreement with the value given in Table I for a 5% complication rate. Abbatucci et al (14) agree on a limit of 5,000 rad in 25 fractions when 3 to 5 cervical vertebrae are irradiated.

However, myelitis induced by a lesser amount of radiation when the patients were treated concurrently with actinomycin-D has been reported (15). A dose of 4,000 rads, 20% less than the dose listed in Table I for 5% complications, delivered to the spinal axis at 200 rads per fraction, 5 days a week, together with actinomycin-D treatment was sufficient to cause impairment of the ability to walk, and bladder and bowel incontinence.

GROWTH IMPAIRMENT

A reduction of bone, muscle and gland development may follow radiation therapy to or near the affected part in childhood (16). One study of 81 patients with Wilms' tumor treated with irradiation and chemotherapy showed 70% of the children developed axial deformities (17). These changes resulted from impairment of epiphyseal enchondial growth of the irradiated vertebral bodies. Growth retardation especially for children of about 2 years of age receiving cranial or cranial and spinal irradiation has been reported (18).

CANCER INDUCTION

Success in the treatment of childhood cancers by radiation or radiation and chemotherapy has permitted long term survivors, some of whom have developed second malignant neoplasms attributable to the treatment. Li (19) has reported that from the study of 410 survivors of childhood cancers, the incidence of new cancers amongst those previously treated was 20-fold higher than for the general population. Of a group of 102 children with second malignant neoplasms, 65% were attributable to radiation and 25% to genetic causes (20).

GENETIC RISKS

Genetic deficiencies induced by radiation or radiation-chemical treatment are very difficult to assess. Only damage appearing in the first generation can be assessed at present, and this represents a small part of the potential damage. With that acknowledged limitation, the reports indicated that no serious genetic damage from therapy has been passed to progeny by survivors of childhood cancer, although inherited tendencies to the incidence of cancers such as retinoblastoma, neuroblastoma and Wilms' tumor are transmitted (21). Likewise abnormal offspring were not observed from 93 pregnancies resulting from male or female parents previously treated by radiation for Hodgkin's disease (22). These findings are buttressed by the failure to demonstrate inherited damage due to radiation in over 70,000 Japanese children conceived after their parents had been exposed to atomic bombs (23). An extended discussion of the genetic effects of low level irradiation by Selby appears in these proceedings.

EVALUATION OF DOSE

The physical evaluation of dose in radiation therapy is done on a reasonably consistent basis in different institutions. The Radiological Physics Center reviews radiation measurements and dose calculations at institutions participating in interinstitutional clinical trials. It was found that about 88% of the institutions reviewed deliver the radiation dose intended within $\pm 5\%$ (24, 25, 26). In a time when radiation therapists are uncertain of the tolerable radiation doses in combined radiation-chemical therapy, it is important that reports of clinical findings in the literature be based upon clear and reproducible dose standards. Table II shows findings reported by the Radiological Physics Center and Tables III and IV indicate the types of problems found at participating institutions. A further discussion of the kinds of discrepancies found and inferences for quality assurance are found in a later paper in this conference by the same author.

TABLE II. Summary of activities, February 1976

Number of institutions visited	174
Number of machines reviewed	352
% calibration within $\pm 3\%$	78%
	(275/352)
Number of machines x protocols reviewed	768
% tumor dose within $\pm 5\%$	88%
	(678/768)

Table III. Measurement errors.

Error	Number	Max. error
Chamber correction factor	47	12%
Timer error	38	9%
Field size dependence	34	7%
Source movement mechanism	4	16%
Anomalous source decay	3	6%
Distance indicator	4	5%
Light and radiation field coincidence	58	15mm
Symmetry of beam	33	20%

Table IV. Calculative errors.

Error	Number	Max. error
Attenuation factor	94	1.5%
f-factor or C_λ	43	6%
Tray factor	39	14%
Off-axis correction, irregular fields	37	13%
Wrong % depth dose	49	20%
Backscatter factor	63	7%
Rad (muscle)/rad (H_2O)	134	1%

CONCLUSION

An indication has been given of the changing and slippery ground upon which the radiation therapist stands as the number of radiation treatments in combination with chemotherapy increases and the awareness of radiation effects such as second malignant neoplasms, impairment of development, fetal damage and genetic changes become more clear. The pressure upon the physicist for increased precision in the control and knowledge of the radiation dose delivered in therapy not only to the tumor but elsewhere in the patient may be supported in clinical findings.

Supported in part by grant CA-10953 awarded by the National Cancer Institute.

REFERENCES

1. S. J. Cutler and J. L. Young, ed, Third National Cancer Survey: Incidence Data (DHEW Publication, NIH, 1975) p. 100.

REFERENCES (Continued)

2. P. Rubin and G. Casarett, San Francisco Center Sumposium, 6th 1970, Radiation Effect and Tolerance, Normal Tissue; Basic Concepts in Radiation Pathology. Proceedings: Editor J. M. Vaeth (S. Karger AG, 1972), p. 1.
3. C. E. Danjoux, Int. J. Radiat. Oncol. Biol. Phys. 5, 441 (1979).
4. T. L. Phillips and K. K. Fu, Cancer 37 (supp 2), 1186 (1976).
5. R. Patwardan and L. L. Doss, Mo. Med. 75, 616 (1978).
6. B. T. Steele and D. S. Lueman, Clin. Nephrol. 11, 272 (1979).
7. G. A. DoPico, A. L. Wiley, Jr., P. Rao and H. A. Dickie, Chest. 75, 688 (1979).
8. J. S. Schneider and J. E. Edwards, Chest 75, 560 (1979).
9. N. D. Lorenzo, A. Nolletti and L. Palma, Surg. Neurol. 10, 281 (1978).
10. W. M. Wara, A. R. Irvine, R. E. Neger, E. L. Howes, Jr. and T. L. Phillips, Int. J. Radiat. Oncol. Biol. Phys. 5, 81 (1979).
11. K. Morita and Y. Kawabe, Radiology 130, 227 (1979).
12. T. L. Phillips and F. Buschke, Am. J. Roentgenol. 105, 659 (1969)
13. W. M. Wara, T. L. Phillips, G. E. Sheline and J. G. Schwade, Cancer 35, 1558 (1975).
14. J. S. Abbatucci, T. Delozier, R. Quint, A. Roussel and D. Bume, Int. J. Radiat. Oncol. Biol. Phys. 4, 239 (1978).
15. P. Littman, J. G. Rosenstock and C. Bailey, Med. Ped. Oncol. 5, 145 (1978).
16. W. B. Dawson, Clin. Radiol. 19, 241 (1968).
17. E. J. Riseborough, Clin. Orth. 128, 101 (1977).
18. S. M. Shalet, C. G. Beardwell, B. M. Aarons, D. Pearson and P. H. Jones, Arch. Dis. Child 53, 491 (1978).
19. F. P. Li, Cancer 40, Suppl, 1899 (1977).
20. A. T. Meadows, G. J. D'Angio, V. Mike, A. Banfi, H. Curtis, R. D. T. Jenkin and A. Schwartz, Cancer 40, 1903 (1977).
21. F. P. Li and N. Jaffee, Lancet 2, 707, Sept. 21, 1974.
22. G. E. Holmes and F. F. Holmes, Cancer 41, 1317 (1978).
23. R. W. Miller, Pediatrics, 41, 257 (1968).
24. R. Golden, J. Cundiff, W. Grant, III and R. Shalek, Cancer 29, 1458 (1972).
25. W. Grant III, Med Phys. 1 (1), 41 (1974).
26. R. J. Shalek, P. Kennedy, M. Stovall, J. H. Cundiff, W. F. Gagnon, W. Grant, III and W. F. Hanson, National Bureau of Standards 75th Anniversary Symposium Proceedings, Page 111 (1976).

RISK/BENEFIT CONSIDERATIONS IN RADIOLOGY

E. C. Gregg
Case Western Reserve University, Cleveland, OH 44106

ABSTRACT

Consideration will be given of the basic radiobiologic effects of ionizing radiations in estimating risks and benefits resulting from the medical uses of such radiations. Even though "worst case" conditions are assumed, such as a linear non-threshold dose-effect relationship, the genetic and somatic risks for the doses usually encountered in medicine appear quite minimal relative to other environmental agents. Data will be presented and analyzed regarding the impact of these considerations on the individual, society, occupationally engaged personnel and accelerator design.

CELL STERILIZATION

When ionizing radiation is incident upon human cells, the most probable events are division delay and death of the cells.[1] For very large amounts of radiation - say many thousands of rads of absorbed dose - death is prompt with the cytoplasm becoming "sticky" resulting in the cessation of most cellular activity. For exposures of hundreds of rads and less, most of the cells will continue to function normally in producing key enzymes and proteins until the time of division but be unable to complete division. Some cells may divide and the daughters fail to divide while the nuclei of others may divide but the outer cell wall remain intact. In many cases, a multi-nucleated cell can be produced which ultimately dies and lyses away. These processes may be considered a genetic death or cell sterilization which does not become obvious until the cell attempts division. Thus rapidly dividing cells such as those in the lining of the gut, the marrow and the sperm will show the effects quite early while others may not show damage until challenged to divide as in the skin when cut. The time delay may be as short as 10 hours in the marrow or as long as years in the case of nerve cells. Irradiation of rapidly dividing cells in both culture and *in vivo* has shown that the dose-survival curve is generally logarithmic with the possible exception of a shoulder at low doses and that about 150 rads are required to sterilize half of the original number of cells (LD_{50}). This dose may be translated into a probability of killing four cells out of one thousand cells with one rad of absorbed dose. Conversely, if one million cells receive one rad of radiation, about 4000 cells will be sterilized. However, if the cells have a 10 hour doubling time, the remaining 996,000 cells will produce the missing cells in about 3 minutes. Albeit a rough calculation, such considerations coupled with the enormous number of cells dying in the body from natural causes would indicate that cell sterilization from one rad is quite negligible.

One possible exception to this is the production of cataracts in which the dead cells are retained and accumulated in the eyes over many years. Many hundreds of roentgens are usually required with an average latent period of 8 years to produce a visible opacity in the lens. Likewise, whole organs can also be affected by cell sterilization but may ultimately recover through replacement. For example, it has been demonstrated that radiation doses of 400 to 500 rads to human gonads will not necessarily induce permanent sterility but rather temporary infertility followed by a return of fertility. Contrarywise, the tissues in the developing embryo and fetus are quite sensitive in that exposures on the order of 10 rads may produce a child with some form of abnormal organ development in perhaps 5% of the live births. Obviously, there is a limited supply of cells available, each with key information and the killing of a few critical cells at a particular time or the production of transformed cells affects the further development of the child. The organs that are affected the most are those under development at the time of exposure.[2]

It is to be noted in passing that cell sterilization is also a risk in radiation therapy during which as much as 5000 photon rads may be delivered to a tumor. One type of risk is the possibility that not all the tumor cells will have been sterilized. Conversely, another risk is the possibility that too many of the wrong (normal) tissues have been destroyed leading to seriously debilitating sequellae. The patient and his advocate must take all such possibilities into account before deciding on the type of treatment. In most cases, the benefit is a known quantity, namely, tumor cure.

CHROMOSOME ABERRATIONS

When cells are irradiated, "breaks" may subsequently be observed in the chromosomes. Although no direct evidence is available, many investigators feel that such gross chromosome aberrations are directly related to and possibly responsible for lethality. Further, these aberrations are not unique. Chromosome "breaks" are not only observed in normal tissue cells but no aberration has been produced by radiation that has not also been seen in unirradiated controls. Measurements have established that the probability of producing a break is about .004 per rad which is very close to the probability of producing cell death.[3] Furthermore, variation of those parameters that change the sensitivity of cells to the lethal effects of radiation (i.e. oxygen consumption) also affect in a similar manner the probability of producing aberrations. It is highly probable that the large visible chromosome defects discussed here do lead to sterility, however, smaller and unobservable effects may also occur that do not lead to cell death but which may change the inheritable characteristics of the cell. This resulting cell could then constitute a mutation of the original cell line.

PRODUCTION OF MUTATIONS

For missense mutants of mammalian cells, the genetic damage

from a mutagenic agent is heritable and should be revertible by further treatment with a secondary mutagen. Those cells for whom reversion has not yet been proved are usually classed as variants but could be deletions (which do not revert) or double mutations. Interestingly, no agents have been found to produce a mutation that has not been observed in the normal population. They merely increase the rate of production of such changes. Because of the difficulty of identifying changes in mammalian cells per se, mutations observed to date have been limited to those affecting the basic biochemical processes in the cells. Examples are induced resistance to radiation which involves the utilization of oxygen and repair mechanisms, increased resistance to IUdR, induced resistance to 8-azaguanine, production of glycine deficiency, etc. The probability of producing such a mutation of a mammalian cell averages about one in a million per rad which is about 1/4000 of the probability of inducing sterilization. Thus, for every mutant produced, about 4000 rapidly dividing cells are sterilized.

GENETIC EFFECTS

If now the gonads of mammals - including man - are irradiated, any mutated germ cell or ovum can unite with its mate during conception and ultimately produce an aberrant offspring. Either or both type cells can have been irradiated with the probability of producing a mutation doubled if both are exposed. Russel and others[4,5] have scored the mutations appearing in the progeny of irradiated mice and found a probability of two in ten million per rad of producing any one specific mutation when irradiating either partner. Both male and female mice seemed to be equally sensitive to the mutational effects of radiation. An additional observation was that if more than 7 weeks intervened between irradiation of the female mice and conception, the number of mutations dropped to zero - implying of course complete repair of the genetic damage. A much lower rate of repair was seen in the males. This phenomenon, of course, can also be considered to be a dose rate effect. The mutation frequency of a specific locus in male mice at 1 rad/min was 30% less than that at 100 rad/min and seemingly remains constant as the dose rate is lowered. On the other hand, this decrease continues in female mice to approach zero at 0.01 rad/min. This effect has not yet been observed in humans but most likely occurs.

Regarding genetic risks for humans, radiation induced mutations manifest themselves in later generations as prenatal death, hereditary diseases, malformations and other deteriorations of the level of health. There are some 1000 suspected varieties of dominant and 750 varieties of recessive mutations in nature along with a number of other types such as x-linked, chromosomal, etc. Nevertheless, x-ray induced mutations constitute only about 4% of the known varieties and there is no proven or even known case of a radiation induced mutation in humans because of the large number of such occurring naturally. Rather limited data on such mutations[6] indicates that the amount of radiation required to double the natural mutation rate for those classes of mutations also produced by x-rays is between 50 and 150 rems to either partner. While the natural mutation rate is 9 aberrant offspring per 100 individuals[7] (Table I), only the first four classes are induced by radiation. Assuming

Table I.

Estimates of the Frequency of Genetic Disorders in Birth Cohort as Cases per 100 Liveborn

	STEVENSON (1959)	UNSCEAR (1962,1966)	BRITISH COLUMBIA Minimal	BRITISH COLUMBIA Adjusted
Dominant	3.32[a]	0.95	0.06	0.08
Recessive	0.21	0.21	0.09	0.11
X-linked	0.04	0.04	0.03	0.04
Chromosomal	-	0.42[b]	0.16	0.20[c]
Congenital malformations	1.41	2.50	3.58	4.28
Other multifactorial	1.48	1.50	1.58	4.73
Unknown	-	-	0.60	2.70

[a] Includes trivial as well as serious anomalies.

[b] Includes Down's syndrome (0.15), other autosomal trisomies (0.05), Klinefelter's syndrome (0.17), Turner's syndrome (0.03) and Cri-du-chat syndrome (0.02) but excludes XXX females (0.12) and individuals with translocations (0.50).

[c] All but about 3% are due to Down's syndrome.

the British Columbia data to be the most complete,[8] we see the probability of producing spontaneously one aberration in any of these four classes is about 0.4/100. Use a doubling dose of 50 rems for a worst case calculation, we see that the probability of producing an aberration by x-rays in any one individual is then 0.8×10^{-4} per rem. Since there are about 1800 loci for both dominant and recessive mutations, we arrive at a probability of 0.4×10^{-7} per locus per rem which is quite close to that for the mouse.

It is to be emphasized that if humans are similar to mice with respect to radiation induced mutations, the genetic risk will be much less at low dose rates than that extrapolated from high dose data.

CARCINOGENESIS

The fact that radiation can induce cancer has been known for many decades, however, the basic cause is still unknown. Fortunately (or unfortunately), data exist from past tragedies that allow an estimate of the probability of radiation carcinogenesis.[6] These are shown in Table II. It is to be noticed that children are more

Table II.

Cancer Statistics*

Primary Site	Prob. of Occurrence (x 10⁴/yr.)	Fractional 5 yr. Survival (F_a)	Prob. of Fatal Malignancy (x 10⁴/yr.)	Prob. of Induction (Pra) (x 10⁶/yr./rem)
Marrow (Leukemia)	1.0	0.13	0.87	1.0
Bone	0.1	0.20	0.08	0.2
Brain (& CNS)	0.5	0.30	0.35	1.0
Lung	3.8	0.08	3.50	1.0
Female Breast				
Ages 20-34	1.1	0.60	0.44	6.0
Ages 35-49	10.4	0.60	4.20	2.0
Thyroid	0.4	0.80	0.08	1.0† / 6.0**
Colon	3.0	0.34	1.98	
Stomach	1.0	0.09	0.91	
Tongue	0.2	0.27	0.15	1.0‡
Liver	0.2	0.30	0.14	
Pancreas	0.9	0.02	0.88	
Prostate	2.0	0.40	1.20	

*Averaged for all races, sexes, and ages except as noted.

†Adults

**Children

‡For total of remaining tissues.

sensitive to the induction of thyroid cancer and leukemia than adults. Likewise, young women are more sensitive to the induction of breast cancer than older women. Interestingly, recent analysis of all available data on irradiation of children in utero showed that the risk of inducing a malignancy was approximately the same as that for adults.[9]

One important point to note is that these data in Table II are valid only if the whole organ is irradiated and the dose is averaged over the whole volume of the organ. For example, if only one breast were exposed to a uniform dose, the probability (per rem) of carcinogenesis would be only one-half of that listed. Secondly, the listed probability of induction is only for fatal cancers. For the

probability of simply inducing a tumor in a given organ without
regard to fatality, the listed probability should be divided by
the one minus the fractional five year survival. However, in this
discussion, we shall be concerned only with the induction of fatal
malignancies with the understanding that the mere induction of
tumors will be about twice as large since the cure rate averages
about 50% for all tumors combined. Lastly, it is to be pointed out
that for any one exposure, the latent period can be as long as 25
years. It should also be stressed that this latent period is not
unique for radiation and is similar for most carcinogens. Thus,
if an individual receives an acute exposure of 1 rem to the bone
marrow, the probability of the occurrence of a fatal leukemia is
about one per million per year for the following 25 years totaling
25 per million in a lifetime. For all sites, the National Academy
of Sciences[6] data indicate that 1 rad of whole body irradiation will
produce between 50 and 180 fatalities from all malignancies in a
million individuals over the first 25 to 27 years after irradiation.
For most of the data used herein, we have assumed a probability of
10^{-4} fatalities over the subsequent 25 years per rem exposure.
Regarding dose-rate effects, the above data on radiation carcinogenesis were obtained with dose rates ranging from the very intense
blast of an A bomb through normal therapeutic and diagnostic procedures to low dose rates from internally deposited radionuclides.
With few exceptions, most dose-effect relationships were best fit
by a straight line that extrapolated through zero. Further, the
exposure doses ranged from a few to many thousands of rem. We shall
thus assume linearity of effect with absorbed dose and the absence
of dose-rate effects and/or repair. This, of course, should produce
the largest risks when extrapolated to very low doses for low LET
radiation. There is some doubt that this will hold for neutrons
where seemingly the RBE increases as the dose rate diminishes.
This will be discussed later.

While many scientists feel that carcinogenesis is most likely
due to radiation induced mutations, it is to be pointed out that
the probability of producing cancer is on the order of 10^{-15} per
rad per cell when one accounts for all the cells in each organ.
Since the probability of mutagenesis in proliferating mammalian
cells is on the order of one per million per rad per cell, the
relation between the two effects is far from clear. However, it
remains that to produce a cancer by radiation, one also mutates and
sterilizes an enormous number of normal cells. This obviously makes
very difficult any attempt to relate mutagenesis and carcinogenesis.
For multiple exposures, to a first approximation one may simply add
the individual probabilities involved for each procedure. However,
for greater accuracy, one must account for the fact that the average
lifetime of an individual is longer than the 25 year latent period
and that the exposures are usually spread over a long time.[10]
Simple addition of the doses over the life of the individual obviously produces a "worst case" calculation.

RISK

It is obvious from the previous discussion that the most serious risk to the average person from ionizing radiation is that of the induction of cancer from the medical use of x-rays. As seen in Table III, exposures from the medical use of radioisotopes is negligible in comparison. Table IV lists the lifetime risk of a

Table III.

Annual Whole-Body Dose Rates (mrem/year) in the United States

Source	Dose Rate	Genetically Significant Dose Rate
Environmental		
Natural	102	90
Global Fallout	4	4
Nuclear Power	0.003	.003
Medical		
Diagnostic X-Rays	72	20
Radiopharmaceuticals	1	0.2
Occupational	0.8	0.8
Miscellaneous	2	2

fatal malignancy resulting from one exposure to a variety of normal diagnostic procedures. Ignoring the mammographic procedures for young women (prescribed only for symptomatic patients), it may be seen that the lifetime risk hovers about 10^{-5} per examination. This is to be compared with a 50 year risk of a fatal cancer occurring spontaneously of 0.08. In other words, the risk of cancer occurring naturally in any one individual is 8000 times greater than that due to one exposure from an average diagnostic examination. It is apparent that many such x-ray examinations can be tolerated before any appreciable risk will result. The same is true of the medical use of radioisotopes and other types of exposures to ionizing radiations for diagnostic purposes.[11] Under any circumstance, however, it is advisable to keep the dose as low as practicable keeping in mind the most sensitive organs in the field.[12]

Regarding genetic risks, Table V lists the gonadal dose delivered by some routine diagnostic examinations.[13] Assuming an average gonadal dose of 200 millirems for an abdominal examination of a female, the probability of producing a child with a detectable aberration becomes 1.6×10^{-5}. This is about six thousand times smaller than the probability of any type aberration occurring

Table IV.

Risks of Carcinogenesis for Various Diagnostic Procedures

Examination	Tissues at Risk	Skin Dose/Film (roentgens)	Number of Films	Average Absorbed Dose (mrem)	Fraction Exposed fa	Risk per Examination (x 10⁶)
Skull Radiograph 65 kVp 2.2 mm Al	Brain Marrow Bone	0.33	2	178 68 88	1.00 0.13 0.10	4.0
Skull 20-Sec. CAT Scan 120 kVp	Brain Marrow Bone		5 (slices)	2700 1100 1400	1.0 0.13 0.10	70.0
Chest Radiograph 65 kVp 2.2 mm Al	Lung Marrow Bone Other Tissues	0.045	2	52 40 50 36	1.0 0.36 0.25 0.02	1.5
Lower Abdomen KUB 70 kVp 2.4 mm Al	Marrow Bone Other Tissues	0.67	2	322 422 265	0.51 0.37 0.07	5.3
Upper Abdomen 20-Sec. CAT Scan 120 kVp	Marrow Bone Other Tissues		5 (slices)	2700 3500 2200	0.18 0.13 0.03	16.0
Mammography Lo Dose Film 35 kVp, 0.75 mm Al 34-50 years 20-34 years	Breast Breast	1.3 1.3	2 per breast 2 per breast	910 910	1.0 1.0	30.0 130.0
Mammography Xerox, 45 kVp 1.5 mm Al 34-50 years 20-34 years	Breast Breast	2.0 2.0	2 per breast 2 per breast	2000 2000	1.0 1.0	66.0 287.0
Dental Typical 75 kVp 12" FSD	Soft Tissue Bone Marrow Thyroid	0.97	4	1440 350 80 40	1.0 0.01 0.02 0.02 1.0	3.0

Table V.

Estimated Gonadal Dose in mrem from Various Radiographic Examinations

Type of Examination	Male 1970	Female 1970
Skull	<0.5	<0.5
Cervical spine	<0.5	<0.5
Chest		
Radiographic	<0.5	1
Photofluorographic	2	3
Thoracic spine	3	11
Shoulder	<0.5	<0.5
Upper GI series	1	171
Barium enema	175	903
Cholecystography or cholangiogram	<0.5	78
Intravenous or retrograde Pyelogram	207	588
Abdomen, KUB, flat plate	97	221
Lumbar spine	218	721
Pelvis	364	210
Hip	600	124
Upper extremities	<0.5	<0.5
Lower extremities	15	<0.5
Other abdominal exams.	857	524
All other	<0.5	6

(Gonad Doses and Genetically Significant Dose from Diagnostic Radiology. USDHEW Publ (FDA) 76-8034, April, 1976)

spontaneously. On the other hand, the average genetically significant dose rate to the general population from medical x-rays has been estimated at about 20 millirem/yr. This is to be compared with a genetically significant background rate of 65 millirem/yr. It must be pointed out that not all the spontaneous mutations in the first four categories in Table I are due to radiation alone. Many other factors such as increased temperature, viruses, chemicals, etc. also contribute. In fact, one dose of 65 millirems to the overall population would account for only about 0.1% of the naturally occurring mutations in the x-ray sensitive classes.

It would appear that the added genetic risk to an individual from one diagnostic examination and the added risk to the general population from the current medical use of x-rays are quite small compared to those risks occurring naturally.

Regarding radiation therapy of cancer, it is important to note that the treatment itself may also induce cancer. Generally this is ignored because of the shorter life expectancy of the patient but for some patients who have a choice of treatments it may be an important consideration. Consider now the treatment of a solid tumor in the abdomen by high energy x-rays where the tissue attenuation may be neglected and where the tumor dose is usually on the order of 5000 rads. However, because of "beaming" determined by treatment planning protocols, the normal tissue dose around the tumor will usually be about 1500 rads. Now for this type field, only about 25% of the marrow and about one-half of the critical internal organs will be exposed to the reduced primary radiation. This will produce a probability of creating a fatal cancer by the direct beam of 1.2×10^{-3} per year neglecting brain, female breast and thyroid.

In addition, the remaining marrow and critical organs will be subject to scatter radiation. From the work of Rawlinson and Johns,[14] this may be shown to be approximately 200 rads average tissue dose for either Co(60) or 25 MeV which will produce an additional probability of a malignancy of 0.2×10^{-3} per year, again neglecting the same organs as above. Photon head leakage would add only 5 rads to these tissues which is far less than the uncertainties in the assumptions and may be neglected. This means that due to the treatment itself, the probability of creating a malignancy sometime in the 25 years after treatment is about 1.4×10^{-3} per year which is close to the "doubling dose" for spontaneously occurring fatal tumors. It is obvious that while our model is reasonably representative of many treatments, this calculation will depend critically on the location of the tumor and type of patient. For a more complete overview, the above probability of inducing a fatal cancer should be compared with a 5×10^{-3} per year chance of dying from any cause averaged over the population of the U.S. older than 50 years of age.

Consider now an x-ray tube head operating at a potential high enough to produce neutrons - say 25 MeV. We shall now assume a neutron induced leukemia probability of 28×10^{-6} per year per rad of marrow dose. For induction of fatal leukemias, this drops to 23×10^{-6} per rad-year and is independent of dose.[15] The use of the neutron dose in rads for malignancy calculations then eliminates any need for RBE (or Quality Factor) considerations. It is important to remember that the increasing RBE for neutrons as the dose is diminished as proposed by Rossi and Mays[15] is due to the assumption (or analysis) of a dose-squared relation for the dose-effect curve for low dose low LET photons only as determined from the Nagasaki bomb data. Throughout this paper we have assumed a dose rate for photon induced malignancies (Table II) that is also independent of dose and which allows a linear extrapolation from high dose to low dose. This is also a reasonable interpretation of the data in the BEIR I Report. Nevertheless, should the Rossi-Mays model be shown to hold at low photon doses, this would mean that the biologic effects due to the photons are smaller at these low doses than those implied by Table II and our calculations are again "worst case".

According to Swanson,[16,17] the neutrons from a 25 MeV linear accelerator will increase the integral photon dose in gram-rads by about 0.3% inside and 0.7% outside the treatment volume. We then see that there will be an 8% increase in the probability of producing a tumor by the treatment field and a 20% increase in that due to the radiation outside the field. Thus, for the combined effect of photons and neutrons, we shall have a probability of producing a tumor of 1.3×10^{-3} per year by the treatment field and 0.24×10^{-3} per year by the leakage and scatter producing a total of 1.54×10^{-3} per year.

Currently, because of the apparently increased and really unknown RBE of neutrons, a lowering of the allowable neutron head leakage is under consideration which would cause extensive (and expensive) machine modifications. It is to be pointed out that if the neutron head leakage in the previous example should be completely eliminated by large amounts of shielding, this will cause a reduction of only 3% in the total probability of producing a malignancy. This seems to be a rather small (negligible) return for such an expensive change in machine design. It would appear that perhaps a more pertinent question concerns the value of treating cancer with accelerators capable of producing neutrons that increase the risk of malignancies by 10%. It would seem that this too is negligible on the basis that a 10% change is much smaller than the uncertainties involved in the malignancy calculations. Nevertheless, this is obviously a medical decision involving the evaluation of improvements (benefits) in treatment occurring because of the higher photon energies. While the previous calculations are worst case and admittedly involve a number of approximations, nevertheless, they can be scaled with reasonable confidence and thus have some value in guiding future decisions.

BENEFITS

While the risks are relatively easy to specify and quantitate, the benefits are not. For those procedures leading to tumor detection and possibly cure, one can relate the benefits to the improvement in cure rate resulting from the diagnostic procedure. However, most of the radiographic procedures are concerned with less fatal end points which lead to alleviation of pain, improvement of the quality of living, and a possible increase in longevity. Very few are related to detection of tumors. Thus, most of the benefits from individual medical examinations are highly personal and difficult to quantitate and should be evaluated by the knowledgeable patient and his medical advocate. Some individuals will accept almost any risks due to radiation exposures in order to alleviate pain while others will stoically accept pain to avoid such risks.

For example, many women refuse x-ray mammography today because they fear the risk of inducing cancer more than the benefits to be gained from early detection. This is obviously their personal choice but usually arises through lack of knowledge about or appreciation of the risks and benefits involved. Part of this is due to an almost fanatical opposition to nuclear power that has resulted in wildly exaggerated or overemphasized effects of radiation reported in newspapers, magazines and television. Unfortunately, some individuals have already suffered because of reaction to induced fear.

For the individual then, it would seem that any benefit-cost considerations are quite subjective and possibly misleading. A perhaps better criterion to use for judgement is simply the fractional increase in risk of inducing a malignancy by the radiologic procedure relative to the probability of any type malignancy occurring naturally. This type risk may be obtained by dividing the absolute risk per examination listed in Table IV by 8×10^{-2} which is the probability of dying from any malignancy over a 50 year period. This fractional increase in risk is about 5×10^{-5} for 80% of the routine radiologic examinations listed in Table VII. This means that most examinations could be done about 20,000 times before the risk of a malignancy from the examination would be equal to that of one occurring naturally (i.e. the "doubling" dose).

Although by far most radiologic examinations are not concerned with the detection of cancer, consideration of cancer detection may be useful in quantitating the societal benefits of medical x-rays. However, to simply detect cancer in an individual is not sufficient since all cancers will ultimately be found. More important is early detection since it has been the feeling of the medical community for the past several decades that earlier detection of cancer will improve survival. However, while the PAP test has confirmed this feeling rather conclusively and mammography somewhat less certainly, no data for other tumors has been presented to firmly establish this hypothesis. In fact, most surveys for lung, brain and stomach cancers have been shown to have little effect on overall cure rates. Of course, many (most?) soft tissue tumors may be detected by conventional means only after they have achieved a certain size and already metastasized. Regardless, location and delineation of a tumor are also important for treatment. Thus, if a tumor is suspected because of some non-localizing test - say, an immunologic test - more radiation at increased risk can then be used to subsequently locate and possibly size the tumor. Such considerations will strongly affect benefit-risk ratio considerations by the individual involved.

For evaluation of societal benefit-risk ratios, consider first mass surveys for breast cancer. If a million women over 35 receive one x-ray mammographic procedure using low dose film such that they receive a total breast dose of 900 millirems, we would detect about 1000 breast cancers at a cost of at most 2 cancers induced sometime over the following 25 years by the procedure itself. Now, it has been estimated that there will be an increase of about 17% in the 5 year survival due to earlier detection through mammography. Thus 170 additional women would be salvaged at a cost of at most 2 individuals producing a benefit-cost ratio of 85/1. For women under 35, this ratio would be about 1 due to lower incidence and increased sensitivity. Thus such surveys would appear justified if confined to older women but many people will not support even this because of the implication of the possible production of a small number of malignancies in a given population. Since such cancers occur naturally, it is a human tendency to blame the diagnostic procedure for any one or all of them.

On the other hand, a society may decide that a particular survey is valuable in spite of the individual risks. In 1968, about 40 million chest fluorographies were carried out in Japan. The results of such a survey are presented in Table VI[18]. Not shown

Table VI.

Results of Chest Radiography of 40 Million Individuals in Japan in 1968 (Kitabatake et al., 1973)

Disease Detected	Number Detected
Curable TB	38,629
Curable Lung Cancer	758
Incurable TB	5,818
Incurable Lung Cancer	2,271
Benign Pulmonary Disease	1,000,000

are calculations indicating the possibility of inducing 46 leukemias by the radiation exposures which should be compared with 97,000 spontaneous leukemias. Also estimated were 7 possibly radiation induced lung cancers and 150 estimated genetic deaths over the first 10 generations. Of interest is the fact that the average marrow dose in these chest exposures was estimated to be about 35 millirems which is to be compared with 4 millirems in the United States. Nevertheless, since the incidence and mortality rates for tuberculosis have diminished considerably in Japan since 1940, it is widely accepted in Japan that mass chest fluorography has made a great contribution to the prevention and control of tuberculosis. Of course, the same problem exists in this case as in mammography; namely, since most of the TB would have been discovered eventually, of what real value is early detection? It is to be noted in passing that the authors claim to have discovered 758 cases of "curable" lung cancer. This is highly suspect since it implies a cure-rate for lung cancer of 25% which is to be compared with 8% in the United States. No criteria for "curable" was given.

Another method of evaluating the societal benefits derived from the medical uses of radiation is to consider the Resource-Loss Model.[19] In this model, one attempts to determine the time lost in economic productivity due to accidents, illness, or death and the improvement in same due to diagnostic radiologic procedures. While such a model does assume that an individual's value to society may be measured in terms of his contribution in time to the nation's productivity and that all individuals are equally valuable - with which many will argue - it does provide a rough method for estimating a benefit-cost ratio. By expressing the reduction in lost-time in dollars gained and comparing with the cost of the examinations in dollars to create such reductions, one can then obtain a dimensionless ratio. Table VII shows the number of radiographic examinations performed in the United States and their cost in 1970. The

Table VII.

Resource-Use Costs Model

Type of Radiographic Examination	Number (million)	Cost ($) per Examination
Chest (thorax)	65	22
Upper abdomen	15	22
Lower abdomen	17	39
Upper extremities	10	17
Lower extremities	12	22
Head, neck, and other	10	22
Gastrointestinal series	6.6	50
Barium enema	3.5	50
All other fluoroscopic examinations	2.5	40
Dental radiography	68	12

total cost for chest examinations is seen to be 1.43 billion dollars. On the other hand, Table VIII shows the estimated dollar savings in lost-time due to chest examinations only. This leads to an obvious benefit-cost ratio of 10/1. Similar ratios will result for most of the other procedures. The risks due to the radiation exposures per se were neglected in the above considerations because of their low average probability of occurrence.

SUMMARY

It would seem that benefit-risk quantitation can have some value in guiding health-care services or surveys for large populations where the end points are reasonably clear. However, such is of little value for the individual where the benefits are highly

Table VIII.

RESOURCE-LOSS BENEFITS MODEL

Estimated Work-Loss Prevented from
Diagnostic Chest X-Ray Examinations

	Work-Days-Saved		Number of Examinations (Millions)	Dollar Benefit per Exam ($50 x days)	Benefit (10^9 dollars)
	Range	Average			
None		0	55.3	0	0
Minimal	1-20	10	5.2	500	2.6
Moderate	21-40	30	2.6	1,500	3.9
Major	41-80	60	1.3	3,000	3.9
Total	81-200	140	.6	7,000	4.2
			65.0		$14.6 billion

subjective. Rather, one should use the risks as a guide in arriving at decisions regarding the wisdom of a particular procedure.

Nevertheless, it would seem that the actual risks to the patient and general public from radiologic procedures and medical uses of radiation are quite small compared to similar risks occurring continuously and spontaneously in our environment. It would also seem that current public fear about radiation exposures is quite exaggerated as judged by both the hysteria in the media and by the expansion in Federal and State regulations over the last decade. For example, considering the very low risks and uncertainties in the biologic data calculated for "worst case" conditions, it seems rather trivial to "certify" x-ray machines to the extent proposed, to control collimation of the beam, to specify exposure doses for various procedures, and to be excessively concerned about a 10% to 30% increase in dose due to repeat examinations. It is also obvious that quality control of film processors has a greater impact on costs because of the silver in the emulsions than on carcinogenesis. It would seem that an informed public coupled with recommendations on safe practice from reputable agencies and threats of malpractice suits should reduce the possibility of biologically significant overexposures. To be sure, the exposure doses should be kept as low as reasonably practicable but exceptional circumstances may demand larger doses than usual. No one has yet related diagnostic accuracy with dose or number of views so it would seem somewhat futile to regulate them. However, it is important to note that the incidence of false positives will increase as the radiation dose is lowered because quantum fluctuations (and other noise) can create images that resemble those objects being detected (i.e. a tumor). This can be extremely important when positive readings result in painful biopsies. Increasing the dose to eliminate false positives due to noise fluctuations usually results in a larger benefit than cost. Likewise, since most missed diagnoses (true negatives) are due to inattention or equivalent on the part of the reader, it follows that increasing the exposure dose will have little effect on the diagnostic error rate. Also, multiple readings can improve the error rate without increasing the radiation dose[20]. Similarly, multiple views can also improve the error rate but at the expense of more dose since some hidden tumors may be found because of a different line of sight (e.g. a tumor that may be hidden by a rib in one view and not in the other). Examination of Table VIII will show that we may gain (save) about 5 work days on the average per chest examination. Since the total body dose per examination is about 45 millirems, calculations by Cohen and Lee[11] indicate that such a dose will reduce the life expectancy by about 0.5 days. Since we gain 5 days at the expense of 0.5 days, this can be interpreted as a benefit-cost ratio of $5/0.5 \simeq 10$ for the individual having the chest examination. It also seems that the risks would still be negligible if the average doses should double or triple and one must ask as a taxpayer if such regulations are really worth the cost of implementation and would not the money (and effort) be better spent elsewhere? In this case, a cost-benefit analysis could be very useful.

An exception to the above discussion is the risk to occupationally engaged personnel. At the present time, such a person can legally receive a dose of 5 rems per year for a lifetime. In the simplest case of a 25 year active working lifetime, an average risk could be that resulting from 125 rems total body exposures. Since the risk will extend into the period beyond retirement, a worst case calculation will lead to a probability of 0.013 of producing a fatal cancer sometime in a 50 year period with the exposure occurring in the first 25 years. This is to be compared with a 0.08 lifetime probability of dying from a naturally occurring malignancy. This is an increase of 16% and could be of concern to the individual should he be made aware of it. Fortunately, most individuals engaged in the delivery of radiation for diagnostic and therapeutic purposes receive far less than the 5 rems per year now allowable.

REFERENCES

1. E. J. Hall, Radiobiology For The Radiologist, 2nd Edition (Harper and Row, 1968).
2. R. Rugh, Radiology 82, 917-200 (1964).
3. M. M. Elkind and G. F. Whitmore, The Radiobiology of Cultured Mammalian Cells (Gordon and Breach, 1967).
4. W. L. Russel, Recovery and Repair Mechanisms in Radiobiology (Brookhaven Symposia in Biology No. 20, 1968), pp. 179-189.
5. F. Lyon, P. G. Papworth and R. J. S. Phillips, Nature New Biology 238, 101-104 (1972).
6. National Academy of Sciences, The Effects on Populations of Exposures to Low Levels of Ionizing Radiation (Report of the Advisory Committee on the Biological Effects of Ionizing

Radiations, November, 1972).
7. B. J. Trimble and J. H. Doughty, Ann. Hum. Genet. (London) 38, 199-223 (1974).
8. K. Sankaranavayanan, The Third European Congress of the International Radiation Protection Association (Amsterdam, 1975).
9. E. E. Pochin, Br. J. Radiol. 49, 577-579 (1976).
10. E. C. Gregg, Radiology 123, 447-453 (1977).
11. B. L. Cohen and I. S. Lee, Health Phys. 36, 707-722 (1979).
12. C. L. Nash, E. C. Gregg, R. H. Brown and K. Pillai, J. Bone Jt. Surg. 61-A, 371-374 (1979).
13. USDHEW, Publ. (FDA) 76-8034 (April, 1976).
14. J. H. Rawlinson and H. E. Johns, Med. Phys. 4, 456-457 (1977).
15. H. H. Rossi and C. W. Mays, Health Phys. 34, 353 (1978).
16. W. P. Swanson, Stanford Linear Accelerator Center PUB-2322 (November, 1979, Rev.).
17. R. C. McCall and W. P. Swanson, Stanford Linear Accelerator Center PUB-2292 (March, 1979).
18. M. D. Kitabatake et al., Radiology 109, 37-40 (1973).
19. National Academy of Sciences, EPA 520/4-77-003 (1976).
20. E. C. Gregg, P. S. Rao and H. L. Friedell, Invest. Radiol. 11, 249-257 (1976).

METHODS OF RISK REDUCTION IN DIAGNOSTIC RADIOLOGY

Stewart C. Bushong
Baylor College of Medicine, Houston, Texas 77030

INTRODUCTION

We know that the radiation doses which we experience in diagnostic radiology are low. On a population basis they are exceedingly low. We also know that the suspected biological effects of these exposures are exceedingly low and that the risk of latent radiation injury to either patient or personnel from diagnostic x-ray procedures is nil. Nevertheless, there are a number of administrative procedures and technical devices which can be employed to good advantage in reducing radiation exposure to patients and personnel and thereby affecting a reduction in radiation risk with little or no loss of diagnostic information. In general, those actions taken with the primary purpose of reducing patient dose will also reduce the dose to occupationally exposed personnel.

PATIENT PROTECTIVE METHODS

ROUTINE QUALITY ASSURANCE

One of the largest sources of unnecessary patient x-ray exposure is perhaps that resulting from repeat examination. Such additional examinations are called retakes for which there are many causes. It is not absolutely clear what is the main cause for retakes but certainly a large percentage is due to inadequate equipment performance. Several authoratative studies of retakes have been reported (1-3) and collectively they suggest that the majority of retakes are due to operator error. Equipment malfunction contributes to less than 10% of retakes. Nevertheless, inadequate equipment performance can be reduced by a routine quality assurance program emphasizing radiation control measurements.

Several states currently require routine radiation control and quality assurance surveys. Depending on the type of facility, the required frequency is usually one to three years. The Joint Commission on Accreditation of Hospitals requires annual surveys. Table 1 lists the information specified by the JCAH for such a survey. Other published recommendations calling for periodic quality assurance surveys suggest necessary measurements and observations, and these are often employed to supplement the requirements of the JCHA.

TABLE 1. Measurements and observations to be included in a JCAH directed quality assurance survey.

A. Film Quality
 1. Processing control
 2. Exposure reproducibility
 3. Linearity (mR/mAs)
 4. Peak tube potential
 5. Timer accuracy
 6. Grids
 7. Film-screen contact
 8. System resolution (film-screen combination and fluoroscopy)
 9. Tomography
   a. fulcrum position
   b. cut thickness
   c. resolving power
   d. uniformity of exposure over entire motion cycle
B. Fluoroscopic Imaging Quality
 1. Resolution of fluoro image intensifier chains
 2. Electronic system noise
 3. Automatic brightness control
C. Radiology Viewing Facilities
 1. Illuminator uniformity
D. Patient Protection
 1. Beam quality
 2. X-ray field localization
 3. Fluoroscopic table top output
E. Personnel Protection
 1. Inspection of protective drapes and side shields
 2. Fluoroscopic inspection of protective drapes and side shields
 3. Testing of interlocks
 4. X-ray on indicator lights
 5. Bucky shield operation

IMAGE RECEPTOR SELECTION

The principal image receptor employed in diagnostic radiology is film. Original radiographic film consisted of a photographic emulsion coated onto a glass plate - hence, the origin of "x-ray plate." Glass was replaced by cellulose nitrate which was replaced by cellulose acetate which in turn is being replaced by polyester.

Originally the photographic emulsion was deposited on only one side of the base. Today nearly all radiographic films are double emulsion - one on each side of the base. This change resulted in effectively halving patient dose.

Other advances in the photographic emulsion have increased its sensitivity with a corresponding reduction in patient dose. Such advances, however, have been largely overshadowed by developments ancillary to the radiographic film - intensifying screens, xeroradiography and carbon fiber materials.

Radiographic Intensifying Screens: Our all American inventor, Thomas A. Edison, became involved in x-ray research shortly after Roentgen's discovery was announced. By 1900, he had evaluated hundreds of phosphors for use as a radiographic intensifying screen before settling on calcium tungstate as most appropriate. This was done in 1898 although it was some 15-20 years later before it was introduced into routine practice. That single development has perhaps been responsible for more patient dose reduction than any other.

The new radiographic intensifying screen phosphors were first described in 1972[4] and have rapidly gained acceptance in clinical radiology. The materials of interest are oxysulfides and oxybromides of lanthanum, gadolydium and yttrium. Other materials, barium fluorochloride for instance, though not truly a rare earth, have also been made available as a faster screen. Table 2 reports the principle types of new generation radiographic intensifying screens. On a relative sensitivity scale if a value of 1 is assigned to conventional calcium tungstate screens this new generation of intensifying screens have speeds from 2 to 8.

Table 2. Representative new faster radiographic intensifying screens.

Suppliers	Identification	Phosphor
3M	Alpha	Gadolinium and lanthanum oxysulfide
Kodak	Lanex	Gadolinium and lanthanum oxysulfide
DuPont	Quanta	Barium fluorochloride
General Electric	Blue Max	Lanthanum oxybromide
U.S. Radium	Ratex	Yttrium oxysulfide

There are two concerns with the use of this new generation of intensifying screens. First, their cost is two to three times that of conventional screens. This makes it rather difficult to recommend their adoption into existing facilities. Most would agree that due to physical wear, calcium tungstate screens have a useful life of perhaps five years. With proper planning, therefore, the new generation of intensifying screens should slowly replace existing conventional screens

For new facilities rare earth screens may be the material of choice even though the cost is high. A careful analysis will show that a complete evaluation of the long term use of this material may indeed result in less cost. If a facility is designed from the beginning for use with rare earth ingensifying screens two obvious savings will be affected. First, the radiographic workload can be assumed to be no more than one half of that which would otherwise occur. Thus, the required protective shielding for that facility can be reduced by one half value layer or approximately $\frac{1}{2}$ lb/ft^2 if lead is used. The construction savings may be considerable. Secondly, since the radiographic workload is reduced, so is the thermal stress on the x-ray tube. This will undoubtedly result in longer tube life. The degree of tube life lengthening will depend somewhat on the manner in which the reduced workload is accomplished. If it is done by reduction of exposure time while maintaining former techniques of mA and kVp, the extended life may not be significant. If the reduction is accomplished by reduction in mA while maintaining the former kVp and exposure time, then the lengthened tube life would be expected to be great.

A disadvantage to the use of rare earth screens, especially in existing facilities, where new and old screens may be employed simultaneously, is the need to match the rare earth screen with an appropriate radiographic film. Most rare earth screens emit light in the green region of the spectrum, and therefore, must be matched to green-sensitive film. This is unlike the conventional calcium tungstate screens which are blue emitting and must be matched with blue sensitive film. Mismatching screens and films will reduce considerably any designed exposure reduction.

Xeroradiography: Conventional radiography is based on the formation of a latent image by a photographic emulsion and wet chemistry processing to produce the visible image. Xeroradiography is quite different. It is based on the formation of an electrostatic latent image by a photoconductive material and a gray processing technique to produce the visible image. Its name, xeroradiography, comes from the Greek (*xeros:* dry; *graphin:* to write) and Latin (*radius:* ray).

Xeroradiography was invented in 1939 by Chester Carlson, a physicist, whose rights to the process were exploited around 1974 by the Hayloid Corporation. This company subsequently became Xerox Corporation. Although many years were spent by Xerox in developing the process for medical imaging, it was not until 1956 that the first commercially available system was produced.

The basic element of the xeroradiographic process is the image receptor. The image receptor is a plate of aluminum approximately 23 x 36 cm and 2 mm thick. This aluminum plate serves as the base for the x-ray-sensitive photoconductive material, selenium, which is deposited carefully with a controlled thickness of 130 μm. The selenium is a semiconductor, that is, it behaves not as an electrical insulator nor as an electrical conductor but somewhere in between. It is also photoconductive; in the dark it behaves as an insulator, but, when exposed to light or x-rays, it is a conductor of electrons.

There are two pieces of apparatus associated with xeroradiography. The first, the conditioner, prepares the image receptor for x-ray exposure. The second, the processor, converts the electrostatic latent image into a visible image through a dry processing technique.

The principal characteristic of the Xerox image is edge enhancement. Edge enhancement is the ability to amplify the contrast at the interface between two structures even when there is only minimal subject contrast. Toner is robbed from one side of the edge and laid down more heavily on the other side, resulting in enhancement of the edge. Edge enhancement amplifies the contrast at the edge and causes an apparent density difference on each side of the edge. It is this edge enhancement that is characteristic of xeroradiography. Xeroradiography has very low inherent contrast, as shown in the characteristic curves of Figure 1.

Xeroradiography has found principal application in mammography, skeletal radiography and some pediatric studies. Xeromammography results in patient exposures ranging from 0.5 to 1.5 rads/view to the entrance tissue. This is somewhat higher than the 0.2 to 1.0 rads experienced using screen-film but considerably lower than direct exposure mammography. Although the patient dose may be somewhat higher using xeroradiography, some contend that the image is far superior. There is considerable scientific literature regarding patient dose in mammography and risk reduction programs (5-14).

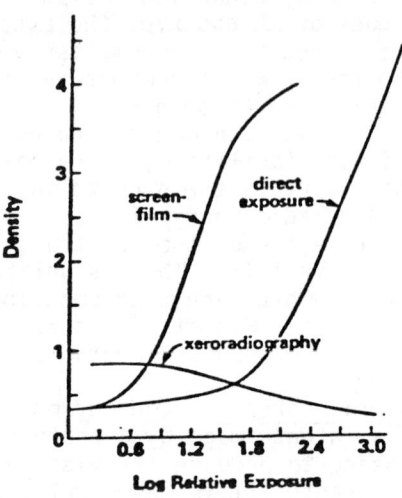

Figure 1. Characteristic curves for the three imaging modalities employed in mammography. (Courtesy S.C. Bushong, Radiologic Science for Technologists, 2nd Edition, C.V. Mosby Co., 1980.)

<u>Carbon Fiber Material:</u> One of the materials the United States developed early in its space exploration program was carbon fiber(15). This material was developed for nose cone applications because of its exceeding strength and heat resistance. It consists principally of graphite fibers ($Z_C = 6$) in a plastic matrix that can be formed to any shape or thickness. To its advantage, this carbon fiber material can be employed with no loss of system resolution and no increase in system noise. This material may contribute to image fog, but not significantly. For Bucky radiography, the combination of a carbon fiber cassette front and tabletop results in a total patient dose reduction of approximately 50%(16-17). Used in conjunction with rare earth screens, therefore, patient doses of 25% or less of those experienced just a few short years ago are possible.

Use of carbon fiber not only reduces the patient exposure but may also result in longer x-ray tube life because of the lower radiographic techniques required. Unfortunately, this material is quite expensive and therefore will enter routine radiologic practice slowly.

RADIOGRAPHIC TECHNIQUE CHARTS

In order to produce consistently high quality radiographs, it is absolutely essential that a technique chart be developed for each x-ray generator. Several popular textbooks provide clear instructions for producing a proper technique chart(18-21). Other papers have stressed the importance of technique charts in quality radiograph(22-24). Generally there are four types of technique charts, each determined by the nammer in which they are applied: a) body habitus; b) variable kVp; c) fixed kVp; and d) automated exposure.

The body habitus technique chart is perhaps the most difficult to develop and it requires the most precision on the part of the technologist. Each patient must be classified as hypersthenic, sthenic, hyposthenic and asthenic, and the body part measured. Radiographic contrast optimization is obtained by adjusting kVp and mAs according to the requirements of the chart.

The variable kVp technique chart is sometimes referred to as a fixed mAs chart since the mAs remains constant for any given body part. Use of this chart also requires measurement of the body part. Selection of the appropriate kVp is determined by this measurement. Nominal technique changes of 2 kVp/cm increment are experienced.

The fixed kVp technique chart is perhaps most widely recommended and employed. This technique presumes that there is an optimum kVp for each body part which will provide an adequate radiographic contrast. The mAs is varried according to the measurement of the thickness of the body part.

The automated exposure is an adaption of the fixed kVp technique. Automated exposures require electronic phototiming circuits and, therefore, are less likely to result in technique error. For automated exposures the operating console is programed for a fixed kVp for each type of radiographic examination. That sets the contrast scale. The mAs is then automatically selected through the phototimed circuit to provide the proper density. Body part measurement is unnecessary. Automated exposures are becoming more widely adopted with new equipment purchases.

X-RAY BEAM LIMITATION

Perhaps the most effective method for reducing patient exposure is to be certain to irradiate only that tissue which is diagnostically important. In this regard, diagnostic x-ray procedures have something of an advantage over many nuclear medicine procedures. Radioisotope application is always total body irradiation; x-ray application is nearly always partial body irradiation. Effective x-ray beam restriction falls into two categories: a) collimation of the beam; and b) use of specific area shielding.

X-Ray Beam Collimation: For many years collimation of the x-ray beam was accomplished by cones, cylinders and diaphragms. While these devices are effective, they are difficult to use because the positioning must be precise so as not to limit the desired extent of the image - a condition called cone cutting. These devices continue to be employed in some special application, but for routine examination the variable aperture light-localizing collimator is used. Such a device is shown schematically in Figure 2.

Figure 2. Schematic diagram of a representative variable aperture light localizing collimator. (Courtesy, Radiologic Science for Technologists, C.V. Mosby, Co. 1980.)

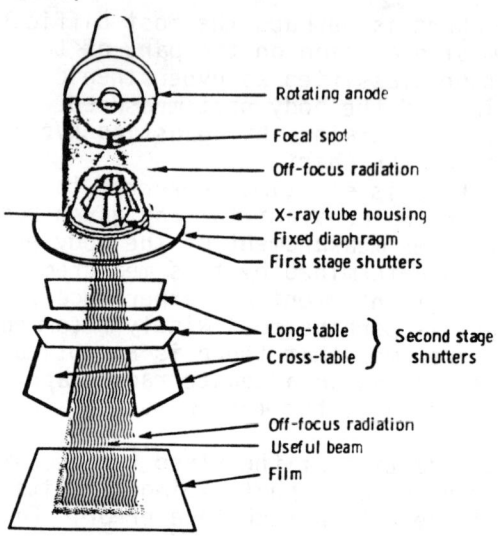

New x-ray apparatus is required to be equipped with positive beam limitation (PBL), an automatic light localing collimator, but this does not prevent the technologist from reducing the field size still further by collimation. By employing minimum collimation not only does one reduce the patient dose but the image quality will be increased because scatter radiation will also be reduced.

SPECIFIC AREA SHIELDING

X-ray examinations result in a partial body exposure while most of our radiation protection guides and radiation response information are based on whole body exposure. Use of specific area shielding is indicated when a particularly sensitive tissue or organ is in or near the useful beam. Two organs, the lens of the eye and the gonads, are frequently shielded from the primary radiation beam. There are two kinds of specific area shielding devices: the contact shield and the shadow shield.

When using contact shields the shielding device is positioned directly on the patient. Lens shields are always of the contact type. Studies have shown[25-27] that dose reductions on the order of 90% are possible when lens shields are used during multidirectional tomography of the head and neck. Such shielding devices cannot be used when such use will interfer with the production of a quality image. That is usually always the case in computed tomography examinations of the head.

Gonad shields can be of either the contact or the shadow shield type. Gonad contact shields can be purchased commercially or made from a properly cut piece of protective material. Shapes such as hearts, diamonds, triangles, and squares have been employed effectively[28-33].

The shadow shield is equally as effective as the contact shield and is more acceptable for use with adult patients. Use of such devices, however, requires careful attenuation on the part of the technologist. The shield must shadow the gonads without interfering with adjacent tissue. Improper positioning of the shadow shield can result in a repeat examination and increased patient dose[34].

The subject of gonad shielding is sufficiently important to require emphasis. Its use has been the subject of a recent lengthy Bureau of Radiological Health report[35] which proposed the following concepts:
   a) Gonad shielding should be considered for all patients who are potentially reproductive. As an administrative procedure this would include all patients under the age of 40 and perhaps even older males.
   b) Gonad shielding should be employed when the gonads lie in or near the primary beam.
   c) Proper patient positioning and beam collimation should not be relaxed when gonad shields are in use.
   d) Gonad shielding should only be used when it does not interfere with obtaining the required diagnostic information.

SELECTION PROCESS

It is becoming increasingly more obvious that a considerable radiation risk reduction is possible if more attention is paid to the clinical conditions attendant to the x-ray request. Thoughtless ordering of x-ray examinations by clinicians undoubtedly adds measureably to our medical radiation burden. Education of clinicians is the most appropriate remedy but secondary measures are available to the radiologist. The radiologist should participate in the selection of the examination and the screening of patients before examination.

Examination Selection: The technologist has practically no control over what some consider the largest source of unnecessary medical radiation risk - unnecessary x-ray examinations. This is almost exclusively the radiologist's responsibility.

Unfortunately, this source of added risk presents a serious dilemma for the radiologist and the clinician. Many x-ray examinations are knowingly requested when the yield of helpful information may be extremely low or even zero. When such an examination is performed, the benefit to the patient may in no way compensate for the radiation hazard. If the examination is not performed, the clinician and the radiologist may be severely criticized and then subjected to legal action should the patient's ultimate management result in failure, even though the examination in question would have contributed little to effective patient management. In such situations the radiologist is found caught between the proverbial "rock and a hard place".

Routine x-ray examinations should not be performed when there is no precise medical indication. Substantial evidence shows that such examinations are of little benefit because they are not cost effective and the disease detection rate is very low. Examples of such examinations are:
   a) Mass Screening for Tuberculosis. There is considerable documentation[36-41] that general screening has not been found effective and better methods of tuberculosis testing are now available. Some x-ray screening in high risk groups (medical and paramedical personnel), service personnel posing a potential community hazard (food handlers, teachers, etc.)

and special occupational groups (miners and workers having contact with beryllium, asbestos, glass, silica, etc.) may be appropriate.

b) Hospital Admissions. Chest x-rays for routine hospital admission when there is no clinical indication of chest disease should not be performed[42,43]. Among patients who would be candidates for such examinations are those admitted to the pulmonary or surgical service or the aged.

c) Pre-employment Physicals. Chest and lower back x-ray examinations are not justified because the yield of previous injury or disease is nil.

d) Periodic Health Examinations. Many physicians and public health officials now question the utility of the annual executive physical and its attendant x-ray examinations, especially fluoroscopic examination.

e) Mammography Screening. There has been considerable investigation into the efficacy of mass mammography screening[44-45] resulting in some rather precise recommendations. Prior to age 40 a baseline mammogram is acceptable in the asymptomatic patient. Regular screening of such patients below the age of 50 is not recommended. On the other hand, regardless of age if the patient is symptomatic or presents a strong family history of breast cancer, routine screening is acceptable.

Patient Selection: Patient selection is certainly an appropriate method of risk reduction available to a radiology service. Although few x-ray examinations are ordered by radiologists, they can and should participate in the selection of patients for examination through screening each request. It is essential that all requests for x-ray examinations be presented in writing with sufficient clinical history to allow the radiologist to judge the merit of the request and perhaps even alter or substitute for the examination. Considerable discussion of this aspect of radiation risk reduction has occurred recently[55-57].

Most important in this category are pregnant and potentially pregnant patients. Safeguards against the accidental irradiation of an early pregnancy are administrative problems. This situation is particularly critical during the first month of pregnancy, when such a condition may not be suspected and when the fetus is maximally sensitive to radiation exposure. After a couple of months, the risk of irradiating an unknown pregnancy becomes small because the patient is generally aware of her condition. If the state of pregnancy is known, then under many circumstances, the radiologic examination should not be conducted.

A number of techniques can be employed to reasonably ensure that irradiation of an unknown pregnancy does not occur. In the words of the International Commission on Radiation Protection (ICRP)[58]:

The ICRP has for a number of years called attention to the embryonic and fetal sensitivity to ionizing radiation. The possibility of pregnancy must be taken into account by the attending physician when he is deciding on examinations that involve the lower abdomen and pelvis of women of reproductive capacity. The commision has pointed out that the ten-day interval following the onset of menstruation is the time when it is most improbable that such women could be pregnant. Therefore, it is recommended that all lower-abdomen and pelvic radiological examinations of women of reproductive capacity which are not of importance in connection with the immediate illness of the patient be limited to this period, when pregnancy is improbable. The examinations that will be appropriate to delay until the onset of the next menstruation are the few that could without detriment be postponed until the conclusion of a pregnancy, or at least until its later half.

This recommendation is called the "ten-day rule". Of course, the x-ray examination should be conducted if the health of the mother or the fetus would be compromised by failure to perform the examination when requested. However, every care should be taken, when appropriate, to shield the fetus from the primary beam and from scatter radiation. Table 3 is a list of some x-ray examinations that should be scheduled according to the ten day rule. When the ten day rule cannot be accommodated and the examination is conducted, it should be done with precisely collimated beams and carefully positioned protective shields.

Some radiation scientists do not agree with implementation of the ten day rule though most would agree that it is the safest approach to patient management. The administrative protocols that can be employed to effect the ten day rule vary from simple to complex with the degree of success proportionally observed. There are three levels of administration - elective booking, patient questionnaire and posting. Posting is the easiest and probably the most appropriate control measure in large general hospitals. Directed elective booking is probably only administratively possible in small community hospitals where there is good communication between the clinician and the radiologist.

Table 3. Some x-ray procedures which should require patient scheduling according to the ten-day rule.

Lumbar spine
Pelvis and abdomen
Hip and femur
Urography
Pyelography
Urethrocystography
Pelvimetry
Hysterosalpingography
Barium Enema

PERSONNEL PROTECTIVE MEASURES

The level of radiation exposure received occupationally by radiology workers is exceedingly low. Table 4 summarizes such levels for technologists and radiologists in four Houston hospitals over the past few years. As seen, average occupational exposures are approximately 500 mrem/yr for both radiologists and technologists.

Table 4.
Average occupational exposure (mrem/year) of radiology personnel in four general hospitals in Houston, Texas

	1967-1968	1969-1970	1971-1972	1973-1974	1975-1976	1977-1978	Average
Hospital A							
Radiologists	407	380	590	1138	1143	657	688
Technicians	315	389	334	207	103	965	255
Hospital B							
Radiologists	295	631	864	367	302	282	447
Technicians	170	311	285	361	176	427	280
Hospital C							
Radiologists	790	520	416	457	829	448	553
Technicians	337	603	259	260	266	305	357
Hospital D							
Radiologists	894	2219	1895	616	214	106	954
Technicians	667	957	472	241	57	32	412

Four areas principally contribute to such low occupational radiation exposures in clinical radiology - equipment design, barrier shields, protective apparel and some administrative procedures. Some aspects of equipment design have been discussed in the previous section relating to patient protection. Other aspects are covered very well in documents published by the NCRP[59] and the BRH[60]. The remaining discussion will center on the latter three items.

BARRIER SHIELDS
Fully 95% of all occupational exposure in diagnostic radiology occurs during fluoroscopy and portable radiography. During fixed radiography, personnel are usually provided with fixed barrier shields. Most of our guidance for the fabrication of fixed barrier shields has been developed by the NCRP[61]. However, a number of recent publications[62-66] suggest that some modifications of the NCRP recommendations are in order.

Barrier shields are of two principal types, primary and secondary. A primary barrier is one which is intended to intercept the primary x-ray beam while the secondary barrier is not designed for primary beam attenuation but rather for scatter and leakage radiation. Primary barriers for general purpose radiographic systems will usually require lead as the shielding material. Secondary barriers can often be accommodated by other materials than lead[67-71].

Some specialty facilities such as mammography and dental installations employ low energy x-ray beams and may have very low workloads. This allows the use of conventional shielding materials even for primary barriers. Other facilities, such as CT scan installations, do not generate primary beams since the image receptor always intercepts the useful beam. Furthermore, the x-ray beam is so finely collimated that the intensity of scatter radiation is very low. Conventional building materials can oftentimes be employed in such facilities as these.

Many facility designers now consider the control booth barrier as a secondary barrier, and therefore, prescribe an appropriate thickness of either gypsum board of plate glass as an acceptable protective shield. Studies[72] have shown that never is the useful beam directed at the control booth barrier during normal operation of conventional radiographic installations. Such an approach is often justified by in-room measurements which show the level of scatter radiation on the tube side of the protective console barrier to be extremely low. At a distance of 2 meters from the scattering patient the intensity of radiation is reduced by approximately 6 orders of magnitude which shows that an exceedingly high workload would be required in order to approach the MPB at the operating console position. The smaller the examination room, of course, the more effective the protective shielding is required.

PROTECTIVE APPAREL

Since nearly all occupational exposure is obtained during fluoroscopy and portable radiography, it is essential that protective apparel, lead or lead equivalent aprons and gloves, be used during such procedures. Table 5 shows the attenuation properties of the three thicknesses of protective apparel that are commonly available. Most would recommend the 0.5 mm lead equivalent protective apron as an appropriate compromise.

Table 5 Some physical characteristics of protective lead aprons.

Equivalent thickness (mm Pb)	Weight (pounds)	X-ray attenuation (%) by kVp of operation		
		50 kVp	75 kVp	100 kVp
0.25	3.2 to 9.5	97	66	51
0.50	6.4 to 11.0	99.9	88	75
1.00	12.8 to 22.0	99.9	98.7	94.4

ADMINISTRATIVE PROCEDURES

Attention to the cardinal principals of radiation protection - time, distance and shielding - is probably the most important aspect of the control of occupational radiation exposure in radiology. During fluoroscopy, radiologists are trained to employ minimum beam-on time. This may require sequencing the deadman switch rather than engaging the switch continuously. The principal purpose of the five minute reset timer on the fluoroscope is to emphasize to the radiologist the requirements for maintaining a minimum x-ray beam-on time.

It is often found appropriate to maintain a log of fluoroscopy procedures. This would serve to minimize both occupational exposure and patient exposure. Such an administrative procedure is particularly helpful during special procedures, cardiac catheterizations and C-arm fluoroscopy by orthopedists. Some physicians engaged in these activities are not adequately trained in the area of radiation control and, therefore, the use of a log serves to emphasize this responsibility of theirs. Such a log should contain information for identification such as date, patient's name, physician's name and procedure, and also information for dose identification such as fluoroscopy time and technique and radiographic exposures and technique.

During fluoroscopy the technologist should step back from the examining table when her presence is not absolutely essential. The exposure rate at the side of the examining table is usually in the range of 300-500 mR/hr but by stepping back an additional three feet, one moves to a lower exposure level of perhaps only 50 mR/hr or less.

Portable radiography requires similar precautions. Each portable x-ray machine should have assigned to it a protective apron and the apron should be worn by the technologist when doing portable radiography. The exposure cord on the portable x-ray unit must be at least 6 feet long and the technologist should be instructed never to allow the useful beam to be pointed at the operator.

A particularly important aspect of occupational radiation control is that associated with personnel monitoring. A properly instituted personnel monitoring program provides each occupationally exposed employee with information regarding the effectiveness of their work habits in maintaining a low exposure profile. Collectively, personnel monitoring records can also indicate the nature of the radiation environment and any abrupt changes in the environment brought on by equipment malfunction. Never should personnel radiation monitoring records be used to attempt to predict late radiation effects. Such monitoring is far too imprecise and as indicated by Table 4 above, accumulated radiation exposures are near background levels.

Three types of personnel radiation monitors are available - the pocket dosimeter, the film badge and thermoluminescent dosimeters. The pocket dosimeter is useful for monitoring visitors and temporary employees in radiology but because of some difficulties with charting, analyzing and evaluating the data obtained, they are not recommended for routine personnel monitoring of x-ray workers.

The film badge has been around for four decades and is, indeed, the main stay of most personnel monitoring programs. It may still be the most appropriate monitor for busy radiology departments. However, TLD is rapidly replacing the film badge in many applications. TLD has the distinct advantage over the film badge of being temperature and humidity independent. This allows the TLD monitor to be worn for longer periods of time. Indeed, many x-ray facilities are converting from monthly film badge monitoring to quarterly TLD monitoring. Quarterly monitoring has the distinct advantage of requiring considerably less record keeping activity. For most facilities, quarterly monitoring can be easily justified on the basis of previous radiation exposure histories, identifying those employees who routinely receive less than ¼ of the MPD.

There is one difficulty associated with personnel monitoring that continues controversial - where to wear the personnel monitor. Most would agree that during fluoroscopy and portable radiography, when protective apparel is worn, the personnel radiation monitor should be positioned outside the protective apron at collar level[73-85]. The rationale behind this approach is that when the radiation environment is perturbed by protective apparel, one should monitor that portion of the body suspected of receiving the most limiting percentage of the MPD. The MPD of 5,000 mrem/yr applies not only to the trunk of the body but also to the head and neck, to the lens of the eyes, bone marrow and gonads. If one positions the monitor under the protective apron in order to record the "whole body dose" one can be assured that the exposure reported will be only approximately 5% of that received by the head and neck. In fact, under most circumstances, the reported exposure will be zero or minimal because the protective apparel performs as it is designed and attenuates as much as 95% of the incident radiation.

Others contend that the monitor is a whole body monitor and therefore, should be worn on the trunk of the body[86-89]. Still others[90] suggest that during fluoroscopy and portable radiography two radiation monitors be assigned; one positioned at collar level, the other at waist level. The records keeping aspect of such a program would be questionable and certainly not at all consistent with the additional effort required.

Many states have not developed regulatory codes specifying that the personnel monitoring device be positioned at collar level during fluoroscopy and portable radiography[91]. These states have developed such codes in the face of conflicting advice from the NCRP. For example, two of the more recent NCRP publications recommend that on the one hand, the monitoring device be worn under the protective apron[92] and on the other hand that it should be positioned at the collar level[93-94]. Undoubtedly the debate will continue.

There is one time where it might be appropriate to provide two personnel monitors and that is during pregnancy. If the previous radiation exposure history of a pregnant employee indicates that the abdominal exposure level could approach 500 mrem during the gestational period, a second personnel monitor should be assigned with instructions for positioning at the waist level under the protective apron. This monitor would be identifed as that for providing an estimate of the fetal dose. Of course, a more appropriate approach for pregnant employees is to reassign them to low exposure duties such as fixed radiography, file room and the dark room.

Occupational radiation exposures in diagnostic radiology are exceedingly low. The development and implementation of a quality radiation control program is essential for continuing such low exposures.

REFERENCES

1. Burnett, B.M., "A study of retakes in radiology departments of two large hospitals", HEW Publication (FDA) 77-8020, 1977.
2. Patrylak, J., Applied Radiology, Jan/Feb., 1978.
3. Goldman, L.W., "Analysis of Retakes: Understanding, managing and using an analysis of retakes program for quality assurance", HEW Publication (FDA) 79-8097, 1979.
4. Buchanan, R.A., Radiology 105:185, 1972.
5. Strax, Philip, American Journal of Radiology 117:686, 1973.
6. Jakobsson, S., Acta Radiologica 14(5), 1975.
7. Bailar, John C., Annals of Internal Medicine 84:77, 1976.
8. Feig, Stephen, Applied Radiology, Jan/Feb., 1976.
9. Nathan, B.E., British Journal of Radiology, 49:586, 1976.
10. Feig, S.A., Radiology 122:1, 1977.
11. Culliton, Barbara, Science 196:853, 1977.
12. Letton, A.H., Cancer 40(1), 1977.
13. Gur, David, Radiology 124:261, 1977.
14. Baxt, J.H., Health Physics 30:91, 1976.
15. Carbon/Graphite Composite Material Study, First Annual Report, 1978, Office of Science and Technology policy, 1979.
16. Ingles, W.R., "Diagnostic Radiation Reduction with Graphite", unpublished report, 1979.
17. Buden, E., "Clinical Experience in Radiation Dose Reduction for Diagnostic Radiology Using Carbon Materials for X-Ray Tabletop and Cassette Front", unpublished report, 1979.
18. Eastman, T.R., Radiographic Fundamentals and Technique Guide, C.V. Mosby, Co., 1979.
19. Cahoon, J.B., Duke University Press, 1974.
20. Cullinan, J.E., Illustrated Guide to X-Ray Techniques, J.B. Lippincott Co., 1972.
21. Jacobi, C.A., Laboratory Manual and Workbook in Radiology Technology, C.V. Mosby Co., 1972.
22. Eastman, T.R., Radiol. Tech. 43:80, 1971.
23. Eastman, T.R., Radiol. Tech. 45:75, 1973.
24. Eastman, T.R.,"Technique Charts: the key to radiographic quality" 46:365, 1975.
25. Cassady, J. Robert, BRH/DEP 70-27, Nov., 1970
26. Krohmer, J.S., Radiology 103:447, 1972.
27. Littleton, Jesse, Radiology 129:3, 1978.
28. Bishop, Harry A., California Medicine 90:20, 1959
29. Godderidge, Cecilie, Applied Radiology 3:4, 1979.
30. Brown, Reynold, Radiology 99:2, 1971
31. Magnusson, Wolfgang, Acta Radiol., 37:288, 1952.
32. Fischel, R.E., Acta Radiol., 12:396, 1972.
33. Purdy, J.A., Radiology 117:226, 1975.
34. Hernandez, R., Radiology 28:3, 1978.
35. Specific Area Gonad Shielding, HEW Publication (FDA) 76-8054, 1976.
36. Boucot, Katharine, JAMA 142:1255, 1950.
37. Holmes, E.M., Am. J. Public Health 640, 1951.
38. Anderson, Robert J., J. Chron. Dis. 2:418, 1953.
39. Barry, M., Brit. Med. J. 1:756, 1965.

40. The Chest X-ray As a Screening Procedure for Cardiopulmonary Disease, HEW Publication (FDA) 73-8036, 1973.
41. Kitabatake, Takashi, Radiology 109:37, 1973.
42. Sagel, Stuart, New England Journal of Medicine 291:1001, 1974.
43. Wilkinson, G. Archibald, Applied Radiology, May/June, 1975.
44. Gur, D., Radiology 124(1), 1977.
45. Rothenberg, L.N., Radiology 117(3), 1975.
46. Vandereit, W.G., American Journal of Roentgenology, 128(5), 1977.
47. Buchanan, J.B., Radiology 123(1), 1977.
48. Andersson, I., Acta Radiologica 18(2), 1977.
49. Mintzer, Richard, Invest. Radiol. 12:465, 1977.
50. Karlsson, M., Acta Radiologica 15(3), 1976.
51. Ostrum, Bernard J., Radiology 109:323, 1973.
52. Muntz, E. Phillip, Radiology 127(2), 1978.
53. Muntz, E. Phillip, Med. Phys. 6(3), 1979.
54. Consensus Development Meeting on Breast Cancer Screening, Bethesda, M.D., Sept. 14-16, 1977.
55. Gikley, Anthony, U.D. Dept. of HEW (FDA) Publication.
56. Brown, Reynold F., BRH #223-75-6015, 1977.
57. Brown, R.F., HEW Publication (FDA) 80-8104, 1980.
58. ICRP, Protection of the Patient in X-Ray Diagnosis, #16, 1970.
59. Medical X-Ray and gamma-ray protection for energies up to 10 MeV. NCRP Report No. 33, 1968.
60. Regulations for the Administration and Enforcement of the Radiation Control for Health and Safety Act of 1968. HEW Publication (FDA) 79-8035, 1978.
61. Structural Shielding Design and Evaluation for Medical Use of X-Rays and Gamma-Rays of Energies up to 10 MeV. NCRP Report, No. 49, 1976.
62. Bushong, S.C., Medical Physics 5:319, 1978.
63. Kelley, J.P., Radiology 104:171, 1972.
64. Gifford, D., Brit. J. Radiol., 48:851, 1975.
65. Witcofski, R.L., Radiology 85:1123, 1965.
66. Rummerfield, Philip, Health Physics 35:718, Nov. 1978.
67. Trout, E.D., Radiology 76:237, 1961.
68. Campbell, Earle M., Radiology 107:213, 1973.
69. Christensen, Ralph C., Health Physics 36:69, 1979.
70. Glaze, Sharon A., Health Physics 36:587, 1979.
71. Christensen, R.C., Health Physics 36:595, 1979.
72. Bushong, S.C., Health Physics 35:431, 1978.
73. Bushong, S.C., Radiol. Health Data and Reports 9, 1968.
74. Bushong, S.C., AAPM Q. 2:36, 1968.
75. Riley, Richard C., Radiology 104:679, 1972.
76. Buchan, R.C., Br. J. Radiol. 40:73, 1967.
77. Faw, R., Br. J. Radiol. 51:557, 1978.
78. Herman, M.W., Br. J. Radiol. 51:225, 1978.
79. Buchan, R.C., Br. J. Radiol. 40:238, 1967.
80. Langmead, Walter A., Br. J. Radiol. 45:473, 1972.
81. Malsky, S.J., Radiology 100:671, 1971.
82. Stacey, A.J., Br. J. Radiol. 47:16, 1974.
83. Van Roosenbeek, E., The Radioactive Patient, p. 26, 1975.
84. Bushong, S.C., Health Physics 17:370, 1969.

85. Bushong, S.C., Br. J. Radiol. 42:632, 1969.
86. Jones, D.E.A., Br. J. Radiol. 40:73, 1967.
87. Jones, B.E., Ann. Occupational Hyg., Vol. 4:104, 1961.
88. Langmead, W.A., Br. J. Radiol. 44:480, 1971.
89. Wiatrowski, W.A., Health Physics 38:434, 1980.
90. Jones. B.E., Phys. Med. Biol. 7:439, 1963.
91. NCRC, Proc. 3rd Annual Nat. Conf. on Radiation Control, 1971.
92. National Council on Radiation Protection and Measurement, 1978, NCRP Report 57, 1978.
93. National Council on Radiation Protection and Measurement, 1966. NCRP Report 32, 1966.
94. National Council on Radiation Protection and Measurement, 1976, NCRP Report 48, 1976.

METHODS OF RISK REDUCTION IN NUCLEAR MEDICINE

James G. Kereiakes, Ph.D., Stephen R. Thomas, Ph.D. and Eugene L. Saenger, M.D., Eugene L. Saenger Radioisotope Laboratory, University of Cincinnati College of Medicine, Cincinnati, Ohio

INTRODUCTION

When radioactive materials are employed in a medical installation, four categories of individuals may be exposed to ionizing radiation: a) patients receiving radionuclides for diagnostic or therapeutic purposes; b) volunteers receiving radionuclides for investigational purposes; c) hospital personnel working with radioactive materials; and d) persons exposed to radiation by being close to patients containing radionuclides.

In all groups but the first, there are no health benefits in addition to the risks associated with their radiation exposures. In the case of hospital personnel working with radioactive materials, the benefits are those associated with other occupational exposures plus the additional intangible benefits that accrue by contributing to the public's health. The limits to their exposure are prescribed in NCRP Reports Nos. 39[1] and 48.[2]

This presentation will be primarily concerned with categories a) and c).

PATIENT

Maximizing patient benefit while minimizing patient risk and discomfort is the goal of the decision-making process in choosing a radiopharmaceutical for a given study.

The first issue to be considered in choosing a radiopharmaceutical for a given study is efficacy. Efficacy of radiopharmaceuticals translates into: a) the degree of target (organ, tumor, etc.) to non-target (other tissues or background) accumulation, retention, or release in a fashion that will provide the information required (target/non-target ratio and kinetics of uptake and release); and b) the compatibility of the radiations emitted from the radioactive drugs with the available detection device (detection efficiency and spatial resolution of the device).

Given that the highest degree of efficacy has been established, the second consideration is patient risk. Risks may arise from adverse reaction to the chemical properties of the agent and include direct chemical toxicity of the agent, sepsis due to microbial contamination of the agent, and pyrogenic responses principally due to contamination of the product with certain microbial byproducts. However, in general, the most significant patient risk relates to the absorbed radiation dose received.

The question of patient discomfort and economic cost must also be considered. Patient inconvenience may arise if the radiopharmaceutical is not available due to production or shipping problems.

The question of patient cost is complex and should not be limited to cost of the radiopharmaceutical drug. Use of an expensive agent that is readily available and hence reduces patient time in the hospital or which requires less expensive equipment may result in a lower cost of the study to the patient than the use of a less expensive agent. Since the cost of the radiopharmaceutical is usually a small part of the procedure cost, it is difficult to justify not using new or improved agents which increase patient benefit and decrease patient risks simply because they cost more than the commonly used agents. An additional consideration, which limits the choice of radiopharmaceuticals for clinical use, is the state of licensing or approval by governmental agencies of new agents. Table 1 provides a partial list of methods of risk reduction for the patient in nuclear medicine.

Table 1. FACTORS ASSOCIATED WITH RISK REDUCTION IN NUCLEAR MEDICINE

A. Requirements of Radiopharmaceutical
    1. Radionuclide identity, content and purity
    2. Radiochemical identity and purity
    3. Content and toxicity of non-radioactive constituents
    4. In-vivo distribution behavior
    5. General safety
    6. Sterlity and apyrogenecity
B. Misadministration of Radiopharmaceutical
C. Radiation Dose
D. Quality Control of Instruments
F. Efficacy Studies

REQUIREMENTS OF RADIOPHARMACEUTICAL FOR USE IN HUMANS

Radionuclide Identity, Content, and Purity

The identity and content of the radionuclide as well as the identity and content of contamination radionuclides must be known prior to administration of a drug to a patient. Where possible, quality assurance data should be verified in the nuclear medicine laboratory and absolute reliance on the primary supplier should not be assumed. Once radionuclide identity and purity have been checked, the activity of the radionuclide present (in the absence of significant radiocontaminants) can be checked by use of calibrated ionization chambers.

Radiochemical Identity and Purity

The chemical identity of radiolabeled agents administered to a human or animal subject should be known and the presence of all chemical forms of the radionuclide other than that which is desired (radiochemical purity) must be assessed. Even when the drug is purchased in final dosage form, the nuclear medicine laboratory should use the best techniques available to verify the radiochemical identity and purity of each material.

Content and Toxicity of Non-Radioactive Constituents

Some radionuclides produced by the (n,γ) reaction contain variable quantities of carrier of the element from which the radionuclide was produced. Similarly, non-radioactive elements may contaminate a radionuclide after their introduction during target processing or radionuclide purification. These non-radioactive constituents must be evaluated relative to potential toxicity and their content in the final product minimized.

In Vivo Distribution Behavior

The single most important quality of a radiopharmaceutical is that it behave in a predictable way _in vivo_. Measurements of _in vivo_ distribution of a radiopharmaceutical in a suitable animal model is essential. Such studies need to be performed prior to qualifying a radiopharmaceutical for use in man.

When basic research justifies evaluation of safety and efficacy of a radiopharmaceutical for purposes of possible clinical use, an Investigative New Drug Application (IND) must be filed with the FDA. Under an IND, a small number of patients should be studied intensively to establish the pharmacology and kinetics of the radioactive drug (phase I studies); followed by an expanded but controlled clinical study to establish safety and indications for use (phase II); typically followed by a larger, less well controlled clinical study to establish a broader basis for evaluating safety and efficacy (phase III).

A New Drug Application (NDA) must be filed with the FDA by the manufacturer if a radiopharmaceutical is intended for (1) widespread use by many clinicians or (2) its use is to be promoted or (3) it is intended for sale. It is required that a thorough review of all the preclinical and clinical data obtained during the IND phase of the agent's development be included in the NDA. Such data are the basis for establishing the safety and efficacy of the agent for use in humans.

General Safety

"General safety" of an agent is evaluated by administering very large doses of the material intended for human use to a normal animal (10-100 times the amount used in man in $\mu Ci/kgm$) and observing the animal over a period of time to determine whether the animal becomes sick or dies. Such "general safety" tests do provide some protection against the introduction of non-specific toxic materials that may not be detected in tests for specific anticipated contaminants.

Sterility and Apyrogenicity

Sterility must be assured for all agents intended for parenteral administration. It is achieved through filtration, chemical treatment, exposure to high intensity radiation fluxes of appropriate wavelength or through a combination of heat and pressure. Sterility is evaluated by testing for the presence of viable organisms. Pyrogenic reactions are rare to non-existent in most present day radiopharmaceutical products. Some reactions have been recorded after administration of radiopharmaceuticals by inhalation, after intrathecal injection of radiolabeled human serum albumin, and after intravenous injection of radiopharmaceuticals containing gelatin. It is doubtful, however, that significant patient reactions have occurred due to the presence of pyrogens in radiopharmaceutical products, as reported reactions are not attributed to pyrogens. Nevertheless, governmental regulations require pyrogen testing for many radiopharmaceuticals and the testing procedure to be employed is rigidly defined in terms of sex, weight, species, and management of the animal to be used in the test.

MISADMINISTRATION

In spite of considerable attention to the choice of a radiopharmaceutical, the final agent chosen may be misadministered and such misadministration may prove to be harmful to the patient.

One consequence related to misadministration of a radiopharmaceutical is radiation injury. There are no truly established medical protocols for its therapy, nor are there NDA-approved, commercially available therapeutic agents for such application. The need for prompt initiation of treatment requires the physician to be familiar with the general principles of such therapy.

Some guidance is provided in a forthcoming NCRP Report on the Procedures for the Management of Contaminated Persons.[3] Techniques are described for reducing the biological effects of administered radioactivity, including (1) increasing the rate of excretion; (2) altering the pattern of biological distribution; and (3) interfering with damage to radiosensitive molecules by the use of radiation protection compounds.

Misadministration reporting requirements (NRC) are to become effective November 11, 1980 (Federal Register, Vol. 45, No. 95, p. 31701).

RADIATION DOSE

With any _in vivo_ radiopharmaceutical procedure, considerations involving the ratio of diagnostic benefit to radiation risk are of concern. In recent years considerable effort has been expended toward the end of quantitating the long-term risks associated with radiation exposure; namely, in determination of the probability of developing benign or malignant disease as a function of time following a given radiation exposure.[4,5] Ideally, the studies have consisted of careful followup on groups of exposed individuals for which reasonably accurate dosimetry data exists. Specific types of disease may be followed, for example, leukemia or thyroid cancer. In most cases where correlations appear, the effects can be adequately described by a linear or quadratic dependence on dose. For these reasons, it is of course desirable to maintain the associated radiation dose to the patient as low as possible during diagnostic procedures.

The radioactive compound with optimal radiological and biological properties should be used for each study, the radioactive half-life of the tracer should approximately equal the time interval between injection and completion of study, and the measurement instrument should have the sensitivity and resolution appropriate to the diagnostic problem. The time used for the study represents a compromise between the time available, based largely on patient condition, and unusual factors relating to the amount of tracer that can be administered. Excretion of the tracer should be promoted when the study is completed or when retention, such as in the urinary bladder, is not a desired part of the study.

Desirable physical characteristics of a radionuclide are given in Table 2.

A review of these characteristics clearly indicate why ^{99m}Tc is so widely used (in approximately 85-90% of all radionuclide procedures in nuclear medicine). Also evident would be the reasons for recommending replacement of ^{131}I by ^{123}I with its more desirable characteristics for diagnostic procedures.

Table 2. DESIRABLE CHARACTERISTICS OF RADIONUCLIDE

1. Organ specific or chemically active
2. Photon decay
3. No alpha or beta decay
4. Short half-life (comparable to study time)
5. Gamma energy $80 \leq E \leq 200$ keV
6. Carrier free
7. Availability

As discussed earlier, the radiation dose depends upon the physical parameters of each radionuclide, the fraction of energy emitted that is absorbed in the tissue of interest, and the biological distribution and retention of the radionuclide. Physical data for most radionuclides are available in the literature, and from these data the fraction of available energy absorbed in various organs can be determined mathematically for defined geometrical shapes and configurations. The reduction in patient dose for ^{123}I (approximately 100 times) based purely on the physical characteristics of the radionuclide, are clearly indicated in Table 3.

Table 3. THYROID DOSES IN PATIENTS OF VARIOUS AGE GROUPS
(rad/υCi, administered)[6]

Radionuclide	Newborn	1 yr	5 yr	10 yr	15 yr	Adult
^{131}I	11.8	8.1	3.8	2.2	1.5	1.1
^{123}I	0.119	0.081	0.038	0.022	0.016	0.011

For an uptake study, 10 μCi of Iodine-123 will give the adult thyroid an absorbed radiation dose of 0.11 rad while 10 μCi of Iodine-131 will give a thyroid dose of about 11 rad. The thyroid of a 5 yr old would receive 0.19 rad (^{123}I) and 19 rad (^{131}I) for an administered activity of 5 μCi.

Use of ^{123}I, wherever possible and particularly for thyroid studies, definitely serves to reduce risk in clinical nuclear medicine, particularly for pediatric patients. In thyroid uptake studies, further dose reduction is accomplished by using a dual-crystal detection technique in contact with the neck[7] instead of the single straight crystal technique at 10 in distance(which would allow reduction of the administered activity). Patient doses from typically administered activities for other radiopharmaceuticals are given in Table 4.

Table 4. TYPICAL PATIENT DOSES[8]

$\leq$ 1 rad

bone imaging	-	^{99m}Tc-polyphosphate
renal studies	-	^{99m}Tc-DTPA
	-	^{131}I-hippuran
lung imaging	-	^{99m}Tc-MAA
liver imaging	-	^{99m}Tc-sulfur colloid
blood pool imaging	-	^{99m}Tc-HSA
thyroid imaging	-	^{99m}Tc-pertechnetate

1-3 rad

kidney imaging	-	^{99m}Tc-iron comples
lung imaging	-	^{113m}In-iron hydroxide
		^{131}I-MAA
liver imaging	-	^{113m}I-colloid
tumor imaging	-	^{67}Ga-citrate
brain imaging	-	^{99m}Tc-pertechanetate
thyroid imaging	-	^{123}I-iodide

$\geq$ 3 rad

blood pool studies	-	^{131}I-HSA
thyroid studies	-	^{131}I and ^{125}I-iodide
brain imaging	-	^{113m}In-DTPA

In nuclear medicine procedures, whole body doses are usually higher than in plain radiographic examinations but are generally less than 0.2 rad. Substantially higher whole body doses in the range of 0.5 to 1 rad are delivered in the following procedures: tumor scanning with ^{67}Ga-citrate and blood pool imaging with ^{131}I-HSA.[8]

Radiation doses received by children are somewhat higher. Common practice is to determine the amount of radioactivity to be administered to a child by multiplying the quantity of radioactive material given to the adult by the ratio of the child's body weight to the adult's weight. The assumption is that the radiation dose to the child will be the same as that estimated for the adult because the concentration of the radionuclide in the organ will be approximately the same. This is not entirely true, however, as the ratio of organ weights may not be the same as the ratio of body weights. Furthermore, the shape of the child's organs may differ from that of the adult and other parameters such as the uptake may be changed. For typically administered activities for the age groups considered, Table 5 provides estimated gonadal doses for both females and males. For the adult, these values appear to be less than 0.5 rad for the scan procedures and radiopharmaceuticals. Estimated doses up to about 1 rad are seen for the younger age groups for ^{99m}Tc-phosphate and ^{99m}Tc-albumin.

Table 5. ESTIMATED GONADAL DOSES FROM SELECTED RADIOPHARMACEUTICALS

Study	Radio-pharmaceutical	Gonads	Gonadal Dose (rad)		
			5 yr	10 yr	adult
bone	^{99m}Tc-phosphate	M	0.724 (3.5)*	1.122 (6.0)*	0.408 (12.0)*
		F	0.403	0.493	0.552
brain	^{99m}Tc-pertechnetate	M	0.219 (3.0)	0.330 (5.0)	0.120 (10.0)
		F	0.135	0.160	0.180
cardiac	^{99m}Tc-albumin	M	0.732 (3.0)	1.100 (5.0)	0.400 (10.0)
		F	0.405	0.485	0.540
kidney	^{99m}Tc-DTPA	M	0.366 (3.0)	0.550 (5.0)	0.140 (7.0)
		F	0.204	0.245	0.189
liver	^{99m}Tc-sulfur colloid	M	0.116 (1.0)	0.156 (1.5)	0.038 (2.0)
		F	0.058	0.062	0.046
lung	^{99m}Tc-MAA	M	0.043 (1.0)	0.057 (1.5)	0.014 (2.0)
		F	0.022	0.024	0.018
thyroid	^{123}I-iodide	M	0.003 (.050)	0.004 (.075)	0.001 (0.1)
		F	0.003	0.003	0.002

*numbers in parenthesis indicate administered activity in mCi

An area of considerable importance in the situation where a pregnant patient has been administered a radiopharmaceutical, is the dose received by the embyro. Table 6 provides an estimated dose to the embyro for scan procedures involving the radiopharmaceuticals listed.

Table 6. ESTIMATED DOSES TO EMBRYO FROM RADIOPHARMACEUTICALS

Radiopharmaceutical	Administered Activity	Estimated Dose To Embryo (rad)
^{99m}Tc-glucoheptonate	3 mCi	0.120
^{99m}Tc-human serum albumin	10 mCi	0.180
^{99m}Tc-macroaggregates	2 mCi	0.070
^{99m}Tc-pertechetate	10 mCi	0.370
^{99m}Tc-polyphosphate	12 mCi	0.432
^{99m}Tc-sulfur colloid	2 mCi	0.064
^{123}I-iodide	100 µCi	0.003
^{131}I-iodide	100 µCi	0.010

For the typically administered activities, doses appear to be less than 0.5 rad (this depends not only on the radiopharmaceutical that is received but also on the stage of pregnancy, particularly where Iodine-131 may be concerned and where incorporation of the radioactive iodine in the thyroid gland of the embyro is a possibility). The thyroid in the embryo starts to form on the eleventh day of pregnancy. However, it is not until the eleventh week that it begins functioning with uptake of iodine. On the eleventh day primitive placenta blood circulation begins.

Particular care should be taken in performing clinical studies involving radioiodine during the second and third trimester of pregnancy (where doses to the thyroid of the fetus may be order of 6-8 rads/µCi of ^{131}I ingested by the mother [9]).

Another factor is whether the mother has a functioning thyroid gland. With no thyroid function, it has been estimated that the dose to the embryo may be about 1.4 times greater than for a mother with euthyroid uptake (about 25%), because of the greater amount of circulating radioiodine.[10]

Much of the biological information needed for dose calculations is inadequate or non-existent. When the literature data are unavailable or unreliable, conservative dose estimates are in order. For radionuclides with short physical half-lives, the retention time in the organ is often assumed to equal the physical half-life. For radionuclides with long physical half-lives, this assumption can result in large overestimates. The fraction of activity contained in an organ is generally estimated from quantitative observations, but if no quantitative information is available, a "best guess" is made. The radiation dose estimates from newly available radiolabeled materials often serve only as crude estimates of the radiation dose to a "standard patient" rather than being estimates of dose to a particular patient.

Therefore, a definite consideration for reduction of risks in nuclear medicine is a better estimate of radiation dose received by patients (particularly pediatric patients) from clinical nuclear medicine procedures. In addition for certain radiopharmaceuticals, such as ^{67}Ga-citrate (which is known for its high degree of nonspecificity in tissue localization), the critical organ may not necessarily be the target organ. It is extremely important that studies providing measured biological information be expanded (again, particularly for pediatric patients). In the recent data involving the administration of ^{67}Ga-citrate for tumor and/or abscess studies in 9 children aged 1.8 to 17.5 years, the critical organ was the metaphyseal growth complex (mean dose - 9.1 rad) as compared to the target organs, liver (mean dose 3.2 rad) and spleen (mean dose - 5.0 rad).[11]

The amount of radioactivity in the organ influences not only the radiation dose received by the patient but also the information content of the study. Radiopharmaceuticals to be used in vivo for diagnostic purposes should maximize the number of detected photons for a given (acceptable) absorbed radiation dose to the patient. For example, the important factors in comparative localization studies are: the difference in activity between the lesion and its background; the amount of activity in the lesion and its background; and the energy of the photopeak as a determinant of the measured contrast for lesions from different depths. For example, consider scanning the liver with sulfur colloid tagged with a formerly used radionuclide (^{198}Au) and presently used radionuclides ^{113m}In and ^{99m}Tc. For a 1500 gram liver, the administered activity to provide an absorbed dose of 1 rad is 19.4 μCi (^{198}Au), 1360 μCi (^{113m}In) and 2170 μCi (^{99m}Tc). Assume that the ratio of activity in the normal liver and the lesion is 10 to 1 for all of these agents. An intrinsic figure of merit (FOM) can be defined for the radiopharmaceuticals which is independent of the geometry of the lesion and surrounding tissues. If the size, shape, and location of the lesion and the consequent effects of attenuation are taken into account, Beck[12] has derived an effective object (FOM). See Table 4 for these values. Based on the figure of merit calculations, the favored radiopharmaceutical for the detection of a liver metastasis would be technetium sulfur colloid. The near infinite biological half-time in the liver of radiocolloids simplifies this choice. Where different rates of excretion occur in normal disease subjects, biological factors must be considered along with physical factors.

However, in order to completely evaluate the entire procedure, the sensitivity and resulotion of the detector system must also be incorporated into the considerations. Table 7 gives the overall FOM for gold colloid, indium hydroxide and technetium sulfur colloid for a liver lesion at different depths for an Anger scintillation camera. The advantage of the technetium sulfur colloid vs the indium and gold colloid derives not from a more favorable target-to-nontarget distribution but rather from the fact that ^{99m}Tc yields a greater number of counts over the normal liver than ^{198}Au per unit of absorbed dose. Also, with regard to the camera, the thin crystal of the camera is more efficient for the 140 keV gamma rays of ^{99m}Tc then for the higher energy gammas of the other two radionuclides. The energy resolution for the ^{198}Au and the ^{113m}In gamma rays permits a better separation of scattered and unscattered photons than for ^{99m}Tc. However, this effect is offset in part by the improved collimation achieved for the 140 keV photons due to decreased septal penetration and increased sensitivity. The above example is illustrative of the selection of a suitable radionuclide as a method of risk reduction in nuclear medicine. However, the example also illustrates the importance of the instrumentation as part of the selection process. The above formulation, based primarily on physical and biological factors, still does not take into account the quantitative visual response of the human observer. Implications for observer performance should also be considered.

Table 7. FIGURES OF MERIT (FOM) FOR LIVER LESIONS CONTAINING ^{198}Au, ^{113m}In or ^{99m}Tc

Radio-nuclide	Effective FOM			Overall FOM		
	surface	1 inch	3 inch	surface	1 inch	3 inch
^{198}Au	0.58	0.46	0.17	0.092	0.11	0.11
^{113m}In	29.0	23.0	7.7	71.0	17.0	8.0
^{99m}Tc	72.0	51.0	12.0	540.0	172.0	42.0

*adapted from reference[13].
[1500 g liver phantom (8 inches thick), 1 inch lesion, with lesion-to-surrounding activity of 10:1]

QUALITY CONTROL OF INSTRUMENTS

The routine monitoring of nuclear medicine instruments, using test procedures that provide a check of the quality and reproducibility of the instruments' performance, is an essential method of risk reduction in any clinical nuclear medicine program. The aim of this monitoring effort is to give the user confidence that the data collected will be relative free of variations caused by fluctuations, or drifts, in the operating characteristics of the instrument. Various accrediting agencies (for example, the Joint Commission of Accreditation of Hospitals, the Social Security Administration Medicare Providers Standards, etc.) and Regulatory Agencies (for example, The Nuclear Regulatory Commission) have recognized the importance of quality control efforts by requiring that a testing procedure be performed and recorded regularly for accreditation or licensing of nuclear medicine services.

Radionuclide Calibrator

If certain tests - such as linearity of response, accuracy (using a certified calibration standard) and geometry effects are performed initially and annually - a calibrator can be used confidently to obtain direct assays of radiopharmaceuticals prior to patient administration.

In addition, before each daily use of the instrument, test of the repeatability of response should be made. Reading variations should be within the manufacturer's specification for repeatability, i.e., ± 2 to 5 per cent, for most calibrators using specified radionuclides. Long-lived reference sources, preferably having energy emission and activity ranges representative of the radionuclide used clinically are commonly used. Sources should be solid or gel form to minimize contamination potential and inadvertent withdrawal for other uses.

Non-Imaging Systems

For well scintillation counters, the repeatability of the instrument can be ascertained in a manner similar to the procedure described for radionuclide type calibrators, by using a long-lived source simulating the actual radionuclides used and using the source in a constant geometry. For uptake probes, a source holder (as shown in Figure 1) providing a reproducible geometry for checking the repeatability of the instrument can be used.[14] This arrangement would also check as to whether the instrument settings such as the high voltage, amplifier again, window setting, etc., have been properly set.

Rectilinear Scanners

For a daily check of the repeatability of this instrument, the same check source and geometry, as described for the uptake probe, can be used. The check source is mounted at the focal plane of the collimator and remains at this position when performing the sensitivity checks. In addition, rectilinear scanner should include film density calibration (weekly), contrast enhancement (monthly), and collimator evaluation (initially and annually).

Scintillation Camera

In addition to the initial acceptance testing procedures and certain procedures (such as pulse analyzer check, Chi-square analysis, energy calibration, energy resolution, linearity, and count rate effects) performed on a less frequent basis, a performance check of the following parameters (which may cause significant degradation in the quality of the scintillation camera images) should be performed on a daily basis: 1) Uniformity - a check to determine the deviation from uniform count density across the field of view of the camera of less than ± 6 to 7 per cent; 2) Spatial Distortion - the ability of the instrument to reproduce linear sources of radioactivity in a manner which conserves all spatial and geometric relationships; and 3) Resolving Power - the ability of the imaging device to produce and display images, discernible

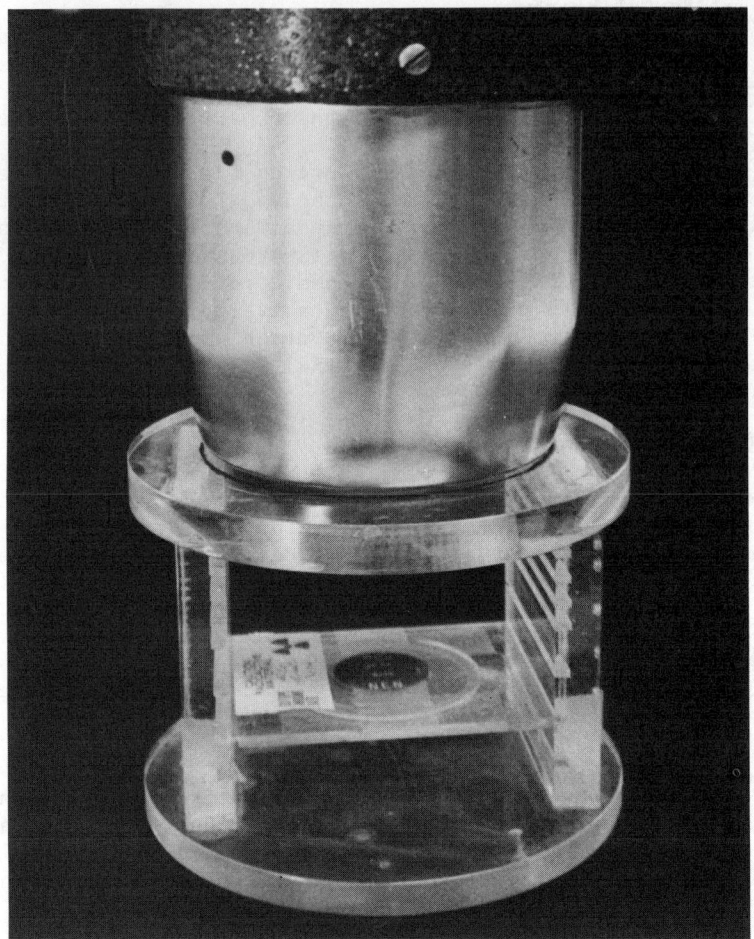

Figure 1. Arrangement for daily sensitivity check of uptake probe.[3]

as separate entities, from an array of radioactive source. The use of a flood source consisting of 2 to 5 mCi of ^{57}Co in gel form is useful for the uniformity check. A bar phantom (consisting of parallel lead bars of width and spacing compatible with the resolution of the camera and embedded in a plastic fixture) along with the flood source is useful for checking the linearity and resolving power.

EFFICACY STUDIES

Questions about the efficacy of a diagnostic test include among other things, the following: a) does the test lead to improved information about the patient with which the physician can reduce

the uncertainty of diagnosis of the disease and b) how does the
information obtained using radiopharmaceuticals compare with the
information provided by other diagnostic modalities.

Improved Radiopharmaceutical

The technetium labeled phosphonates lend themselves to many
possibilities for altering their structure to improve their bone
imaging capabilities. Several improvements have been made with
the most recent being HMDP (hydrophymethylene diphosphate) which
has been synthesized with the hydroxyl group retained in a single
carbon disphosphonate. In a comparative clinical study, ^{99m}Tc-HMDP
was found to be superior to ^{99m}Tc-HEDP (hydroxyethylene disphosphonate) as a bone scanning agent documenting more rapid blood clearance,
significantly better bone delineation, lower soft tissue background
and overall quality. The per cent tag with ^{99m}Tc-HMDP always
exceeded 90%.[15]

However, a clinical comparison between this same agent,
^{99m}Tc-HMDP, and ^{99m}Tc-PPi (pyrophosphate) for myocardial infarction
indicated that ^{99m}Tc-PPl not only has a superior sensitivity for
acute myocardial infarction but also a significantly increased intensity of uptake in positive areas. Thus ^{99m}Tc-PPi remains the
agent of choice for myocardial infarct imaging.[16]

These types of comparative studies serve to determine which
agent provides improved information for the diagnosis of a specific disease.

Comparison With Other Modality

Several comparative studies are currently in progress to ascertain which diagnostic modality (such as computed tomography,
ultrasound, or radiopharmaceuticals) provide more meaningful information for diagnosis of patient disease. In one such study, for
example, one hundred forty-one patients with cerebral or cerebellar
infarction were examined by x-ray computed tomography (XCT) as soon
after the ictus as possible. The examination was repeated in 7 days,
and a radionuclide scan was performed. The major value of XCT in
the evaluation of the stroke patient is that the examination can re-
liably and without delay detect an intraparenchymal hemorrhage and
can, in many instances, easily differentiate vascular from non-
vascular intracranial lesions. These characteristics, when compared with lack of specificity and the latency of radionuclide scan,
indicate that XCT is the preferred technique for noninvasive
investigation of acute stroke.[17]

SUMMARY

Nuclear medicine is a medical specialty in which new procedures,
instruments, and radiopharmaceuticals are being introduced at a
rapid pace. Guidelines are intended to present principles that may
be utilized over a long period of time, whereas, recommendations
need to be updated more frequently. Based on current knowledge, the
following is indicated:

General Recommendation

The main principle guiding investigations of patients is that the amount of radioactivity administered should be the minimum consistent with adequate information from the diagnostic procedure being performed. This will ensure that the minimum radiation dose is delivered to the patient.

Adult Patients

Experience has shown that most diagnostic tests can be carried out successfully with amounts of radioactivity that give rise in adult patients to organ doses of about 1 rad, and usually not greater than 5 rad, per investigation. However, the value of the test to the patient's well-being and/or the seriousness of the disease being investigated may often outweigh possible long-term radiological hazards. In the latter case, a higher administered activity may be acceptable.

Pediatric Patients

The activities to be administered may be calculated approximately by adjusting the activity given to adults on a weight or body surface area basis so that the normalized activity administered is comparable. In general, the doses to the organs should be of the same order as or if possible less than those received by adults during the same procedure to hold to a minimum the hazard of somatic effects of ionizing radiation. Particular care is required to ensure that the radiation doses received by the gonads are as low as possible in view of the possibility of damaging the genetic material in the germinal epithelium of the children.

Because of high radiation dose, ^{131}I should not be used for routine thyroid function testing in children. Similarly, in children suspected of enzymatic defects in iodine metabolism, or in whom estimates of regional thyroid function are needed, studies of uptake and turnover of radioiodine may be indicated. In such circumstances, the radionuclide of iodine, or analogs used, should give the minimal radiation exposure.

Pregnant Women

Investigations carried out on pregnant women often involve radiation doses to both the mother and the fetus. Consideration must be given to the amount of radiation as well as the quantity of radioactivity transmitted across the placenta and to the resulting fetal uptake. In view of the findings summarized in NCRP Reports 39[1] and 54[18] relating to radiation protection of the fetus and the fact that radiation doses of the order of a few rads may be associated with an increased incidence of leukemia and childhood malignancies, it is important to keep the fetal doses below these levels and to carry out only such investigations as are imperative during pregnancy.

Elective procedures, especially those involving radiation doses in excess of 0.5 rad (whole body dose) or with agents having a propensity for localization in the conceptus, e.g., radioiron incorporated in erythropoietic cells of the fetus and colloids that concentrate in reticuloendothelial cells of the placenta, should be avoided whenever possible during pregnancy.

The whole body dose delivered to the fetus in placental imaging studies is 100 to 200 times lower than that delivered in conventional obstetric radiography and pelvimetry. Next to ultrasound, radionuclide techniques appear to provide the method of choice for placentography.[8]

Therapeutic Studies

Therapeutic studies with radioactive drugs should be avoided during pregnancy unless abortion of the pregnancy is planned. In order to minimize the possibility of genetic hazards after radiation therapy of non-pregnant females in the child bearing years, the patient should be advised to postpone possible pregnancies for at least several months to permit such repair to genetic damage as may have occurred.

Use of New Agents

Physicians are encouraged to utilize new nuclides, when they become available, which provide improved image quality and which result in lower radiation doses or decreased examination times. Old agents that result in higher radiation doses than new tracers should be replaced by the newer agents as soon as their effectiveness is demonstrated and problems in instrumentation and availability are solved. When new tests providing equivalent or superior diagnostic information and lower radiation exposures become available, they should be adopted, and the older test discontinued.

PERSONNEL

During the period of growth of nuclear medicine, ^{99m}Tc has become the predominant radionuclide used in approximately 85-90% of all administered radionuclides. It is significant that, due to the lower patient exposure resulting from the use of ^{99m}Tc as compared with most other radionuclides, the quantity injected per procedure has changed from typical quantities of tens of μCi's to tens of mCi's. As a result, the potential exposure of nuclear medicine personnel has increased due to the usage of ^{99m}Tc. Considering all aspects, handling the larger quantities of ^{99m}Tc has also resulted in additional requirements for shielding facilities (see Figure 2)[19], also for additional personnel monitoring devices such as finger badges and wrist badges in addition to the normally used whole body badges. Methods of risk reduction to personnel definitely include the routine use of these devices.

An understanding of how radiation exposure occurs is basic to the success of efforts to achieve lower personnel exposures. Most nuclear medicine personnel believe they receive most of their radiation exposure from elution. However, these materials should always be shielded and

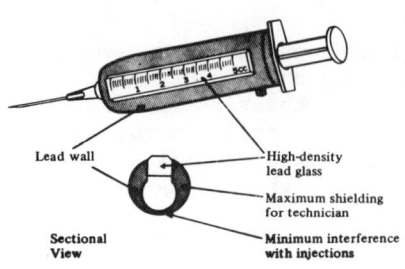
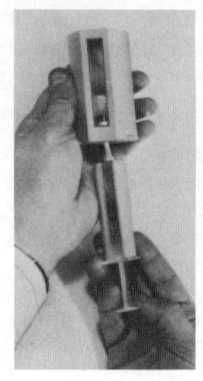
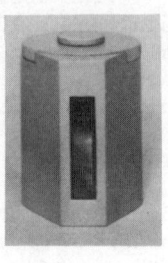

Syringe Shield

Vial Shield

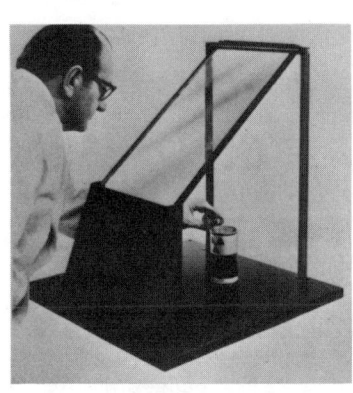
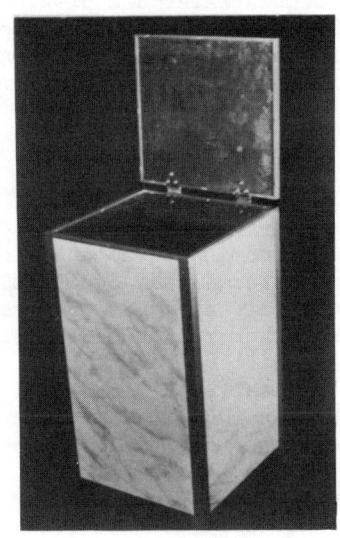

Work Shield **Waste Shield**

Figure 2. Practical Lead Shielding for a Nuclear Medicine Laboratory (adapted from reference 19).

when this simple precaution is taken the exposure to the handler
is very low. In analyzing the ways in which nuclear medicine
personnel are exposed to radiation while performing various procedures, it is convenient to determine the amount of exposure in
three broad categories: dose preparation and assay, injection and
imaging. The results of studies for some common clinical nuclear
medicine procedures are tabulated in Table 8. The data are for
procedures of average difficulty on typical adult patients. Syringe
shields were used when performing injections.

In addition some of the generators presently in use contain
Curie amounts of radionuclides and should be properly shielded for
the safety of nuclear medicine personnel.

The significant difference in total exposure from bone scans
obtained with a rectilinear scanner as compared with a camera (0.09
vs 0.57 mR) is an interesting example of specific equipment affecting radiation exposure. The additional exposure results primarily
from the large distance from patient to console (where the technologist spends most of the time), in the case of the scanner, compared to the short distance from the patient - while frequently
repositioning the patient and camera in obtaining a series of views
to cover the whole body using the camera.

Table 8. TYPICAL EXPOSURE TO PERSONNEL FROM SELECTED PROCEDURES[19]

Procedure	Typical Activity Injected (mCi ^{99m}Tc)	Typical Exposure at Body Position mR			TOTAL	% of Exposure from Imaging
		Dose Preparation & Assay	Injection	Imaging		
Brain	20	0.04	0.02	0.22	0.28	79
Cerebral Blood Flow	20	0.04	0.02	0.03	0.09	33
CBF & Brain	20	0.04	0.02	0.25	0.31	81
Liver & Spleen	4	0.01	0.01	0.03	0.05	60
Bone Scan (Rectilinear Scanner)	15	0.02	0.01	0.06	0.09	67
Bone Scan (Camera)	15	0.02	0.01	0.54	0.57	95
Thyroid	2	0.02	0.01	0.04	0.07	57
Myocardium	15	0.01	0.01	0.02	0.04	50
Angio	10	0.02	0.01	0.04	0.07	57

In the last column of Table 8 the percentage of exposure from
imaging is listed. Generally, these data reveal that for most of
the procedures the exposure from imaging is a major fraction of the
exposure from the entire procedure. The exception is the cerebral

blood flow study. The imaging for a cerebral blood flow study usually requires only a few minutes.

To evaluate the exposure rate from handling unshielded material versus use of a syringe shield, measurements (using thermoluminescent dosimeters) were made with a hand-simulated arrangement. The results of measurements (for 20 mCi ^{99m}Tc) are given in Table 9.

These measurements indicate that the exposure rate at the highest point (immediately adjacent to the liquid) is 22,000 mR/h from 20 mCi in a 2 cc volume. The measurements were designed to provide information on the relationship between the dose at the most exposed point and other locations on the fingers where a "ring" badge may be worn. These measurements indicate that the most exposed point, tip of index finger, received 156 times more exposure than at back of ring finger, typical ring position. Thus, if a ring badge is worn on the ring finger facing the back of the hand, the radiation exposure to the most exposed point on the fingers could be as much as 156 times greater. This correction of ring badge results should be considered when personnel monitoring results are reviewed. Because of these considerations, in many laboratories, the ring badges are worn on the index finger facing in toward the thumb whenever that location would not interfere with required assignments. When the dosimeter is worn on the index finger, the finger tip exposure may still be underestimated by a factor of 20 to 55 depending on location and whether or not a syringe shield is used.

Devices and Techniques for Reducing Radiation Exposure

In general, one should avoid all unnecessary exposures to radiation. The time-honored advice in this regard is to control exposure time, distance and shielding. The control of exposure time may be very important in reducing exposure of nuclear medicine personnel to ^{99m}Tc radiations. This is particularly true if shielding is neglected. By thoughtful planning of techniques and procedures, it is sometimes possible to reduce markedly the exposure of laboratory personnel. The termination of exposure time may often be achieved by interposing shielding between the source and potential exposee; the use of syringe shields will materially reduce exposure to the finger tips of those who fill syringes or perform injections. A point which is often not fully appreciated is that unshielded syringes may also contribute significantly to exposure of the whole body. When good practice is followed, a vial of the ^{99m}Tc solution will reside in a lead shield and be drawn directly into the shield syringe (see Figure 2). When working with special preparations or for other reasons handling ^{99m}Tc, a shielded work station should be used (see Figure 2). A shielded waste container should be provided in each room where radioactive materials are prepared or injected. Ideally, a shield such as that shown in Figure 2 should be used which shields the radiation in all directions and which contains a plastic lined cardboard waste box, which is simply closed and sealed until transferred to an authorized

Table 9. EXPOSURE RATE TO THE HAND FROM 20 mCi ^{99m}Tc (2 cc Volume)[19]

Position	Exposure Rate (mR/hr)	Shielded (Syringe Shield) Exposure Rate (mR/hr)	Shielded Factor Unshielded/Shielded
tip of thumb	170	110	1.5
tip of index finger	22,000	330	67
tip of 2nd finger	12,000	93	129
center of index finger	1,000	7	157
base of index finger	390	14	28
base of 2nd finger	430	20	22
base of ring finger	160	16	10
4th finger	90	12	7.8
back of ring finger	140	39	3.6
palm	130	8	16
back of palm	52	4	13
wrist	9	1	9.0
back of wrist	9	2	4.5

radioactive waste receiver with minimal handling. This helps reduce the possibility of bacterial contamination, puncture wounds from hypodermic needles and contamination with radioactive materials.

Particular attention should always be given to shielding around primary stock containers of radionuclides, including ^{99}Mo - ^{99m}Tc systems. It must be emphasized that the exposure rates which are permitted for shipments in transit are not suitable for long-term exposure to personnel. It was shown earlier that when good general radiation safety practices are employed regarding shielding, etc., a major portion of the exposure of nuclear medicine personnel occurs during imaging procedures. In some cases, exposure time during imaging may be reduced by selection of equipment which requires less time. The distance from patient to attending personnel can often be increased without detriment to patient care. Another technique which can sometimes be employed is to place a lead apron over the abdominal area to shield radiation which originates in the bladder or nearby organs. There are two thicknesses of lead apron commonly available: 0.25 mm lead equivalent and 0.5 mm lead equivalent. These thicknesses of lead reduce exposure by a factor of 2, or a factor of 4, respectively. Also portable shields are used in some nuclear medicine laboratories. With proper attention to radiation safety, nuclear medicine departments should be able to reduce their total departmental whole body exposure to approximately 0.05 mR per millicurie of ^{99m}Tc injected.[19]

SPECIAL HEALTH PHYSICS CONSIDERATIONS

For specific health physics considerations related to clinical nuclear medicine, the physicist is referred to Nuclear Regulatory Commission (NRC) Regulatory Guide 10.8 "Guide for the Preparation of Applications for Medical Programs" (January 1979)[20]. This guide describes the type and extent of information needed by the NRC to evaluate an application for a specific license for the possession of byproduct material (reactor-produced radionuclides) and its use in human beings.

Therapy (Iodine-131)
1. keep I-131 in lead shield at all times (if possible)
2. open container in fume hood (now have portable hoods)
3. personnel wear gloves
4. patient in private room (if possible); or if room with other patient, other patient beyond child bearing age
5. use of disposable items
6. radiation survey at specified distances to determine limits of time for attending personnel (radiation or non-radiation worker) and visitors
7. no pregnant personnel attending; no children as visitors
8. surveying of items to be disposed
9. patient excreta into lavatory
10. release of patient (less than 30 mCi)
11. survey of patient's room prior to reassignment
12. instructions to nursing staff
13. home instructions to patient and families upon release of patient
14. possible bioassay procedures for personnel

Radioactive Gases (Xenon-133)

Xenon-133 is used for ventilation imaging in clinical nuclear medicine. The following procedures are recommended for use of xenon-133.

1. use hood for storage of xenon-133
2. use available shielding materials
3. special apparatus for administration and collection of xenon-133
4. dilution through exhaust system (considering total activity used per week and air supply and exhaust from area) so as not to exceed concentration averaged over 1 year of 3×10^{-7} µCi/ml (unrestricted areas)
5. use absorption of exhausted air in charcoal traps (periodic survey of exhaust of trap)
6. emergency procedure in case of accidental release of xenon-133

REFERENCES

1. Basic Radiation Protection Criteria. National Council for Radiation Protection and Measurements Report No. 39, NCRP, Washington, D.C., (1971).
2. Radiation Protection for Medical and Allied Health Personnel. National Council for Radiation Protection and Measurements Report No. 48, NCRP, Washington, D.C., August (1976).
3. Procedures for the Management of Contaminated Persons. National Council for Radiation Protection and Measurements Report, Washington, D.C., (in preparation).
4. The Effects on Populations of Exposures to Low Levels of Ionizing Radiation (BEIR Report). Report of the Advisory Committee on the Biological Effects of Ionizing Radiations, National Academy of Sciences, New York, November (1972).
5. Calculation of Reactor Accident Consequences: Appendix VI, Reactor Safety Study, WASH-1400 (NUREG 75/014), U.S. Nuclear Regulatory Commission, Washington, D.C., October (1975).
6. Kereiakes, J.G., P.A. Feller, F.A. Ascoli, S.R. Thomas, M.J. Gelfand and E.L. Saenger. Pediatric Radiopharmaceutical Dosimetry. in Radiopharmaceutical Dosimetry Symposium, HEW Publication (FDA) 76-8044, Rockville, Maryland (1976).
7. Branson, B., H.N. Wellman and J.G. Kereiakes. An Ultra-sensitive ^{123}I Thyroid Uptake System Utilizing Peak: Scatter Organ Depth Correction. Int. J. Applied Rad. and Isotopes 22(8):502, (1971).
8. Webster, E.W., N.W. Alpert and G.L. Brownell. Radiation Doses in Pediatric Nuclear Medicine and Diagnostic X-ray Procedures. in Pediatric Nuclear Medicine, ed. by A.E. James, H.N. Wagner and R.E. Cook. W.B. Saunder, Philadelphia, Pennsylvania (1974).
9. Book, S. and M. Goldman. Thyroidal Radioiodine Exposure of The Fetus. Health Phys. 29:874 (1975).
10. Shalek, R.J. and M. Jahns. Personal Communication,(1980).
11. Thomas, S.R., M.J. Gelfand, J.G. Kereiakes, G.S. Burns, R.C. Purdom and H.R. Maxon. Dosimetry Considerations for the Liver, Spleen and Metaphyseal Growth Complexes in Children Undergoing ^{67}Ga-citrate Scanning Procedures. Presented at Soc. of Nucl. Med. Annual Meeting, Atlanta, Georgia, June 26-29 (1979).
12. Beck, R.N. A Theoretical Evaluation of Brain Scanning Systems. J. Nucl. Med.: 2,314 (1961).
13. Radiation Protection in Nuclear Medicine. National Council for Radiation Protection and Measurements Report, SC #32 (Draft), October 22 (1979).

14. Kereiakes, J.G. and R. Van Tuinen. Quality Control Procedures for Nuclear Medicine Instruments. in Handbook of Medical Physics, CRC, Boca Raton, Florida (to be published 1980).
15. Silberstein, E.B. A Radiopharmaceutical and Clinical Comparison of ^{99m}Tc-Sn-HMDP and ^{99m}Tc-Sn-HEDP. Radiol.(submitted)
16. Wakat, M.A., H.M. Chilton, B.T. Hackshaw, R.J. Cowan, J.D. Ball and N.E. Watson. Comparison of ^{99m}Tc-pyrophosphate and ^{99m}Tc-hydroxymethylene disphosphonate in Acute Mycardial Infarction: Concise Communication. J. Nucl. Med. 21(3), 203-206 (1980).
17. Campbell, J.K., O.W. Houser, J.C. Stevens, H.W. Wahner, H.L. Baker and W.N. Folger. Computed Tomography and Radionuclide Imaging in the Evaluation of Ischemic Stroke. Radiol. 126:695-702 (1978).
18. Medical Radiation Exposure of Pregnant and Potentially Pregnant Women. National Council for Radiation Protection and Measurements Report No. 54, NCRP, Washington, D.C., July (1977).
19. Barrall, R.C. and S.I. Smith. Personnel Radiation Exposure and Protection from Technetium-99m Radiation. in Biophysical Aspects of the Medical Use of Technetium-99m. American Assoc. of Physicists in Medicine, Monograph No. 1, AAPM, 111 E. Wacker Drive, Chicago, Illinois (1976).
20. Guide for Preparation of Applications for Medical Programs. Regulatory Guide 10.8, U.S. Nuclear Regulatory Commission, Washington, D.C., January (1979).

METHOD OF RISK REDUCTION IN RADIATION THERAPY

Robert J. Shalek
The University of Texas System Cancer Center
M. D. Anderson Hospital and Tumor Institute
Houston, Texas

INTRODUCTION

In considering risk reduction, one might ask whether it is radiation risk reduction for the patient or legal risk reduction for the physician or the physicist. Fortunately, whatever one does toward radiation risk reduction usually reduces the risk for all concerned. In this discussion only the reduction of risk to the patient will be considered.

CHOICE OF DOSE PRESCRIPTION

In Figure 1, an idealized relationship between local tumor control and complications is shown (redrawn from Rubin, 1). The full

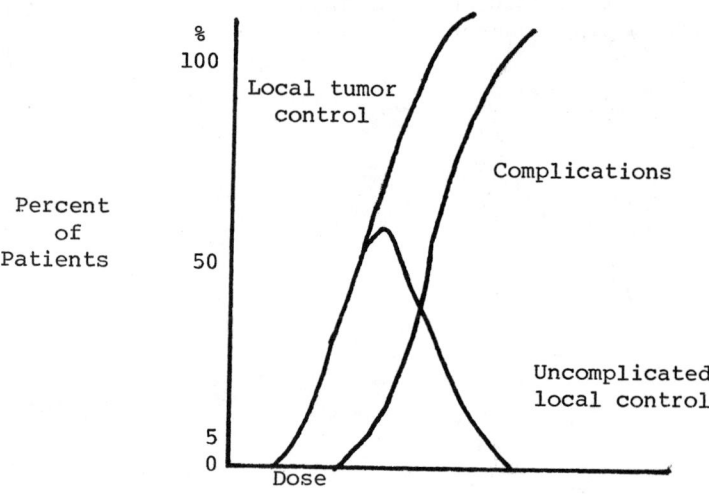

Figure I. Tumor control and complications versus radiation dose.

shape of the curves for local tumor control and for complications is
not known for any particular treatment site and treatment technique,
however, if the curves have any validity, local tumor control without complications passes through a maximum as radiation dose is
varied. For particular treatments radiotherapists know the upper
boundaries of dose which can be tolerated with acceptable complications. A therapist can choose a radiation dose which would give
zero complications, but with a low chance of local tumor control.
Such a choice reduces the radiation risk to the patient and the legal risk to the therapist, but increases the patient's risk from his
disease. A therapist may try for higher cure rates by increasing
the dose prescription if he can deal with the treatment complications
medically and with the attendant anxieties of patients and referring
physicians. Combined radiation and chemical treatment will change
the tumor control and the complications response in Figure 1 rendering a therapist's prior experience with radiation alone an uncertain
guide. He then becomes dependent upon experimental therapy, his own
or that of others. If he relies on the literature for standards of
acceptable dose prescription he is also depending upon the consistency of his delivery of dose with that of the author.

FULFILLMENT OF DOSE PRESCRIPTION

A radiation treatment usually has three parts: (a) the dose prescription (b) the treatment plan in fulfillment of the dose prescription and (c) the application of the plan to the patient. In
many institutions the therapist takes responsibility for the 1st and
3rd items and the physicist takes responsibility for the second.

The treatment plan consists of the radiation measurements and
calculations necessary to fulfill the dose prescription. There are
many steps between the national radiation standard and the duration
of a radiation treatment. The details of these stpes are described
in handbooks and other publications (2,3,4,5,6). Here, many of the
steps and quality assurance procedures will be mentioned without
elaboration together with more general recommendations.

National standards and their dissemination. National radiation standards rely upon radiation measurement devices which depend
upon either the measurement of temperature, charge, length or mass
as at the National Bureau of Standards (NBS) in the United States or
upon a reliable comparison to such absolute measurements as in many
developing countries. A characteristic of national standards of all
countries is their agreement to within 1% with the standards of other
countries. This consistency is achieved under the auspices of the
Bureau International des Poids et Mesures (BIPM) in Sevres, France.
Thus, there is a structure for consistency in radiation measurements
the world over.

Within a country, Regional Calibration Laboratories maintain secondary radiation standards derived by comparison with the national standards. Such standards maintained with high quality ionization chambers agree with the national standards to within 1%. The Regional Calibration Laboratories disseminate radiation standards by comparing their secondary standards to user's field instruments.

Field instrument then have a calibration factor that permits radiation measurements at the calibration energy to within about 1.5% of the national standards. In radiation chamber comparisons done on site at 39 institutions, the Radiological Phsyics Center (RPC) agreed with the chamber calibration factors in clinical use that were traceable to NBS to within 1% ±0.2% standard deviation as shown in Table I (7). Ten years ago reviewing physicists occasion-

Table I. Chamber factors derived by field intercomparison RPC/Institution).

	Number	Mean	Standard deviation
One step from calibration lab	39	1.01	0.02
More than one step from calibration lab	37	1.01	0.04

ally found institutions with chamber factors that were 10% or more discrepant.

Calibration of radiation therapy machines. Field instruments are used to calibrate radiation therapy machines. As indicated in "Dose Evaluation in Radiation Therapy," by this author in these proceedings, of 352 machines reviewed, 78% had calibrations in clincial use that agreed within 3% with that of the reviewing physicist. Subsequent mailed thermoluminescent dosimeters (TLD) to these institutions indicates agreement with the clinical calibration in use with a standard deviation of about ±2%.

With photon and electron beams of energies above 4 MeV, systematic discrepancies of 1 to 2% enter into the machine calibration depending upon the material of the ion chamber and the photon or electron energy (6). These differences will cause institutions to differ in the fulfillment of dose prescription.

At this time there are wide differences between various institutions in the periods between checks of radiation output from therapy machines. Some machines, particularly linear accelerators are checked daily. On the other hand some cobalt units may be used for years without a check. A case can be made for checking the output of every radiation therapy machine at least once a week. All types of machines including cobalt units can show sudden changes of output without other symptoms or signals of trouble. If such a change occurs at an unknown time within a one week period, a reasonable adjustment can be made to the treatment of current patients undergoing 4 to 6 weeks of therapy. But if the period between checks is longer it may not be possible to make a satisfactory compensation for an output change.

<u>Other physical factors relating to the correct delivery of dose.</u>
Gagnon (7) has considered various technical factors affecting the fulfillment of dose including chamber factors, transmission through blocking trays, wedge transmission factors, coincidence of the radiation field and light field, beam symmetry, monitor end effect, timer error, and depth dose factors. The results of checking 357 machines at various institutions for coincidence of the radiation field are illustrated in Table II.

Table II. Coincidence of radiation field and light field

Type of machine	Number of Machines surveyed	Mean[a] discrepancy (mm)	Maximum discrepancy (mm)	Percent with discrepancy <3 mm
All	357	2.5	15	83
All ^{60}Co	231	2.5	15	89
Modern ^{60}Co[b]	152	2.0	6	95
Other ^{60}Co	79	3.5	15	65
All linacs	99	2.5	5	90
All betatrons	14	3.0	7	71
1MV Van de Graaff	13	4.0	8	8

[a] To the nearest 0.5 mm.
[b] AECL Theratron 80 and 780, Eldorado 8 and 78, and Picker M Series.

From these studies present acceptable and practical criteria for agreement are recommended as shown in Table III.

Table III.

Parameter	Acceptable agreement
Chamber calibration factor	2%
Machine calibration	3%
Wedge transmission factor	2%
Coincidence, light and radiation field	3 mm
Beam symmetry	3%, any 2 points equidistant from central ray
Depth dose	2%
Fulfillment of tumor dose prescription	5%

Fulflillment of tumor dose prescription. The criterion of 5% for fulfillment of tumor dose prescription adopted initially by the RPC appears to be a practical choice for most treatments. For complex treatments such as those for Hodgkin's disease, the 5% criterion can be met with difficulty. Bar graph distributions are shown for uncomplicated treatments in Figure 2 (8). These findings

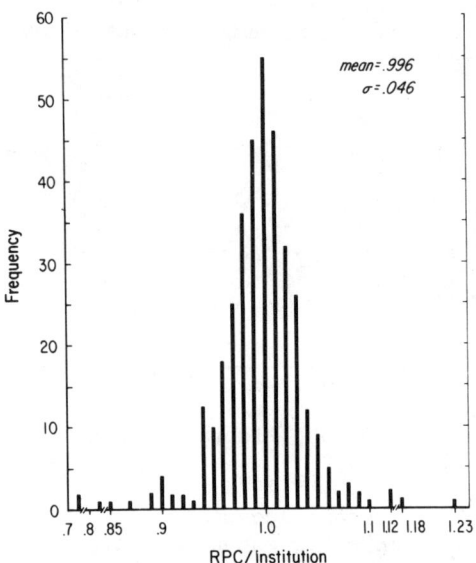

Figure 2. For uncomplicated treatments the frequency of occurrence versus the ratio of the fulfillment of tumor dose estimated by the RPC to that stated by the institution. Irregular fields (mantle, etc.) and tangential breast treatments are not included. Each of the 352 treatment machines reviewed are counted once.

resulted from initial physics reviews during the period 1968 to 1976.

Application of the plan to the patient. Knowledge of the tumor position in the body and surrounding organs is gained by palpation, radiography, computed tomography scanning (CT), and ultrasound scanning. Simulation of the treatment upon a diagnostic machine that has similar geometry to the major treatment machine helps assure that treatment radiation arrives where intended and does not arrive where not intended. Verification of these hopes is also done upon the major treatment machine by film exposed beyond the patient. Of particular importance is avoidance of overlap of treatment beams at normal structures. Insensitive film such as Kodak RP/V Therapy Verification Film may be left in place during an entire single radiation treatment, thus recording events such as organ or patient movement during treatment (9).

CONCLUSION

It is generally accepted that radiation tumor doses delivered should be within 5% of that prescribed. It is also generally taken that no harm will come to a patient if the dose to a particular organ is within 10% of that considered tolerable. I was aware of that statement 30 years ago and I assume that it has an even longer history. There are suggestions from time to time that both of these criteria are too wide. With modern measuring instruments, diagnostic methods and calculation techniques, it is possible to reduce the tumor dose criteria to 4% and perhaps to 3%. There is also some clinical data which suggests that local tumor control may depend upon very precise delivery of radiation dose. Shukovsky has published data indicated that local control of squamous carcinoma of the supraglottic larynx may depend sharply upon dose differences as small as 5% (10). Thus we are in a time of tightening dose standards which may have justificaion in clinical findings.

Supported in part by grant CA 10953 awarded by the National Cancer Institute.

REFERENCES

1. P. Rubin and G. Casarett, Ther. Onc. 6, 1 (1972).
2. Hospital Physicists Association, Phys. Med. Biol. 14, 1 (1969).
3. American Association of Physicists in Medicine, Phys. Med. Biol. 16, 379 (1971).
4. American Association of Physicsits in Medicine, Med. Phys., 2, 110 (1975).
5. J. B. Massey, Manual of Dosimetry in Radiotherapy, International Atomic Energy Agency Vienna Technical Report 119 (1970).

6. National Council on Radiation Protection and Measurements. Dosimetry of X-ray and Gamma-ray Beams for Radiation Therapy in the Energy Range 10 keV to 50 MeV. In press. (1980).
7. W. F. Gagnon, L. W. Berkley, P. Kennedy, W. F. Hanson and R.J. Shalek, Med. Phys. 5, 555 (1978).
8. R. J. Shalek, P. Kennedy, M. Stovall, J. H. Cundiff, W. F. Gagnon, W. Grant, III and W. F. Hanson, National Bureau of Standards, NBS SP456, 111 (1976).
9. A. G. Haus and J. E. Marks, J. App. Photo. Eng. $\underline{2}$, 11 (1976).
10. L. J. Shukovsky, Am. J. Roentgenol. Radium Ther. Nucl. Med. $\underline{108}$, 27 (1970).

RADIATION TERATOGENESIS: FETAL RISK AND ABORTION

Robert I. Brent
Stein Research Center
Thomas Jefferson University
Philadelphia PA 19107

INTRODUCTION

In spite of the fact that we have a great deal more to learn about radiation teratogenesis and teratogenesis in general, there have been many experiments and observations about the effects of radiation on the developing embryo. A complete review will not be presented, and the reader is referred to recent reviews on this subject.[1-5]

Prior to the blastocyst stage, the embryo is a multicellular organism with an insensitivity to the teratogenic and growth-retarding effects of radiation and the greatest degree of sensitivity to the lethal effects of irradiation[6-8] (Figs. 1-3). During early organogenesis, the embryo is very sensitive to the growth retarding, teratogenic and lethal effects of irradiation, but has the ability to recover somewhat from the growth-retarding effects in the postpartum period. During the early fetal period, the fetus has diminished sensitivity to multiple organ teratogenesis, retains central nervous system sensitivity, is growth-retarded at term, but recovers poorly from the growth retardation in the postpartum period.[6,9-11] During the later fetal stages, the embryo is not grossly deformed by radiation but can respond with permanent cell depletion of various organs and tissues if the radiation exposure is high enough.[5,12] One can postulate many mechanisms for the effects of irradiation, which include cell death, mitotic delay, disturbances of cell migration, alteration in macromolecular structure, and many others. Until we know more about the mechanisms involved in embryopathology, it is difficult to determine which mechanisms are most important in the process of radiation-induced embryopathology. Furthermore, the same pathogenic mechanisms may not be primarily operative at all stages of gestation. Radiation-induced cell death may be minimally important at one stage of gestation of the embryo's ability to replace the killed cells. At another stage of gestation, cell death may be a primary factor because the embryo has lost the ability to replace dead cells and that fetus may be permanently cell depleted.

Other radiation-induced effects that have been invoked to explain embryopathology are cytogenetic abnormalities and somatic mutations.[13,14] Cytogenetic abnormalities may be responsible for preimplantation death in the irradiated mammalian zygote,[8,11,13] but point mutations are less likely to be a contributing factor to abnormal morphogenesis. Of course, neither phenomenon has been adequately studied at every stage of mammalian gestation.

Radiation effects may apppear at once and result in cell

death, embryonic death, or teratogenesis. Other effects may not be obvious immediately and can only be measured or ascertained in the postpartum or adult period. Neuronal depletion, infertility, tissue hypoplasia, neoplasia, or shortening of life span are phenomena whose significance can only be evaluated in the postpartum or adult organism.[1,5,15-20]

The neurophysiological and behavior changes in adult organisms that have been irradiated in utero are the most difficult to evaluate. The difficulties arise for several reasons: 1) it is not easy to eliminate postnatal environmental effects as contributing factors; 2) reported findings are frequently not reproducible and are not dose-related; 3) behavioral changes may not be able to be correlated with the neuroanatomical changes, and 4) animal behavior tests may have minimal application to the human situation. This subject is reviewed by Furchtgott[22] and Brent[3]. Except for the work of Piontkovskii,[23,24] all behavioral studies of animals or humans exposed to radiation during gestation do not exhibit any measurable changes if the exposure is below 25 rads.

HUMAN RADIATION TERATOGENESIS

The classical effects of radiation on the developing mammal are gross congenital malformations, intrauterine growth retardation, and embryonic death. Each of these effects has a dose response relationship and a threshold exposure below which there is no difference between the irradiated and the control population. Since human pregnancies predominantly consist of a single embryo, it would be unusual to see the classical triad of effects, although it is conceivable that if the dose and timing were appropriate, a stillborn, growth-retarded, malformed embryo could result.

Growth retardation and central nervous system effects, such as microcephaly or eye malformations, are the cardinal manifestations of intrauterine radiation effects in the human. The occurrence of microcephaly is such a significant component of the effects of intrauterine radiation that a separate "Teratogen Update" has been written about this subject.[25] The reports of several authors indicate that microcephaly is the commonest malformation observed in humans randomly exposed to high doses of radiation during pregnancy.[26-34] In Goldstein and Murphy's reports, 19 of 75 irradiated embryos were microcephalic or hydrocephalic children, having received an estimated dose of greater than 100 rads as a minimum. Almost all the microcephalic children were mentally retarded. The following malformations were also reported: two children with hypoplastic genitalia, one child with cleft palate, one child with hypospadius, an abnormality of the large toe, and an ear abnormality. Many of the children had intrauterine growth retardation and there were various abnormalities of the eyes, including microphthalmia, cataracts, strabismus, retinal degeneration, and optic atrophy. The unique finding was that no visceral, limb or other malformations were ever found unless the child exhibited intrauterine growth retardation, microcephaly (congenital malformations of the brain), or readily apparent eye malformations. Dekaban reported that 22 infants were exposed between the 3rd to 20th week of human gestation were microcephalic, mentally retarded or both (Fig. 4). The estimated protracted exposure was 250 R and all of the malformed infants exhibited growth retardation.

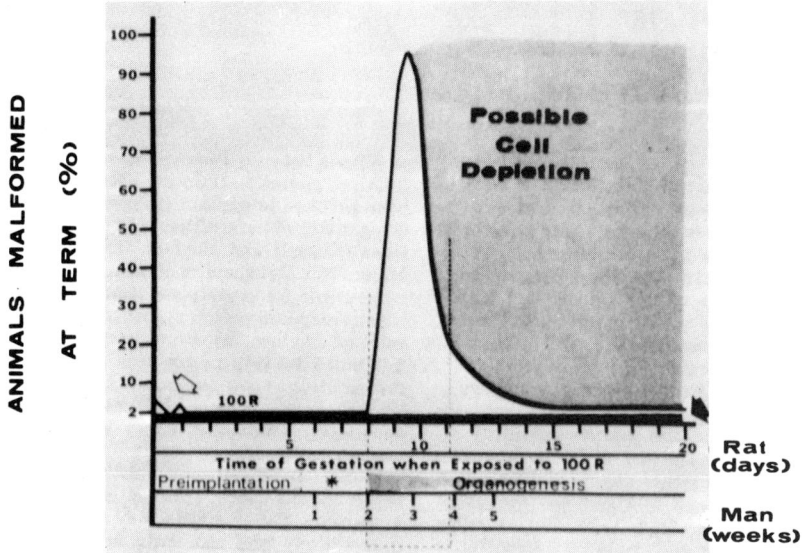

Fig. 1 This graph depicts the relative incidence of gross congenital malformations in the rat following an exposure of 100 R. The arrow on the right side of the ordinate points to the 2% control incidence of congenital malformations seen in this species. The incidence of malformations before the 9th day is the same as in the controls. The light arrow on the left side of the ordinate points to a slight increase in malformations on the 1st day. This was inserted because of the work of Russell in a particular strain of mice. A very large increase in malformations occurs during the early organogenetic period. Note that this corresponds to the 3rd and 4th weeks of human pregnancy. This high incidence of gross malformations falls off rapidly as organogenesis diminishes. Note that organogenesis to some degree (CNS) continues to term. Also note that although gross malformations may not be produced during the late fetal stages with 100 R, an irreversible loss of cells occurs. The significance of these cell losses is under study. The asterisk (*) is placed at the stage of implantation to indicate that although malformations are not readily produced at this stage, growth retardation can be induced.

The most frequent abnormalities were 1) small size at birth and stunted growth; 2) microcephaly; 3) mental retardation; 4) microphthalmia; 5) pigmentary changes in the retina; 6) genital and skelatal malformations, and 7) cataracts (Fig. 4). All of the embryos reported by Dekaban received hundreds of rads. The patients were treated with radiation for various reasons, including

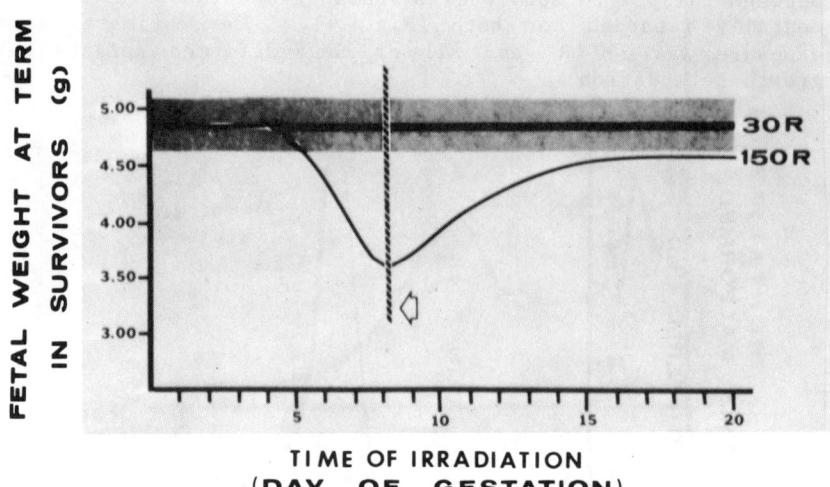

Fig. 2 The term fetal weight in the Wistar colony of rats in our laboratory averages 4.8 g on the 22nd day when delivered by cesarean section that morning. Note that 150 R causes growth retardation just after implantation but before the stage is sensitive to teratogenesis (arrow pointing to vertical line). From the time of implantation until term, 150 R produced some degree of growth retardation. Note that 30 R does not appear to produce significant deviations in growth, although it may be that all experimental groups are too small to show differences in weight at this low dose.

dysmenorrhea, metrorrhagia, myomata, arthritis or tuberculosis of the sacroiliac joint, and malignant tumors of the uterus or cervix. In several instances, radiation was initiated without knowing the patient was pregnant.

It is of interest to note that in one of the case reports[35] a typical campomelic dwarf was reported and the cause was attributed to radiation. High dose radiation was delivered from the 2nd to 5th month. This rare recessive syndrome was not described in 1930, and the authors were not in a position to recognize its possible genetic etiology.[36]

Radiation-induced microcephaly, growth retardation, and microphthalmia are represented in Figures 5 and 6.

From a sample of 1,265 subjects exposed in utero at Hiroshima, 183 were analyzed by Miller[30] and Wood and others.[31,32]
Seventy-eight of these fetuses were less than 16 weeks of age at the time of irradiation; 105 were 16 weeks or more. Of 78, 25 were microcephalic (head circumference more than two standard deviations below the mean), and 11 were mentally deficient. Of the 105, seven were microcephalic as defined, and four were mentally deficient. The incidence of microcephaly increased with increasing exposure. In 14 of the offspring with smaller than normal head circumference

who were also mentally deficient, 10 were $\geq$ 2 S.D. below the mean height for age. In 16 children with small heads who were not mentally deficient, there was not a marked reduction in stature. Tables 1 and 2 summarize some of the characteristics of the patients exposed in utero before the 16th week of gestation.[30,32,37] Severe mental retardation was not observed in any patients that received less than 50 rads while in utero.[38] In a summary of the microcephalic data, Blot[37] noted that, while there was no increased risk for microcephaly in the population exposed in Nagasaki below 150 rads, there was an increased risk in the population exposed in Hiroshima at much lower doses. Blot pointed out that 30% of the radiation in Hiroshima was due to neutrons. Thus, a 20-rad exposure consisting of 30% neutrons (RBE 10) could expose the embryo to 74 rem of radiation. It should also be pointed out that 10-20 rads of low L.E.T. radiation will not increase the incidence of microcephaly in experimental animals.

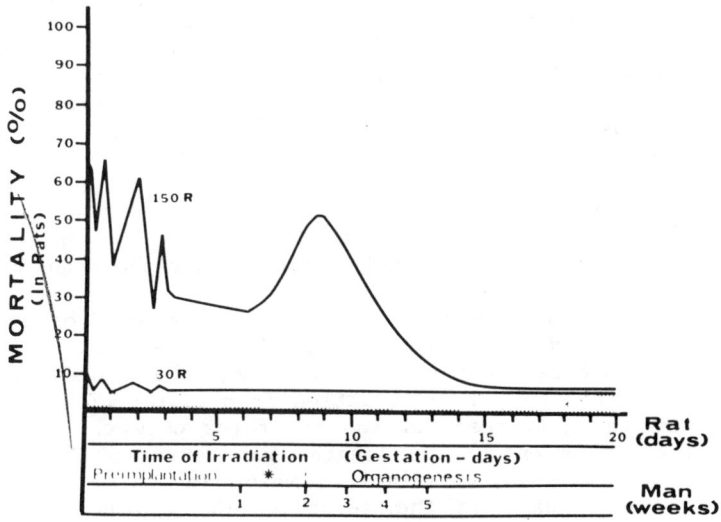

Fig. 3 The lethal effect of radiation in rats is greater on the 1st day. It appears that the LD/50 shifts at different times of the day during early gestation, possibly because the cells are dividing synchronously, therefore, the zygote will vary in its radiosensitivity, depending on the stage of the cell cycle. Note that the embryo becomes somewhat resistant in the implantation stage and then becomes sensitive to the lethal effect of radiation during early organogenesis. A 30 R dose apparently does increase the resorption rate when radiation takes place on the 1st day. The superimposition of this lethality curve for rats onto the human embryonic development timetable may not be appropriate and is for comparison purposes only, but it allows one to estimate at least roughly the stages at which the human embryo might be most readily killed by high doses of radiation.

Analysis of the human data reveals some interesting and important facts. Growth retardation, microcephaly, and mental retardation are predominant observable effects following acute exposures greater than 50 rads (low L.E.T. radiation). No report of a bonafide radiation-induced morphological malformation has been reported in a human that has not exhibited growth retardation or a central nervous system abnormality. One might question why the central nervous system seems to be more sensitive in the human than in experimental animals in whom many organ systems are malformed by irradiation. The explanation for this apparent discrepancy is that the central nervous system maintains its sensitivity to radiation throughout gestation and into the neonatal period, while the other organ systems have much narrower periods when obvious morphological alterations can be produced[1-4] (Fig. 1). Secondly, the period of exquisite sensitivity to multiple system malformations is quite small in the human (2nd to 4th week) when compared to the rat (9th to 13th day). In the human, all organ systems can be readily malformed by high doses of radiation during 5% of pregnancy. Thirdly, human exposures have occurred at random during pregnancy and the exposure is controlled for purposes of therapeutic irradiation (100's of rads), or not controlled, as at Hiroshima and Nagasaki. Therefore, the exposures that occur in the human during the period of maximum sensitivity will be infrequent and/or will result in a high incidence of abortions, while the great majority of exposures will occur during the fetal stages when the central nervous system is unable to repair radiation-induced neuronal death. Thus, the nature of radiation effects in the human and the apparent discrepancies with animal data can be explained by the manner in which human populations have been exposed.

There are rare instances in which human embryos have been studied immediately after exposure to high doses of irradiation. Driscoll and others[39] were able to study the acute effects in two human fetuses exposed to radiation from radium with which their mothers were being treated for cancer of the cervix. The fetuses, 15 cm and 21 cm in crown-rump length, were examined 2 and 10 days after the beginning of irradiation, which lasted 48 hours in the first case and 4 days in the second. The crowns of the heads received about 800 R and 1600 R, respectively.

Destruction of primitive proliferative and migratory cells in the brains and of granulopoietic cells in the hematopoietic tissue occured in both, but evidence of acute necrosis of lymphoid and mesenchymal cells was still visible only in the smaller fetus exposed for 48 hours. Mesenchyme cell necrosis extended as far as the kidney, where the dose may have been of the order of 50 to 100 rads in this fetus. In the larger fetus exposed for 4 days, more degenerating ova were seen than in comparable unirradiated subjects. These observations provide a link between human laboratory animal data, suggesting that patterns of cellular radio-sensitivity in man are similar to those in other mammals.[15]

Irradiation of the human fetus from diagnostic exposures below 5 rads have not been observed to cause congenital malformations or growth retardation,[40-44] but all such epidemiological studies are not negative.[45,46]

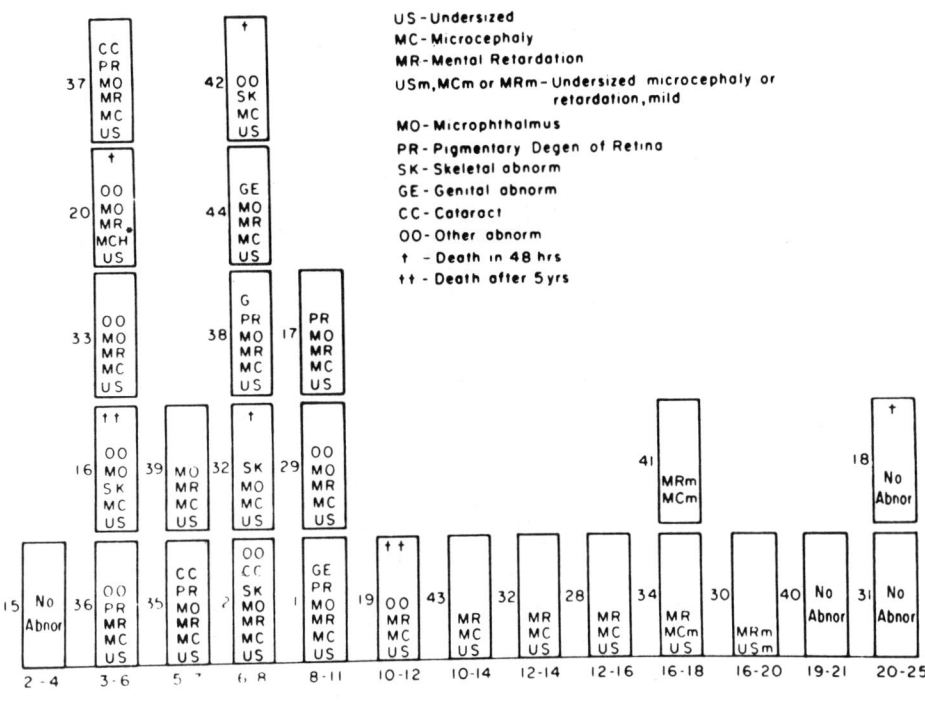

Fig 4 The spectrum of malformations in 26 human infants in utero. Note that all infants receiving therapeutic doses of radiation were growth-retarded if they were irradiated between 3 and 20 weeks of gestation. Note that in no instance is there an associated malformation in structures than the nervous system without either microcephaly or mental retardation (Dekaban, '68, with permission from the Journal of Nuclear Medicine.)

These are extremely difficult studies to perform, and it appears that the animal data support the contention that gross congenital malformations will not be increased in a human pregnant population exposed to 5 rads or less. This contention is further strengthened by the fact that most human exposures to extensive diagnostic radiation studies are fractionated and/or protracted. This type of exposure is likely to be less effective in producing malformations than is an acute exposure.[47,48]

Although the animal and human data support the conclusion that no increase in the incidence of gross congenital malformation, intrauterine growth retardation, or abortion will occur with exposures below 5 rads, that does not mean that there are definitely no risks to the embryo exposed to lower doses of radiation. Whether there exists a linear or exponential dose-response relationship or a threshold exposure for genetic, carcinogenic, cell-depleting, and shortening-of-life-span effects has not been determined. In establishing maximum permissible levels for the embryo at low exposures, we estimate the risk at 1 rad on the basis of a linear relationship (Table 3).

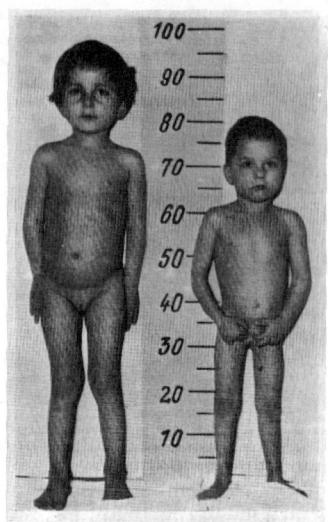

Fig. 5 The smaller child received in utero radiation during the 3rd to 4th month of gestation. The skin dose to the abdomen was 900 rads and was delivered for the purpose of sterilization of the mother because she had metatastic breast carcinoma. The child was full term but weighed only 1900 g. He had microcephaly and cerebral atrophy. Growth retardation persisted into childhood as evidenced by comparison with a child the same age who is in the 50th percentile. There was shortening of the left tibia and an exostosis on the right tibia. The eyes had decreased vessel size and pallor of the left disk. There were abnormal motor movements, weakness, and severe mental retardation.

COUNSELING PREGNANT WOMEN EXPOSED TO RADIATION AND ESTIMATING THE RISKS

Radiation effects in various mammalian embryos are more similar than the effects of most other teratogens or embryopathic agents because radiation has a direct effect on the developing embryo,[8,17,49-52] and variations in placental transport and maternal metabolism do not significantly alter the results of irradiating the embryo. Thus, one can more readily transfer the results of radiation experiments with pregnant mammals to the human than with any other teratogen.

The biologic effects of embryonic radiation are summarized for exposures of 10 rad and 100 rad in Tables 4 and 5 for various species and different stages of gestation. Table 6 lists the estimated LD/50, minimum malforming dose, minimum lethal dose, minimum dose to produce growth retardation, and other parameters for the human embryo, based on extrapolations from animal data.

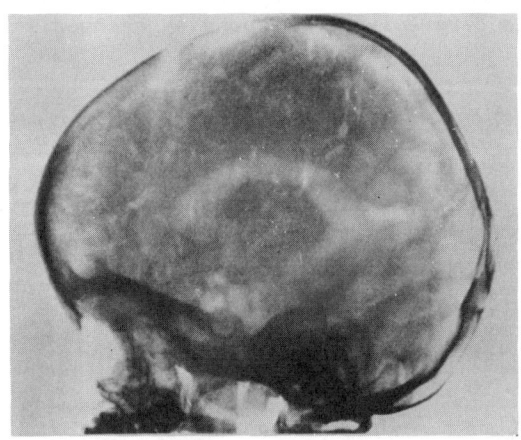

Fig. 6 Lateral view of the skull of the patient in Figure 5. The encephalogram revealed microcephaly and porencephaly. The mother received 900 rads of radiation to the abdomen. Based on the kilovoltage of the X-ray machine and the filtration, the estimated exposure to the embryo was 200-300 rads. The embryo could be as young as 9 weeks or as old as 20 weeks at the time of irradiation, based on the meager history that is available.[53]

Table 7 lists the effects of low exposures to developing mammalian embryos. The data indicate that continuous exposures below 2,000 mrads per day have no effect on numerous parameters such as fertility, growth, mortality, or the incidence of congenital malformations.

In the human, diminished body growth, head size, and mental development have been observed after 50 rads to the mother during the earlier months of gestation, and some disturbances of growth may occur after as little as about 25 rads. Blot and Miller[38] report that small head size was observed in children receiving 10 rads while in utero, but there was no mental retardation associated with this exposure and there were other important considerations. This exposure consisted of a significant neutron component which has a greater relative biological effect. Secondly, the groups were very small, and thirdly, there were other serious environmental factors that could have contributed to disturbances of fetal growth. Even if one considers this effect to be etiologically related to radiation exposure, the total human data from Hiroshima and Nagasaki do not support a significant effect attributable to radiation in the groups that received below 10 rads in utero. In experiments with laboratory mammals, in which more precise observation of dose and stage of development is possible, doses as low as 25 rads have produced some impairment of neurologic function and behavior. Alterations in the morphologic development of some brain neurons and certain other cellular changes have been observed after as little as 10-20 rads in fetal and infant rats, but tests thus far have not revealed corresponding changes in function.

TABLE 1. *Frequency of small head circumference at ages 10–19 years according to city, gestational age, and radiation dose (Blot '75)*

Dose rad	Gestational age (weeks)			
	Hiroshima		Nagasaki	
	0–17	18+	0–17	18+
Not in city or distally exposed	–	31/764	–	10/246	–
0–9	4(1)/63+	4/65+	0/1	0/9
10–19	6(1)/54	0/44	0/7	0/6
20–29	6/24	1/14	0/5	2/7
30–39	4/8	0/10	2/4	0/6
40–49	3/11	0/6	0/6	0/3
50–59	9(2)/20	2/24	0/9	0/11
100–149	2/4	0/10	0/2	1/5
150+	5(5)/13	1(1)/8+	8(3)/9	2(1)/9
Unknown	1/7	0/3	0/0	0/0
Total (in city)	40(9)/204	8(1)/184	10(3)/43	5(1)/56

Cases in parentheses give number with small head circumference and mental retardation.
Plus (+) indicates one person with mental retardation without small head circumference.

TABLE 2. *Number of cases and relative risk of mental retardation according to dose category (Blot '75)*

	Hiroshima			Nagasaki		
Dose (rad)	Sample size	Cases[1]	Relative risk[2]	Sample size	Cases	Relative risk
Not in city or distally exposed	830	5(2)	1.0(1.0)	246	4(2)	1.0(1.0)
0–9	145	3(1)	3.4(3.8)	11	0	–
10–49	189	2(1)	1.8(1.5)	45	0	–
50–99	47	3(1)	10.6(11.8)	20	0	–
100–199	29	4(1)	22.9(28.6)	13	0	–
200–299	8	3	66.3(104)	5	1(1)	12.3
300	6	2	55.3(92.2)	7	3	26.4(52.7)

[1] Numbers in parentheses are numbers of cases (included in the totals) whose mental retardation was apparently due to causes other than intrauterine radiation.
[2] Numbers in parentheses are relative risks excluding cases whose mental retardation was apparently due to non-radiation causes.

Innumerable developmental processes are sensitive to radiation, as to other environmental teratogenic agents, and each process has its individual threshold or dose-range below which radiation has no visible effect. In radiogenic microcephaly or impaired body growth, the development of the abnormality depends on the summation and interaction of the interruptions of a large number of processes characteristic of the stage of development. and there are threshold dose-ranges below which these effects are not observed. Furthermore, the embryo does have sophisticated recuperable powers which are present in all mammalian cells.

Based on this information, it would appear that the hazards of exposures in the range of diagnostic roentgenology (20 mrads-

5000 mrads) present an extremely low risk to the embryo, when compared to the spontaneous mishaps that can befall the human embryo, when compared to the spontaneous mishaps that can befall the human embryo (Table 3). Approximately 30-50% of human embryos abort spontaneously. Human infants have a 2.75% malformation rate at term, which rises to approximately 6-8% once all malformations and genetic diseases become manifest. In spite of the fact that doses of 1-3 rads can produce cellular effects and the fact that diagnostic exposure during pregnancy has been associated with malignancy in childhood, the maximum theoretical risk to the human embryos exposed to doses of 5 rads or less is extremely small (Table 3 and 6).

TABLE 3. Estimate of risks of 1 rad exposure (low L.E.T.) to the developing human embryo

Age (days)	Mutagenic effect[1,4,6]	Carcinogenic effect (Stewart, '73)[2] (Stewart et al., '56, '58) (Mole, '79)	Carcinogenic effect ABCC[3] Wood et al., '67c Kato, '71	Gross congenital malformations Death, growth retardation	Permanent cell depletion
1	No data	No data	No data		No effect[5]
14					
18	10^{-7} per locus	10^{-3}	6×10^{-6}	Same as controls	?
28					
50					
Late fetus to term					

[1] Based on an estimated doubling dose for mutagenesis of 100 rads. Assuming a linear dose response curve and no threshold for mutagenic effects.
[2] Stewart's data would indicate that the embryo is 100 times more sensitive to the carcinogenic effect of radiation than the adult. This is a controversial matter and others (Miller, '70; Jablon, '73; Brent '77; Diamond et al., '73) feel that this association may be other than a radiation effect.
[3] ABCC Atomic Bomb Casualty Commission Data on Carcinogenesis do not indicate that the embryo and fetus are at increased risk. The risk presented is the same carcinogenic risk attributed to adults, assuming maximal effect at low doses, namely, a linear dose response curve—and no threshold for carcinogenic effects.
[4] The mutagenic effects have not been studied in the preimplantation period.
[5] During the preimplantation period, the surviving embryos are not reduced in size even when the dose is very high although, at this stage, the embryo is very sensitive to the lethal effects of radiation. The estimate is assumed to be the adult risk, since there was no increased carcinogenic effect in the population of exposed fetuses in Hiroshima and Nagasaki.
[6] Estimate is assumed to be adult risk since there was no increased carcinogenic effect in the population of exposed fetuses.

*Stewart '73-Ref. 54 Stewart et al., '56-Ref. 55· Stewart et al., '58-Ref. 56: Mole '79-Ref. 57: Wood et al., '67c-Ref. 58: Kato '71-Ref. 59: Miller '70-Ref. 60; Jablon '73-Ref. 61· Brent '77-Ref. 4; Diamond et al., '73-Ref. 62.

In my experience, when the data and risks are explained to the patient, the family with a wanted pregnancy invariably continues with the pregnancy. The difficulty that frequently arises is that the radiation risk from diagnostic radiation is evaluated without considering the significant normal risks of pregnancy. Furthermore, many physicians approach the evaluation of a diagnostic radiation exposure with a cavalier attitude. The usual procedures in clinical medicine are ignored and opinion based on meager information is given the patient. Frequently, it reflects the physician's bias about radiation effects or his total ignorance of the fields of radiation biology. We have patient records in our files of scores of patients who have been told to have an abortion following a radiation exposure. In many instances the embryo received no

measurable exposure. In most instances the exposure was well below 5 rads and in several instances the physician's evaluation was so unsystematic that he was not aware that the patient was not pregnant at the time of the exposure. Why is it that a physician ignores the systematic approach of patient evaluation when confronted with a pregnant woman who has been exposed to radiation? Whatever the reason, there is a minimal systematic approach that every patient deserves. The following information should be obtained.
1. Stage of pregnancy of the exposure.
2. Menstrual history.
3. Previous pregnancy history.
4. History of congenital malformations
5. Other potential harmful environmental factors that have occurred during this pregnancy.
6. Mother's and father's age.
7. Type of radiation study. Dates and numbers of studies performed.
8. Calculation of the embryonic exposure by a medical physicist or competent radiologist.
9. Status of this pregnancy: wanted, unwanted.
10. Evaluation of this information. Arriving at decision by both patient and counselor.
11. Placing in the medical record a summary of the information and the fact that patient has been informed that a normal pregnancy has a significant risk of having something go wrong and the counselor is not guaranteeing the outcome of the pregnancy.
12. The use of amniocentesis and ultrasound to evaluate the fetus is an individual decision that would have to be made in each pregnancy.

Our experience has taught us that there are many variables involved in a radiation exposure to a pregnant or potentially pregnant woman. Therefore, it is impossible to provide a routine stereotyped response for each patient. The following examples are some typical cases of radiation exposure that necessitated evaluation.

> A 27 year-old mother, gravida 3, para 2, abortus 0 called on a Friday afternoon because she was 8 weeks pregnant and was scheduled for a therapeutic abortion on Monday morning. Her obstetrician and a pediatric genetic counselor had advised her to have a therapeutic abortion because at the time of conception she had several X-ray examinations of the abdomen, and they were concerned that the embryo would be malformed. No dosimetry had been performed and no evaluation initiated. It took about 10 minutes on the phone to determine that she became pregnant after the diagnostic radiation studies and that her two previous boys had minor problems (hemangioma and pyloric stenosis). We cancelled the abortion and the mother

delivered a normal, full-term girl. She was
adequately warned that we could not guarantee
the outcome of the pregnancy-that there are
27.5 serious malformations per 1,000 births-
as a minimum. She had another determining
factor in that she had a serious problem with
varicose veins and planned a tubal ligation
after either the abortion or the delivery.

TABLE 4. *A compilation of the effects of 10 rads or less acute radiation at various stages of gestation in rat and mouse*[a]

	Stage of gestation (days)				
	Preimplantation	Implantation	Early organogenesis	Late organogenesis	Fetal stages
Mouse	0–4 1/2	4 1/2–6 1/2	6 1/2–8 1/2	8 1/2–12	12–18
Rat	0–5 1/2	5 1/ 2–8	8–10	10–13	13–22
Corresponding human gestation period	0–9	9–14	15–28	28–50	50–280
Lethality	+[b,c]	−	−	−	−
Growth retardation at term	−	−	−	−	−
Growth retardation as adult	−	−	−	−	−
Gross malformations[d] (asplasia, hyperplasia, absence or overgrowth of organs or tissues)	±	−	−	−	−
Cell depletions, minimal but measurable tissue hypoplasia	−	−	−	−	−
Sterility	−	−	−	−	−
Significant increase in germ cell mutations[e]	±	±	±	±	±
Cytogenetic abnormalities	−	−	−	−	−
Neuropathology	−	−	−	−	−
Tumor induction[e,f]	−	−	±	±	±
Behavior disorders[g]	−	−	−	−	−
Reduction in life-span[e]	−	−	−	−	−

[a] Dose fractionation or protraction effectively reduces the biologic result of all the pathologic effects reported in this Table.
[b] (−) no observed effect; (±) questionable but reported or suggested effect; (+) demonstrated effect; (++) readily apparent effect; (+++) occurs in high incidence.
[c] At this stage the murine embryo is most sensitive to the lethal effects of irradiation. With 10 rads in the mouse, Rugh reports a slight decrease in litter size in the mouse (Brent, '77).
[d] Rugh reports exencephalia with 15 and 25 rad in a strain of mice with a 1% incidence of exencephalia. Others have not been able to repeat these results (Brent and Bolden, '67a).
[e] The potential for mutation induction exists in the embryonic term cells or their precursors. Several long-term studies indicate that considerably greater doses in mice and rats do not affect longevity, tumor incidence, incidence of congenital malformations, litter size, growth rat, fertility.
[f] Stewart and others have reported that 2 rad increases the incidence of malignancy by 50% in the offspring. See text for discussion.
[g] Piontkovskii reports behavioral changes in the rat after 1 rad daily irradiation. This work has not been reproduced. See text for discussion.

*Brent '77-Ref. 4: Brent and Bolden '67a-Ref. 8

The case history illustrates the minimal data that were
collected by the physicians before counseling the patient. There
was an added feature in this case. The paternal family was
Catholic and the thought of an abortion was causing much dissention
within the family.

Mrs. John B., a 26 year-old para 1, gravida 2,
abortus 0 woman, had LMP on October 31, 1966. On
November 18, she had the onset of a mild gastroenteritis with pain localized to the RUQ. Although the other symptoms of gastroenteritis disappeared, the pain persisted. Mrs. B had just

TABLE 5. A compilation of the effects of 100 rads acute radiation on embryonic development at various stages of gestation in rat and mouse[a]

	Stage of gestation (days)				
	Preim-plantation	Implan-tation	Early organogenesis	Late organogenesis	Fetal stages
Mouse	0–4 1/2	4 1/2–6 1/2	6 1/2–8 1/2	8 1/2–12	12–18
Rat	0–5 1/2	5 1/2–8	8–10	10–13	13–22
Corresponding human gestation period	0–9	9–14	15–18	28–50	50–280
Lethality	+++[b,c]	+	++	±	–
Growth retardation at term	–	+	+++	++	+
Growth retardation as adult	–	+	++	+++	++
Gross malformations (asplasia, hypoplasia, absence or overgrowth of organs or tissues)	–	–	+++	±[d]	–[d]
Cell cepletions, minimal but measurable tissue hypoplasia	–	–	±	++	+
Sterility	–	–	±	–	++[e]
Significant increase in germ cell mutations[f]	±	±	±	±	±
Cytogenetic abnormalities[g]	±			+	+
Cataracts	–	–	–	+	+
Neuropathology	–	–	+++	++	+
Tumor induction[h]	–	–	±	±	+
Behavior disorders[i]	–	–	+	+	±
Reduction of lifespan[j]	–	–	–	–	–

[a] Dose fractionation or protraction effectively reduced the biologic result of all the pathologic effects reported in this Table.
[b] (–) no observed effect; (±) questionable but reported or suggested effect; (+) demonstrated effect; (++) readily apparent effect; (+++) occurs in high incidence.
[c] Russell reported that 200 rads increased the incidence of XO aneuploidy in 2–5% of offspring in mice with a spontaneous incidence of 1%. 100 rads kills substantial numbers of mouse and rat embryos at this state, but the survivors appear and develop normally.
[d] 100 rads produces changes in the irradiated fetus which are subtle and necessitate detailed examination and comparison with comparable controls.
[e] The male gonad in the rat can be made extremely hypoplastic by irradiation in the fetal stages with 15 rads. In the mouse the newborn female is most sensitive to the sterilized effects of radiation. Much of this research on other animals cannot be applied to the human.
[f] The potential for mutation induction exists in embryonic germ cells or their precursors. The relative sensitivity of the embryonic germ cells when compared to adult germ cells is not known. Several long-term studies in animals do not indicate any exceptional differences.
[g] Footnote a refers to the aneuploidy produced in a strain of mice with a 1% incidence of spontaneous XO aneuploidy. Bloom has reported a much higher percentage of chromosome breaks in human embryos receiving 100–200 rads in utero than in adults receiving the same dose of irradiation. As yet, there have been no diseases associated with this increase in frequency of chromosome breaks.
[h] Animal experiments and the data from Hiroshima and Nagasaki do not support the concept that in utero irradiation is much more tumorigenic than extrauterine irradiation. On the other hand, Stewart and colleagues and many others report that irradiation from pelvimetry (2 rads) increases the incidence of leukemia and other tumors.
[i] A statistically significant increase in percentage of mental retardation occurs with this dose of radiation. On the other hand, normal intelligence has been found in children receiving much higher doses in utero.
[j] Animal experiments indicate that survivors of in utero irradiation have a life-span which is longer than groups of animals given the same dose of radiation during their extrauterine life and the same life expectancy as unirradiated controls.

TABLE 6. Estimation on the acute LD/50 dose, minimal malforming doses, cell depleting dose, and lethal doses for the human embryo based on compilation of mouse, rat, and human data

Age	Approximate minimal lethal dose, rads	Approximate LD/50 rads	Minimum dose recuperable growth retardation in adult, rads[1]	Minimal dose for recognizable gross malformation, rads	Minimum dose for induction of genetic, carcinogenic, and minimal cell depletion phenomena
Day 1	10	70–100	No effect	No effect	unknown
Day 14	25	140	25	–	unknown
Day 18	50	150	25–50	25	unknown
Day 28	> 50	220	50	25	unknown
Day 50	> 100	260	50	50	unknown
Late fetus to term		300–400	50	> 50	unknown

[1] Estimates for maximum dose effective in reducing body weight. Specific organs or measurements may be more or less sensitive.

TABLE 7. Reported effects of low exposures of radiation on the embryo when administered throughout pregnancy

	Organism	Source	Approximate exposure rate per minute (R)	Exposure per day	Exposure per pregnancy	Comments	Effects
Russell et al. ('59)	Mouse	137Cs	0.0086	12.4 R	171 R	1st–18th day	None except shortened breeding period in female
Ronnback ('65)	Mouse	137Cs	0.0017	8.4 R	170 R	During gestation and in some instances 20 days postpartum	None
Vorisek ('65)	Rat	60Co	0.0017	2.5 R	—	Daily during pregnancy	None
Stadler and Gowan ('64)	Mouse	60Co	0.0015	2.2 R		Continuous through 10 generations	None
Coppenger and Brown ('65)		60Co	0.0014	2.0 R	—	Continuous through 11 generations	None
Konerman ('69)	Mice		0.007	10 R	180 R	1st–18th day	None
			0.014	20 R	360 R	1st–18th day	None
				20 R		Day 6–13 only	Increased congenital malformation
Wesley ('60)	Humans	Background		0.3mR	0.1 R	Variation in background radiation	Increased congenital malformation
Genrry et al. ('59)	Humans	Background		0.3mR	0.1 R	Variation in background radiation	Background radiation level not a factor in incidence of congenital malformations
Grahn and Kratchman ('63)	Humans	Background		0.3mR	0.1 R	Variation in background radiation	Background radiation level not a factor in incidence of congenital malformations
Segal et al. ('64)	Humans	Background		0.3mR	0.1 R	Background radiation	No influence
Kriegel and Langendorf ('64)	Mouse	X-ray		2.5 R		Acute dose given daily	No influence
				5 R			No influence
				10 R			Malformations, resorptions, growth retardations
				20 R			
Piontkovskiy ('58, '61)	Rat	X-ray		1 R	20 R	Acute dose given daily	Functional changes in behavior and motor activity (questionable)
Laskey et al. ('73)	Rat	HTO	Continuous 0.01–10 uCi HTO ml of body water	0.003–3 rad/day	0.066–66	Tritiated water continuous exposure	Male testes reduced 10u Ci; no growth or reproductive impairment in F₁; F₂ generation had reduced weight

moved to this city with her husband and one child and this was the first time she had seen her new family physician. The pain persisted on and off for 10 days, and on November 28 and 29 she had a cholecystogram and an upper G.I. series. The diagnostic studies were negative and she was treated symptomatically for several days when the symptoms diasppeared. On December 6, she realized that she had missed her menstrual period and a pregnancy test revealed that she was pregnant.

By the time our laboratory was called, several physicians had recommended therapeutic abortion and the woman was exhibiting significant anxiety. We requested that the local medical physicist estimate the dose to the embryo, and at the same time the number and position of the films and length and position of fluoroscopy were submitted to us. We calculated that the embryo had received approximately 1.1 rad over a period of 2 days. The physicists in their locale estimated the dose by performing dosimetry with a phantom and the equipment utilized for the actual procedure. He reported that the dose for the fractionated exposure was 1.4 rad. The recommendation to the family and physicians involved was that this dose of radiation would not result in embryonic death, embryonic growth retardation, or malformations, and that the woman could continue with the pregnancy. She chose to continue the pregnancy and delivered a 3,400 gm normal boy at 40 weeks of gestation.

Case histories similar to this are transmitted to our laboratory frequently. In most instances, the dose to the embryo is below 5 rads and frequently is below 1 rad. The variations in the approach of the physician in charge are dependent on many factors: 1) whether the pregnant woman is married, 2) whether the pregnancy was planned, 3) the mental status of the mother and/or father, 4) the abortion laws in that state, and 5) the knowledge of the physician regarding radiation hazards to the embryo.

Other case histories illustrate these problems.

A 19 year-old unmarried secretary went to her physician because of abdominal pain. She told him her menstrual periods were regular and the pain was periumbilical and persistent. An upper G.I. series was performed but was unsatisfactory because the young girl had eaten breakfast before the study. When the second study was performed, she mentioned that she was 2 weeks past her scheduled menstrual period and that she could be pregnant. The father of the child was married. The radiation therapist at the hospital recommended a therapeutic abortion because of radiation hazards to the embryo. The estimated dose to the embryo over a period of 3 days was 1.6 rad.

Our laboratory was called and informed of the case history and recommendation. Our conclusion was that this dose of radiation would not result in embryonic malformation, growth retardation, or death, and that the radiation hazard should not be used as the scapegoat to obtain a therapeutic abortion for "social" reasons. The laws of that state did not permit any therapeutic abortions, so the girl flew to another state where the theapeutic abortion was performed.

The spector of radiation hazards, we believe should not be invoked to circumvent a social or legal problem. If the abortion laws are archaic or unfair, physicians should work together to change them. They should not create an implied serious radiation hazard problem, which is not justified by the fact, in order to solve social, psychological, or legal problems.

> A 29 year-old housewife, para 0, gravida 1, abortus 0, presented in her 6th month of pregnancy with the history that she had been to her dentist the week before and one radiograph of her left upper first molar was made. She was anxious and very worried about the effect of radiation on her baby. She was reassured but called back six times asking new questions. The estimated dose to the embryo was practically 0 rads. She continued to be anxious and became more hyperactive. She delivered a 3,100 gm baby boy with a minimal syndactyly of the 4th and 5th finger of the left hand, but who otherwise was normal. A legal suit was almost instituted in this case.

It is surprising the number of cases that are evaluated or brought to trial in which the only radiation exposure of the mother pertains to the head, the neck or chest, and yet there is both clinical and basic science information that indicates that embryopathology is only a consequence of direct embryonic exposure. High doses of radiation to the mother, while shielding the embryo, result in offspring who have the same incidence of congenital malformations as control embryos.[49,52,75]

Although it is our opinion that a dose of less than 10 rads to the implanted embryo does not result in a significant increase in the incidence of congenital malformations, growth retardation, or fetal death, possibly significant tumorigenic or genetic hazards cannot be ruled out. Even if one believed that the tumorigenic (leukomogenic) effects of radiation were real, let us examine how difficult it would be to utilize this information in counseling a patient who has received a dose of perhaps 2 rads during her pregnancy. According to Stewart,[54] the risk of leukemia following this exposure in utero is 1:2,000 vs 1:3,000 in unexposed controls over a 10-year period (Table 8). If one were inclined to recommend therpeutic abortion for this embryo because the probability of developing leukemia is 50% greater than controls, one would perform abortions in 1,999 exposed non-leukemics for every leukemic "saved." It is one thing to avoid radiation because of a potential or conjectured hazard, but it is another matter to recommend therapeutic abortion on this basis. If a physician were inclined to accept this increased probability (1:2,000) as a great enough risk to recommend therapeutic abortion, he would be placed in a serious dilemma, since there are other epidemiologic situations in which the risk of leukemia is greater. In fact, the hypothetical increment risk for 2 rads of <u>in utero</u> radiation is 1 in 6,000 over a 10-year period. It is the combined control risk plus the increment risk that result in a 1 in 2,000 risk for these patients. If one examines Table 8, it is obvious that the risk of leukemia is greater in "unirradiated" siblings of leukemics (1:720) than in patients subjected to diagnostic radiation (1:2,000), according to Stewart's data.

Certainly, it would be untenable to hold the position that all future pregnancies of parents with one leukemic child should be aborted. One can carry this argument to its ridiculous extreme by advocating that all pregnancies should be aborted, since the risk of malformation is approximately 40-60 per 1,000 deliveries, and this does not include the probability of postnatal diseases occurring in these offspring. Some may interpret this as a facetious discussion, but to the clinician and family it is not a game of probabilities. It is a medical problem involving an individual human pregnancy.

The physician will never be able to guarantee the outcome of a pregnancy. The basic logic of the practice of medicine will be undermined when some of its practitioners recommend therapeutic abortion for possible hazards with probabilities far below the expected incidence of disease and malformations in the embryo and infant. In all instances of counseling parents concerning the hazards to the embryo of a particular radiation exposure, the biologic knowledge is only one facet to be considered. The risk of radiation damage is based on the estimated dose and the stage of gestation. The reaction to this risk depends on the age of the parents the number of children in the family, the religion and ethics of the family, and the options available to the family based on the regional laws regarding therapeutic interruptions of pregnancy. Information that is more difficult to acquire pertains to the emotional maturity of the family and whether the pregnancy was planned or unplanned.

There were many instances in the past in which a radiologist recommended abortion for a patient whose embryo received a fractionated dose of 0-5 rads during the 1st trimester of pregnancy, because of the possibility of having a malformed embryo. Frequently, this recommendation was made for unmarried women, primarily to assist them in eliminating unwanted pregnancies. It is this type of "good samaritan" recommendation that will reap retribution when that same radiologist attempts to defend himself against the contentions that a series of diagnostic radiologic examinations caused a particular malformation.

TABLE 8. *Risk of leukemia in various groups with specific epidemiologic and pathologic characteristics in populations followed for 10 to 30 years*

Group	Approximate risk	Increased risk over control population	Occurrence
Identical twin of leukemic twin	1/3	1,000	weeks to months
Irradiation-treated polycythemia vera	1/6	500	10–15 years
Bloom syndrome	1/8	375	<30 years of age
Hiroshima survivors who were within 1,000 meters of the hypocenter	1/60	50	average 12 years
Down's syndrome	1/95	30	<10 years of age
Irradiation-treated patients with ankylosing spondylitis	1/270	10	15 years
Siblings of leukemic children	1/720	4	to 10 years
Children exposed to pelvimetry in utero (gestational exposure)	1/2,000	1.5	<10 years
US white children <15 years of age	1/2,800	1	to 10 years

Modified from Miller ('70).

EXPOSURE FROM RADIATION THERAPY

There is ample evidence to indicate that radiation therapy in the region of the abdomen can result in doses of radiation that will deleteriously affect the fetus. In such a case it is important to confer with either the radiotherapist or a qualified medical physicist in order to determine the total dose delivered to the embryo. If the fetus absorbs 50 rads or more at any time during gestation, there is a significant possibility that the fetus might be damaged. There are, of course, instances in which human fetuses exposed to greater doses have survived[29,76] and appeared normal, but at this dose. the probability of central nervous system damage or other malformations is real and the parents should be so informed. If the dose observed by the embryo during the early organogenetic period amounts to several hundred rads, ther is a reasonable possibility that the embryo may abort. As one proceeds into the 2nd and 3rd trimester. the chance of abortion and malformation declines but irreparable damage to the central nervous system can occur.

When the radiation therapist fails to investigate the possibility of pregnancy or fails to record all the information regarding the pregnancy and the steps taken in arriving at a decision. he places himself in double jeopardy. He may be accused of poor medical practice in a suit over a malformed infant and thereby may be more likely to lose the case even when the radiation may not have been responsible for the abnormal embryonic development.[77]

Let us examine some representative cases.

> A 31 year-old woman was in her 6th month of pregnancy when her physician noted an enlarged lymph node in the anterior cervical region. A diagnosis of Hodgkin's disease was made and she received approximately

> 3,200 rads to the anterior cervical region
> adjacent areas over a period of 4 weeks.
> The fetus was viable at the time of diag-
> nosis and the family wanted the baby. The
> dose of radiation to the fetus was less
> than 25 rads. The mother delivered a
> full-term baby who appeared to be normal.

In this case, the physician supported the wishes of the family.

> A 36 year-old woman, para 4, gravida 6,
> abortus 1, was 1 week past her menstrual
> period, which usually was regular. Exami-
> nation revealed a moderate-sized lesion of
> the cervix. The pregnancy test was posi-
> tive. A biopsy of the cervix revealed a
> carcinoma of the cervix that had invaded
> the muscle layer. A dilation and curettage
> was performed and the patient was treated
> with instillation of radium. In this case,
> the options were presented to the family
> before the biopsy and above-mentioned
> course was taken.

THE USE OF DIAGNOSTIC OR THERAPEUTIC RADIATION IN WOMEN OF REPRODUCTIVE AGE WHEN THE OVARIES OR UTERUS WILL BE EXPOSED

1. In a woman of reproductive age, it is important for the patient and physician to be aware of the pregnancy status of the patient before any type of abdominal X-ray exposure is planned. If the embryonic exposure will be 5 rads or less, the radiation risks to the embryo are miniscule when compared to the spontaneous risks. The patient will accept this information if it is offered as part of the preparation for the X-ray studies at a time that both the physician and patient are aware that a pregnancy exists.

The pregnancy status of the patient can be determined by several means: (a) the X-ray referral slip can request the L.M.P. and the P.M.P. and whether the patient can possibly be pregnant; (b) if the patient is uncertain about her pregnancy status, a pregnancy test should be performed; (c) pregnancy tests could be performed on all hospital admission of women of reproductive age.

2. Because the risks of 5 rad fetal irradiation are so small, the immediate medical care of the mother should take priority over the risks of diagnostic radiation exposure to the embryo. X-ray studies which are essential for optimal medical care of the mother and evaluation of medical problems that need to be diagnosed or treated should no be postponed. Elective procedures, such as employment examination or follow-up examinations, once a diagnosis has been made, need not be performed on a pregnant woman even though the risk to the embryo is very small. If other procedures (ultrasound etc.) can provide adequate information without exposing the embryo to ionizing radiation then, of course they

should be utilized. Of course, there is an initial period when a pregnancy test will be negative and the patient can be pregnant. Furthermore, the menstrual history will be of little use in this circumstance. The risks of 5 rads or less of radiation are extremely small during this period of gestation. The patient will benefit from knowing that the diagnostic study was indicated and should be performed, in spite of the fact that she might be pregnant.

3. In those instances in which elective X-ray studies need to be scheduled, it is difficult to know whether to schedule them during the first half of the menstrual cycle just before ovulation or during the second half of the menstrual when most women will not be pregnant. The risk of diagnostic exposures to the oocyte or the preimplanted embryo is extremely small and there is no data on which to compare the relative risk of 5 rads to the oocyte or the preimplanted embryo.[1,2,5] If the diagnostic study is performed in the first 14 days of the menstrual cycle, should the patient be advised to defer conception for several months, based on the assumption that the deleterious effect of radiation to the ovaries decreases with increasing time between radiation exposure and subsequent ovulation? The physician is in a dilemma because he is warning the patient about a very low risk phenomenon. On the other hand, avoiding conception for several months is not an insurmountable hardship. This potential hazard is quite speculative for the human as indicated the the NCRP report [78] dealing with preconception radiation.

> It is not known whether the interval between irradiation of the gonads and conception has a marked effect on the frequency of congenital changes in human offspring, as has been demonstrated in the female mouse. Nevertheless, it may be advisable for patients receiving high doses to the gonads (over 25 rads) to wait for several months after such exposures before conceiving additional offspring.

Since the patients exposed during diagnostic radiologic procedures absorb considerably less than 25 rads, the recommendation made here may be unnecessary, but it involves no hardship to the patient or physician. Since both the NCRP and ICRP have recommended that elective radiologic examination of the abdomen and pelvis be performed during the first part of the menstrual cycle to protect the zygote from possible but largely conjectural hazards, a recommendation to reduce another possible hazard by avoiding fertilization of recently irradiated ova perhaps should merit equal attention.

4. If a woman is exposed to greater than 5 rads of radiation and then is found to be pregnant, then a determination of the merits of continuing the pregnancy must be decided by the physician, patient, and radiation expert. A decision as to whether to terminate the pregnancy must be decided by the physician, patient,

and radiation expert. A decision as to whether to terminate the pregnancy will depend on: (a) the non-radiation-related hazard of the pregnancy to the expectant mother; (b) the extent and type of radiaiton hazard to the embryo or fetus; (c) the ethnic and religious background of the family; (d) the laws of the state pertaining to legal abortion. and (e) any other relevant consideration. Usually, the radiation risk to the embryo or fetus will not be the predominating factor in arriving at a decision unless one is dealing with exposures in the therapeutic range.

If exposures below 5 rads do not measurably affect the exposed embryos, and others[5] recommend performing diagnostic procedures at any time of the menstrual cycle, if necessary, for the medical care of the patient, why spend so much effort and energy in determining the pregnancy status of the patient?

There are several reasons why the physician and patient should have the burden of determining the pregnancy status before an X-ray or nuclear medicine procedure is performed that will expose the uterus.

First, if the physician is forced to include the possibility of pregnancy in the differential diagnosis, a small percent of diagnostic studies may no longer be considered necessary. Early symptoms of pregnancy may mimic certain types of gastrointestinal or genito-urinary disease.

Second, if the physician and patient are both aware that pregnancy is a possibility and the procedure is still performed, it is much less likely that the patient will be upset if she proves to be pregnant.

Third the careful evaluation of the reproductive status of women undergoing diagnostic procedures will prevent many unnecessary lawsuits. Many lawsuits are stimulated by the factor of surprise and won on the basis of the double jeopardy of the defendant.[3,12,77] In some instances the jury is not concerned with cause and effect, but with the fact that something was not done properly by the physician. In this day and age, failure to adequately communicate can be interpreted as less than adequate medical care. Both these factors are eliminated if the patient's pregnancy status has been properly evaluated and the situation adequately discussed with the patient. Physicians are going to have to learn that practicing good technical medicine may not be enough in this litigation-prone society. Even more important, the patient will have more confidence if the decision to continue the pregnancy is made before the medical X-ray procedure is performed, since the necessity of the proceudre would have bben determined with the knowledge that the patient was pregnant

In summary, this "Teratogen Update" reviews the effects of radiation on the developing mammalian embryo and, especially, the human embryo. Counseling the women of reproductive age who will be exposed to radiation or have been exposed to radiation is frequently performed by physicians in a cavalier fashion. without the benefit of knowing the radiation exposure or the risks. The patient deserves to be counseled about the radiation hazards to the embryo by individuals who are both knowledgeable about the data that are available and willing to obtain the necessary information from the patient. Superficial evaluations of radiation exposures are a disservice to the patient and an example of poor medical care.

References

1. R.L. Brent, Effects of radiation on the foetus, newborn and child, in Fry, Grahn, Griem and Rust, Late Effects of Radiation, Taylor & Francis, London, 1970, pp. 23-60.

2. R.L. Brent, Irradiation in pregnancy in Sciarra Davis' Gynecology and Obstetrics, Vol. 2, Harper and Row, New York, 1972, pp. 1-32.

3. R.L. Brent, Environmental factors radiation. in Brent and Harris, Prevention of Embryonic Fetal and Perinatal Disease, Fogarty International Center Series on Preventive Disease, Vol 3, DHEW Publication No. NIH 76-853, Bethesda, MD, 1976 pp. 179-197.

4. R.L. Brent, Radiations and other physical agents, in Wilson and Fraser, Handbook of Teratology, Vol. 1, Plenum Press, New York, 1977, pp. 153-223.

5. R.L. Brent, and R.O. Gorson, Radiation exposure in pregnancy, in Mosley, Baker, Gorson, Lalli, Latourette and Quinn, Current Problems in Radiology, Vol. 2, Year Book Medical Publishers, Chicago, pp. 1-48.

6. L.B. Russell, X-ray induced developmental abnormalities in the mouse and their use in the analysis of embryological patterns. I. External and gross visceral changes, J. Exp. Zool. 114, 545-602 (1950).

7. L.B. Russell and W.L. Russell, The effects of radiation on the preimplantation stages of the mouse embryo, Anat. Res 108, 521 (1950).

8. R.L. Brent and B.T. Bolden, The indirect effect of irradiation on embryonic development. III. The contribution of ovarian irradiation, uterine irradiation. oviduct irradiation and zygote irradiation to fetal mortality and growth retardation in the rat, Radiat. Res. 30, 759-773 (1967).

9. L.B. Russell, X-ray induced developmental abnormalities in the mouse and their use in the analysis of embryological patterns. II. Abnormalities of the vertebral column and thorax, J. Exp. Zool. 131, 329-395, (1956).

10. L.B. Russell and W.L. Russell, An analysis of the changing radiation response of the developing mouse embryo, J. Cell Comp. Physiol 43, 103-149, (1954).

11. R. Rugh, Major radiobiological cooncepts and ionizing radiation on the embryo and fetus, in Haley and Snider, Response of the Nervous System to Ionizing Radiation, Academic Press, New York, 1962, pp. 3-26.

12. R.L. Brent, Litigation-produced pain, disease, and suffering, an experience with congenital malformation lawsuits, Teratology 16, 1-13, (1977).

13. L.B. Russell and C.L. Saylors, The relative sensitivity of various germ-cell stages of the mouse to radiation-induced nondysjunction, chromosome losses and deficiencies, in Sobels, Repair from Genetic Radiation, Pergamon Press, New York, 1963, pp. 313-342.

14. L.B. Russell and N.H. Major, Radiation-induced presumed somatic muations in the house mouse, Genetics, 42 161-175, (1957).

15. S.P. Hicks and C.J. D'Amato, Effects of ionizing radiations on mammalian development, in Woollam, Advances in Teratology, Vol. 1, Logos Press, London, 1966, pp 196-250.

16. R. Murphee and H. Pace, The effects of prenatal radiation on postnatal development in rats, Radiat. Res., 12 495-504, (1960).

17. R.L. Brent and B.T. Bolden, The long-term effects of low dosage embryonic irradiation, Radiat. Res., 14 453-454, (1961).

18. R. Rugh, Effect of ionizing radiations, including radio-isotopes on the placenta and embryo, Birth Defects, Orig. Article Series 1 64-73, (1965).

19. R. Rugh and M. Wohlfromm, X-irradiation sterilization of the premature female mouse, Atompraxis. 10 511-518, (1964).

20. R. Rugh and M. Wohlfromm, Can x-irradiation prior to sexual maturity affect the fertility of the male mammal (mouse)? Atompraxis, 10 33-41. (1964).

21. D. Cowen and L.M. Geller, Long-term pathological effects of prenatal x-irradiation on the central nervous system of the rat, J. Neuropath. Exp. Neurol., 19 488-527, (1960).

22. E. Furchtgott, Behavioral effects of ionizing radiations, 1955-1961, Psychol Bull., 60 157-199, (1963).

23. I.A. Piontkovskii, Certain properties of the higher nervous activity in adult animals irradiated prenatally by ionizing radiations. The problem of the effect of ionizing irradiation on offspring, Byull. Eksp. Biol. Med. (in Russian), 46 77-80, (1958).

24. I.A. Piontkovskii, M.B. Goldberg and O.E. Miklashevskii, Some peculiarities of the higher nervous activity in adult animals subjected antenatally to the action of ionizing radiation, Part III, Byull. Eksp. Biol. Med. (in Russian), 51 24-31, (1961).

25. R.W. Miller and J.J. Mulvihill, Small head size after atomic irradiation, Teratogen Update, Teratology, 14 355-358 (1976).

26. J. Zappert, Uber roentgenogene fetale Microcephalie, Mschr. Kinderheilk., 34 490-493, (1926).

27. L. Goldstein and D.P. Murphy, Microcephalic idiocy following radium therapy for uterine cancer during pregnancy, Am. J. Obstet Gynec. 18 189-195, 281-283, (1929).

28. L. Goldstein and J. Kratchman, Etiology of ill health in children born after maternal pelvic irradiation. II. Defective children born after post-conceptional maternal irradiation. Am. J. Roentg. 22 322-331, (1929).

29. A.S. Dekaban, Abnormalities in children exposed to x-radiation during various stages of gestation: tentative timetable of radiation injury to the human fetus, J. Nucl. Med. 9 471-477, (1968).

30. R.W. Miller, Delayed radiation effects in atomic bomb survivors, Science, 166 569-574, (1970).

31. J.W. Wood, K.G. Johnson, Y. Omori, S. Kawamoto and R.J. Keehn, Mental retardation in children exposed in utero to the atomic bombs in Hiroshima and Nagasaki, Am. J. Publ. Hlth., 57 1381-1390, (1967).

32. J.W. Wood, K.G. Johnson and Y. Omori, In utero exposure to the Hiroshima atomic bomb. An evaluation of head size and mental retardation: twenty years later, Pediatrics, 39 385-392, (1967).

33. G. Plummer, Anomalies occurring in children exposed in utero to the atomic bomb in Hiroshima, Pediatrics, 10 687-692, (1952).

34. J.M. Yamazaki, S.W. Wright and P.M. Wright, Outcome of pregnancy in women exposed to the atomic bomb in Nagasaki, Am. J. Dis. Child, 87 448-463, (1954).

35. D.P. Murphy and L. Goldstein, Micromelia in a child irradiated in utero, Surg. Gynec. Obs., 50 79-80, (1930).

36. P. Maroteaux, J. Springer, J.M. Opitz, J. Kucera, R.B. Lowry, N. Schimke and S.M. Kagan, Le syndrome campomelique, Presse Med., 22 1157-1162, (1971).

37. W. Blot, Growth and development following prenatal and childhood exposure to atomic radiation, J. Radiat. Res., 16 Supplement 82-88, (1975).

38. W. Blot and R.W. Miller, Mental retardation following in utero exposure to the atomic bombs of Hiroshima and Nagasaki, Radiol, 106 617-619, (1973).

39. S.E. Driscoll, S.P. Hicks, E.H. Copenhaver and C.L. Easterday, Acute radiation injury in two human fetuses, Archs. Path., 76 113-119, (1963).

40. K. Nokkentred, Effect of radiation upon the human fetus, Munksgaard, Copenhagen, 1968, p. 228.

41. A. Tabuchi, Fetal disorders due to ionizing radiation, Hiroshima J. Med. Sci. 13 125-173, (1964).

42. A. Tabuchi, S. Nakagawa, T. Hirai, H. Sato, I. Hori, M. Matsuda, K. Yano, K. Simada, and Y. Nakao, Fetal hazards due to X-ray diagnosis during pregnancy, Hiroshima J. Med. Sci. 16 49-66, (1967).

43. L.J. Kinlen and E.D. Acheson, Diagnostic irradiation, congenital malformations and spontaneous abortion, Br. J. Radiol. 41 648-654, (1968).

44. A. Vilmusen, Environmental factors in congenital malformations, F.A.D.L.'s Forlag, Copenhagen, 1970.

45. O.P. Heinonen, D. Slone, and S. Shapiro, Birth defects and drugs in pregnancy, Publishing Sciences Group, Littleton, MA, 1977, p. 516.

46. L. Jacobsen and L. Mellemgaard, Anomalies of the eyes in descendants of women irradiated with small X-ray doses during age of fertility, Acta Ophthal., 46 352-354, (1968).

47. K.R. Brizzee, and R.B. Brannon, Cell recovery in foetal brain after ionizing radiation, Int. J. Radiat. Biology, 21 375-378, (1972).

48. R.L. Brent, The response of the 9-1/2 day-old rat embryo to variations in exposure rate of 150 R X-irradiation, Radiat. Res., 45 127-136, (1971).

49. R.L. Brent, The indirect effect of irradiation on embryonic development. II. Irradiation of the placenta, Am. J. Dis. Child, 100 103, (1960).

50. R.L. Brent and B.T. Bolden. The indirect effect of irradiation on embryonic development. IV. The lethal effects of maternal irradiation on the first day of gestation in the rat, Proc. Soc. Exp. Biol. Med., 125 709-712, (1967).

51. R.L. Brent and B.T. Bolden, Indirect effect of x-irradiation on embryonic development. V. Utilization of high doses of maternal irradiation on the first day of gestation, Radiat. Res., 36 563-570. (1968).

52. R.L. Brent and M.M. McLaughlin, The indirect effect of irradiation on embryonic development. I. Irradiation of the mother while shielding the embryonic site, Am. J. Dis. Child, 100 94-102, (1960).

53. M. Basic and D. Weber, Uber intrauterine Fruchtschadingung durch Rongenstrahlen, Strahlentherapie, 99 628, (1956).

54. A. Stewart, The carcinogenic effects of low level radiation. A re-appraisal of epidemiologists methods and observations, Hlth. Phys. 24 223-240, (1973).

55. A. Stewart, J. Webb, D. Giles and D. Hewitt. Malignant disease in childhood and diagnostic irradiaiton in utero, Lancet, ii 447, (1956).

56. A. Stewart, D. Webb and D. Hewitt. A survey of childhood malignancies, Br. Med. J., i 1495-1508, (1958).

57. R.H. Mole, Radiation effects on prenatal development and their radiological significance, Br. J. Radiol., 52 89-191, (1979).

58. J.W. Wood, R.J. Keehn, S. Kawamoto and K.G. Johnson, The growth and development of children exposed in utero to the atomic bombs of Hiroshima and Nagasaki, Am. J. Publ. Hlth , 57 1374-1380, (1967).

59. H. Kato, Mortality in children exposed to the A-bombs while in utero, Am. J. Epidem., 93 435-442, (1971).

60. R.W. Miller, Epidemiological conclusions from radiation toxicity studies, in Fry, Grahn, Griem and Rust, Late Effects of Radiation, Taylor & Francis, London, 1970.

61. S. Jablon, Comments, Hlth. Phys., 24 257-258, (1973).

62. E.L. Diamond, H. Schmerler and A.M. Lilienfeld, The relationship of intrauterine radiation to subsequent mortality and development of leukemia in children, A prospective study, Am. J. Epidem., 97 283-313, (1973).

63. L.B. Russell, S.K. Badgett and C.L. Saylors, Comparison of the effects of acute, continuous and fractionated irradiation during embryonic development, in Buzzati-Traverso Special Suppl., Int. J. Radiation Biol., Immediate and Low Level Effects of Ionizing Radiation Conference held in Venice, Taylor & Francis, London, 1959, pp. 343-359.

64. C. Ronnback, Effects of continuous irradiation during gestation and suckling period of mice, Acta Radiol. (Ther.) 3 169-176, (1965).

65. P. Vorisek, Einfluss der kontinuierlichen intrauterinen Bestrahlung auf die perinatale Mortalitat der Frucht, Strahlentherapie, 127 112-120, (1965).

66. R.L. Brent, Medicolegal aspects of teratology, in Biologic and Clinical Aspects of Malformations, Mead Johnson Symposium on Perinatal and Developmental Medicine No. 7, Vail, Colorado, 1975, pp. 65-76.

67. J. Stadler and J.W. Gowen, Observations on the effects of continuous irradiation over 10 generations on reproductivities of different strains of mice, in Carlson and Gassner, Proceedings of an International Symposium on the Effects of Ionizing Radiation on Reproductive Systems. Pergamon Press, New York, 1964.

68. C.J. Coppenger and S.O. Brown, Postnatal manifestations in albino rats continuously irradiated during prenatal development, Tex. Rep. Biol. Med., 23 45-55, (1965).

69. G. Konermann, Die keimesentwicklung der maus nach einwirkung kontinuierlicher Co^{60} gammabestrahlung wahrend der blastogenese, der organogenese und der fetal periode, Strahlentherapie, 137 451-466, (1969).

70. J.P. Wesley, Background radiation as the cause of congenital malformation, Int. J. Radiat. Biol., 2 97-118, (1960).

71. J. Gentry, E. Parkhurst and G. Bulin, An epidemiological study of congenital malformations in New York State, Am. J. Publ. Health, 49 497, (1959).

72. D. Grahan and J. Kratchman, Variation in neonatal death rate and birth weight in the United States and possible relations to environmental radiaiton. geology and altitude, Am. J. Hum. Genet., 15 329-352, (1963).

73. A. Segall, B. MacMahon and M. Hannigan, Congenital malformations and background radiation in northern New England, J. Chron. Dis., 17 915-932, (1964).

74. H. Kriegel und H. Langendorff, Die wirkung einer fraktionierten rontgenbestrahlung auf die embryoanalentwicklung der Maus, Strahlenterapie, 123 429-437, (1964).

75. J.W. Laskey, J.L. Parrish and D.G. Cahill, Some effects of lifetime parental exposure low levels of tritium on the F2 generation, Radiat. Res., 56 171-179, (1973).

76. A.A. Neifakh, Role of the maternal organism in the irradiation illness of fetal mice, Dokl. Akad. Nauk. Biol. Sci. Sect., 116 821-824, (1957).

77. A. Ronderos, Fetal tolerance to radiation, Radiology, 76 454, (1961).

78. R.L. Brent, Medicolegal aspects of teratology, J. Pediat., 71 288-298, (1967).

79. National Council on Radiation Protection and Measurements, Basic Radiation Protection Criteria, NCRP Report No. 39, Washington, D.C., 1971.

A RADIATION RISK EDUCATION PROGRAM - LOCAL

Stewart C. Bushong and Benjamin R. Archer
Baylor College of Medicine, Houston, Texas 77030

INTRODUCTION

We, radiation scientists, have done a miserable job of informing the public about the true risks of radiation exposure. Prior to Three Mile Island, March, 1979, there was already considerable public anxiety over radiation exposure, particularly that associated with nuclear power generation. Since that unfortunate incident, newspapers and magazines have been filled with inflammatory and often totally incorrect reporting of radiation levels and radiation effects. "Thousands of lives lost to radiation", " 'Radiation never safe.' expert says", "Our unborn are endangered by radiation...", "Scientists debate safe levels of radiation for workers". These are representative of the types of headlines that introduce newspaper articles purporting to show that the low levels of radiation exposure experienced in every day life are harmful. Table 1 is a summary of such radiation doses.

It is nonsense for the public hysteria to reach such heights in the presence of a wealth of data that shows such dose levels to be essentially innocuous.

The public has been worked up to a fearful frenzy of radiation exposures associated with nuclear power and nuclear weapons. The population exposure from medical applications of radiation is more than an order of magnitude greater. We must begin a conserted program of public information to alleviate these fears by honest discussion of the real radiation exposures that exist and the true level of bioresponse to be expected from such exposures.

Table 1. Radiation in Our Daily Lives

Cancer Therapy - 5,000,000 mrads and up*
MPD for Radiation Workers - 5,000 mrads/yr*
X-Ray Mammogram 200 to 2000 mrads*
Complete Dental X-Ray Series - 500 mrads*
Pocos De Caldas, Brazil - 7,000 mrads/yr
Natural Background, Denver - 300 mrads/yr
              San Francisco - 120 mrads/yr
              New York - 135 mrads/yr
              Houston - 90 mrads/yr
One Month Vacation in an Orbiting Skylab - 200 mrads
Chest x-ray - 10-50 mrads*
Genetically Significant Dose from Medical X-rays - 20 mrads/yr*
Eating (^{40}K in Food) - 40 mrads/yr
Living in a Brick Home - 35 mrads/yr
Living in Wood Frame Home - 11 mrads/yr
Average dose within 50 mi of TMI - 0.4 mrad
Two Week Vacation Mountain Area - 3 mrads
Cross Country Jet Flight - 1 mrad
Living Next to a Nuclear Power Station - <1 mrad/yr
Consumer products - <1 mrad/yr

*Partial body exposure

In addition to informing the public correctly about radiation exposures and radiation effects, we must make sure the public understands the enormous extent of benefit derived from radiation applications in our society. Our role as radiation scientists and teachers is to properly emphasize the medical benefits of radiation exposure as well as possible effects. Should our medical application of radiation come under restrictive regulation because of public anxiety, undoubtedly the public heatlh and safety would not be served.

We must begin this education program now and at the local level. It is surprising that the number of health practioners who employ radiation in their diagnosis and treatment are so severely misinformed. We must begin by properly educating radiologists, technologists, and other health professionals in the true nature of radiation and its effects.

The public perceives that radiation scientists are in great discord regarding the effects of ionizing radiation. It must be made clear to the public that this discord is a reflection of our lack of knowledge of precisely how safe radiation is rather than how hazardous it is. We know that low levels of ionizing radiation are safe.

FORMAL EDUCATION PROGRAM

Formal training programs have been established at many universities, medical schools and hospitals. In general these formal training programs reach three populations--radiologists, technologists and other health professionals.

Formal Training of Radiologists

There are 355 radiology training programs in the U.S. at this time. Most do not have formal training in radiation biology and those that do provide such training rarely emphasize the effects of low levels of radiation exposure. Radiology residents, in general, receive sufficient information regarding the radiation dose levels experienced in diagnostic radiology. The biological effects of such levels are rarely placed in proper perspective for these physicians in training.

Such deficiency in training programs is understandable. The written examination given by the American Board of Radiology for certification of radiologists rarely has such questions included. In fact, only 10% of the examination covers radiation protection or radiation biology. Furthermore, recommended curriculum guides such as that published by the American Association of Physicists in Medicine[1] includes no recommended instruction in radiation biology and very little radiation protection. Additionally, there are a number of excellent radiobiology texts[2-7] but none deals effectively with late effects of low dose irradiation.

Most substantial information regarding low dose, late effects of radiation exposure is contained in numerous research reports. The BEIR Report[8] and the several U.N. reports[9-11] contain most of the presently available information in synthesized form. We as radiation educators must be aware of this information and pass it along in concise, understandable form to radiologists in training.

Formal Training of Radiologic Technologists

What has been said regarding the deficiencies in radiologists training is magnified ten-fold for technologist training. Each year we train approximately 10,000 technologists but very few of them ever receive adequate instruction in radiation biology. This is principally because of inadequate training of instructors of radiologic technology.

The American Society of Radiologic Technologists recognizes this deficiency. In their curriculum guide[12] radiation biology is superbly emphasized. Table 2 is reproduced from this document and shows the extent of radiation biology knowledge that is expected of radiologic technologists. In general, I think we who educate radiologic technologists fail in delivering this information to them effectively.

Table 2. Suggested Curriculum in Radiation Biology for Radiologic Technologists

I. Development of Radiation Biology: Historical Overview
II. Background Radiation - Radiation Units
III. Factors Influencing the Effects of Irradiation
IV. Direct and Indirect Action: Action of Radiation in Aqueous Systems
V. The Oxygen Effect
VI. The Nucleus - DNA
VII. Genetics: The Effects of Ionizing Radiation in the Nucleus
VIII. Relative Radiosensitivity of the Nucleus and Cytoplasm: Effects in the Total Organism; the Immediately Lethal Effects
IX. Response of Tissues and Organs to Irradiation
X. Response of Whole Organisms to Total-Body Radiation
XI. Radiation Syndromes
XII. Effects on Developing Embryos
XIII. Radiation Effects on Immunity-Radiation Immunology

Formal Training of Other Health Professionals

A number of other health professionals employ radiation in their daily practice yet receive little instruction in radiation protection and radiation biology. Such a list would include cardiologists, orthopedists, dermatologists and gynecologists. These physicians all apply radiation in specific areas of their practice but their knowledge of radiation intensities and radiation effects is minimal and inadequate because most of this information is passed along from inadequately informed preceptors. Nurses are frequently called upon to administer to patients who have received brachytherapy radiation, implants and patients treated with therapeutic doses of radioisotopes such as ^{131}I.

Radiation educators must introduce themselves to program coordinators of the training programs identified above to be sure that somewhere in their training, these health professionals receive formal lectures on radiation biology and radiation protection. This author suggests a minimum of 4 hours of instruction for each. Table 3 shows a suggested lecture outline for hours 1, 3 and 4 which can be presented to all of the above health professionals.

The first lecture would introduce the resident physician to the various types of radiation and their sources, the levels of radiation exposure experienced from natural and man-made sources and some basic information regarding atomic and nuclear physics. The second lecture should review the specific application of radiation to that medical specialty under consideration.

Table 3. Lecture Outline
Four Hour Program for Health Professionals

First Hour
  Introduction and Historical Development
  Atomic and Nuclear Physics
    Atomic Structure
    Nuclear Structure
    Electromagnetic Radiation
  The Nature of Ionizing Radiation
    Ions and Ionization
    Particulate Radiation
    X-Rays and γ-rays
Second Hour
  (Specific for the type of health professional in training)
Third Hour
  Patient Doses experienced in this specialty
    External Beam
    Internal deposition of radionuclides
  Personnel Exposures experienced in this specialty
  Radiation Protection Standards
    Maximum Permissible Doses
    Regulatory requirements
      Source Registration
      Licensure

Fourth Hour
  Fundamentals of Radiobiology
    Biological modifying factors
    Physical modifying factors
  Molecular Radiobiology
    Direct v. Indirect Effect
    Target theory
  Cellular Radiobiology
    Cell Survival Kinetics
    Recovery
  Mammalian Radiobiology
    Early Effects
    Late Effects
      Life Span Shortening
      Local Tissue Effects
      Leukemia
      Cancer
      Genetic Effects
  Risk Estimates

As an example, Table 4 shows what one might suggest for hour two for presentation to dermatologists. Dermatologists require specific instruction in the types of sources they apply - superficial and grenz x-rays and radium primarily. Such instruction must include the fundamentals of dosimetry and treatment planning. The third lecture reviews radiation intensity levels experienced in the various medical specialties, and basic radiation protection programs for minimizing those exposure levels. The final lecture reviews radiation biology with emphasis on low-dose late effects at the whole body level. This final lecture should synthesize exposure levels experienced in each specialty to suspected effects.

Table 4. Lecture Outline
Hour Two for Dermatologists

External Beam Treatments
  X-ray machines
    Design and function
    Superficial
    Grenz rays
    Beam Quantity and Quality
    Percent Central Axis Depth Dose
  Treatment Design
    Tissue Dosimetry
    The Treatment Plan
    Dose-response relationships
Brachytherapy Treatments
  Types of radionuclide sources
  Radium and Radium Equivalent Dosimetry
  Time-Dose relationships
  Use of applicators
  Mold fabrication
  The Treatment Plan

IN-SERVICE TRAINING

Most hospitals have on-going in-service training programs for all the professional staff. These programs should include at least annual lectures by medical or health physicists or radiation biologists. These lectures should cover the various aspects of basic radiation protection and radiobiology as applied to the institution and each should be acknowledged by date and outline in the in-service file. In a large general hospital there are perhaps three groups to be targeted for such in-service training.

In-Service Training of Physicians

I have found it helpful to occupy the lecture slot at one of the monthly hospital physician staff meetings to report to physicians continuing information on radiation levels and radiation effects. It is particularly helpful to keep them informed not only of radiation as it effects their medical practice but also radiation in our daily lives. Physicians, as we all know, are held in high regard in all communities. They are in particularly persuassive positions and can influence the public mood regarding radiation positively but only if they are properly informed.

In-Service Training of Technologists

Technologists are usually the first line of communication with patients in the department of radiology. Radiologists usually have little such contact. Consequently, we must rely on technologists to communicate effectively with the radiology patients. In-service training programs directed to technologists should continually emphasize the radiation protection aspects of their profession and radiation biology. In addition, the radiological physicist is in a unique position to continually up-date the technologists skills in areas of new technological development. Following 70 years of ratehr unremarkable growth we have, in the last decade, seen an explosion of new developments in radiology that are particularly associated with imaging. Diagnostic ultrasound, CT scanning, rare earch screens, carbon fiber materials are only a few of the more prominent such developments. Each has special radiation protection considerations. In-service training of technologists designed to inform them of the physical basis for these developments should include discussions of the characteristic radiation protection aspects of each.

In-Service Training of Nurses

Of all the health professionals, nurses perhaps have most patient contact and, therefore, are in a position to allay any patient fears regarding radiation. This, of course, means that the nursing staff must be educated regarding radiation levels and effects. Annual in-service training programs should cover these topics. In those hospitals where radiation therapy is practiced additional nursing instruction may be necessary. Brachytherapy patients and radioisotope patients require special handling. There is little formal information available in this area and, therefore, the radiation physicist must rely on a discussion of in-house procedures developed for handling such patients.

Table 5 lists typical nursing instructions for managing Gold seed brachytherapy patients. In order for nursing staff to properly understand these instructions, they need to have some information regarding radiation levels. This must be followed by a discussion of radiation effects so that the nursing staff is given a proper balance of what their real risk is in caring for such a patient. Instructions for radium or cesium intracavitary application would be similar.

Table 5. Radiation Safety Procedures for Interstitial Radiation Therapy

GOLD-198 SEEDS
1. The gold seeds are implanted into the patient in surgery.
2. The patient is then transferred to a recovery room and the radiation level is monitored by a representative of the Radiation Safety Office.
3. If the radiation level is above 5 mR/hr at one meter, a sign clearly indicating "Radiation Area" will be posted on the patient's door, and this sign should not be removed until either the sources have been removed or the patient is released.
4. A statement of radiation levels, nursing instructions, and visitor restrictions are posted on the room door. A copy of this form is also placed on the patient's chart. If the radiation level is below 5 mR/hr at one meter, the form is placed in the patient's chart, but no form is placed on the patient's door.
5. The nurses involved are briefed as to special procedures.
6. If the original level was above 5 mR/hr, the patient is monitored daily until the radiation falls below this level, and the visitor instructions on the door are modified accordingly.
7. No pregnant women or persons under eighteen years of age may enter the patients' room.
8. While in the room, visitors must remain at least one meter from the patient's bed. Each visitor is limited to _____ hours per day. (50 mR/day)
9. Additional precautions DO   DO NOT need to be followed regarding food trays, medications, needles, syringes, etc. Instructions:

Continuation Table 5.

10. . After the patient leaves the hospital, the room is again monitored to ensure against possible loss of gold seeds.
11. A statement of the total activity implanted into the patient is kept on file in the Radiation Safety Office.

Patients undergoing radioisotope therapy may require even more careful handling. Table 6 lists instructions for nurses appropriate for such patients. Unlike the brachytherapy patient, the radioisotope patient constitutes a potential contamination hazard in addition to external radiation exposure. In such cases, nursing personnel must be properly informed of the care necessary for handling such patients and all items with which they come into contact.

TABLE 6. Special Nursing Instructions
For Radioiodine Therapy

Radiation Safety Precautions
1. The patient is not permitted to leave the room without a written order from the attending physician.
2. Wear disposable rubber gloves whenever it is necessary to touch the patient or to touch any item in the patient's room. Deposit used rubber gloves in the lined trash container provided in the room. It is not necessary to wear a disposable gown or an isolation mask.
3. Any items brought into the patient's room must remain in the room during the therapy period -- i.e., sphygnamonometer, stethescope, phlebotomy equipment, eating trays, disposable plates and disposable utensels, linen and bed clothes, personal hygiene utensels, thermometer. No trash or linen can be removed from the patient's room during the therapy period.
4. After the therapy is completed, the radiation safety officer will check the entire room for radiation contamination; do not remove anything from the room prior to this time unless approved in writing by the attending physician.
5. To limit radiation exposure to nursing personnel, do not spend more time in the patient's room than is necessary to administer required nursing care.
6. While in the room, visitors should not get within three feet from the patient's bed. Visitors are limited to _____ hours. (50 mrem/day)
7. No pregnant women or persons under 18 years of age may enter the patient's room.

Special Nursing Care
1. Radioiodine therapy requires that the patient take an oral

Continuation Table 6.

dose of radioactive liquid iodine. Some of the iodine is retained in the body, but most of the iodine dose is excreted in the urine in the first 18 hours of therapy. A small amount of radioactivity is present in the patient's saliva for the duration of the therapy.

2. Special medication is written as p.r.n. order in the "Physician's Orders" for nausea. Within the first six hours after swallowing the liquid iodine, the patient's vomitus may contain radiation. If the patinet vomits within the first six hours, treat the vomitus as radioactive and notify the Nuclear Medicine Department for further instructions.

3. Ambulatory patients will use the commode in their room. The commode should be flushed three times after use when Iodine is the radioactive material.

4. Diagnostic samples of blood, urine and feces should only be obtained when authorized by the Radiotherapist.

5. The food tray may be returned to the kitchen in the normal manner.

6. The patient must wear hospital pajamas.

7. Urine is radioactive; spills, bedwetting or any accident with urine are radiation hazards. Wear gloves. Cover with absorbent material and place the absorber in the designated waste container. Notify Radiation Safety Officer immediately.

8. The radiation levels in the room are low enough so that proper nursing care can be administered without nursing personnel being excessively exposed to health-endangering radiation.

PUBLIC INFORMATION PROGRAMS

I must repeat again that we as radiation scientists have failed miserably to properly educate the public regarding radiation, its levels and its effects. We must begin now to engage ourselves as vigorously as individually possible in media programs at the local level. Radio talk shows, television interviews and lectures to community groups are all modalities that can be pressed into public education programs. In the case of written reports such as newspaper interviews, care must be taken to follow-up with the reporter and approve of the written draft before publication. As we all know, a 30 minute interview that is synthesized into a five paragraph report can oftentimes convey quite the opposite impression than that which was intended.

Our national radiation organizations must begin to sponsor public information programs and perhaps even sponsor Washington level lobbyists for this purpose. The aim would not be to influence legislation but rather to insure that a balanced discussion of risk and benefit occurs and that accurate risk information is delivered. The Health Physics Society has taken the first step in this direction by granting to its Midwest Chapter a small sum of money to conduct the Radiation Effects Information Hotline.

The Radiation Effects Information Hotline is a program of information resources made available to the public by WATTS telephone lines. The Board of Directors of the Health Physics Society has recently expanded this program from regional status to national status. The telephone number is 800-942-9440 and anyone having a question about radiation is encouraged to call that number. Volunteers staff the number during most working hours and if a volunteer is not immediately available, a recording is automatically made and that call returned. If the volunteer source cannot provide an immediate answer, the question is recorded for subsequent research following which a return call is made and the answer provided. Figure 1 shows a temporal summary of the first three months operation of this program during which time 207 calls were reviewed. Interestingly, as shown in Figure 2, most of the queries involved medical radiation exposure.

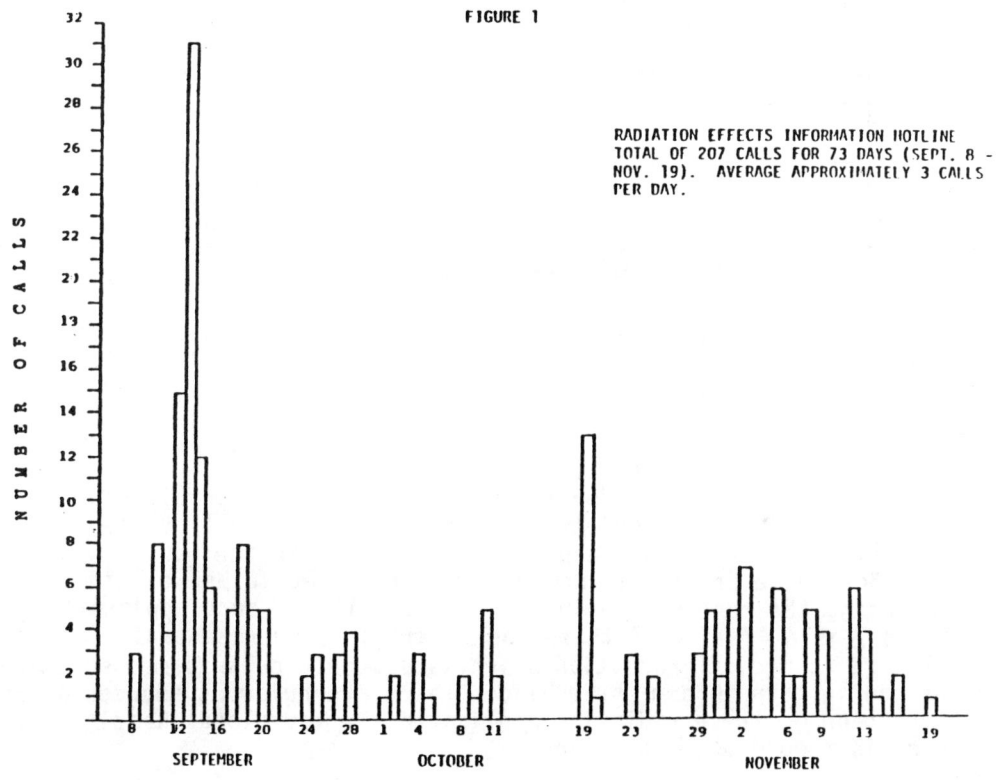

FIGURE 1

RADIATION EFFECTS INFORMATION HOTLINE
TOTAL OF 207 CALLS FOR 73 DAYS (SEPT. 8 - NOV. 19). AVERAGE APPROXIMATELY 3 CALLS PER DAY.

(Courtesy Health Physics Staff of Argonne National Laboratory)

FIGURE 2

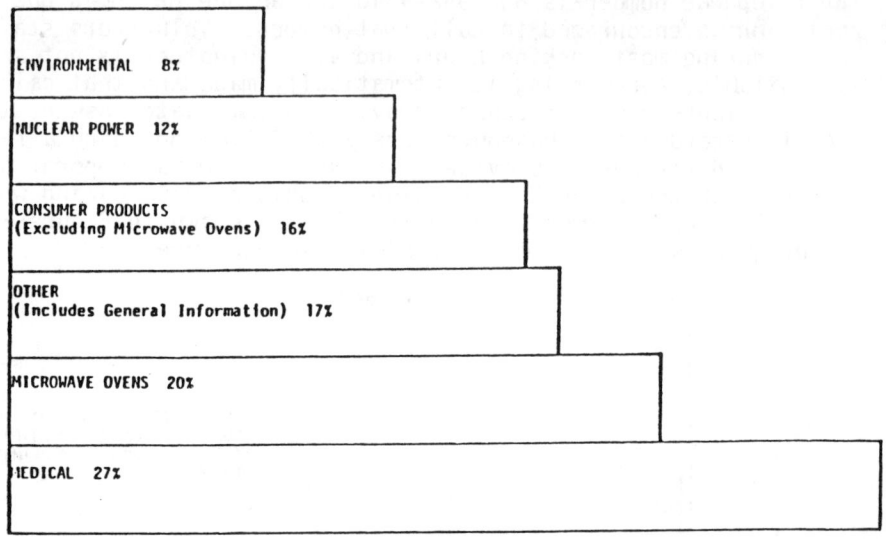

(Courtesy Health Physics Staff of Argonne National Laboratory)

Unfortunately, this program has not been sufficiently advertised and, consequently, is a relatively unknown program. Through our individual efforts it should become better known as we make it known in our communities.

A PROPER BENEFIT RISK EVALUATION

Our local public information program should emphasize the benefits of radiation to society. We are, of course, well versed in the medical benefits of such applications and few in the public would question these benefits. However, we also need to be well informed regarding the research in industrial benefits of such applications. Table 7 is a listing of these applications as representative of those that we as medical radiation scientists should be informed so that we can in turn inform the public. There are numerous sources of information on these radiation applications. Your local hospital library is a good place to start.

Table 7. A Summary of the Benefits of Radiation to Society

A. Research Applications
   - Basic Research
   - Biomedical Research
   - Industrial Research
B. Medical Applications
   - Diagnostic Radioisotopes
   - Therapeutic Radioisotopes
   - Radiation Producing Machines
C. Industrial Applications
   - Tracer Methodology
   - Basic Metals
   - Geophysical
   - Gauging
   - Environmental Monitoring
D. Consumer Applications
   - Food Preservation
   - Wood Products
   - Smoke Alarms
   - Instrument Dials
   - Security Surveillance
   - Static Eliminators
   - Spark Gap Irradiations

Table 8. Life Span Shortening Associated with Various Conditions

Condition	Days
Being unmarried-male	3500
Cigarette smoking-male	2250
Heart disease	2100
Being 30% overweight	1300
Cancer	980
Stroke	700
Motor vehicle accidents	207
Alcohol (U.S. Average)	130
Accidents in home	95
Average job - accidents	74
Drowning	41
Job with radiation exposure	40
Illicit drugs (U.S. aver.)	18
Natural radiation (BEIR)	8
Medical x-rays	6
Diet drinks	2
Reactor accidents-UCS	2*
Reactor accidents-Rasmussen	0.02*
Smoke alarm in home	-10
Air bags in car	-50

*These itmes assume that all U.S. power is nuclear. UCS is Union of Concerned Scientists, the most prominent group of nuclear critics.

We must also have a fundamental knowledge of radiation risk but in particular radiation risk as it relates to other risks in our society - relative risk. Much of this information can be obtained from the various publications of industrial safety such as the National Safety Council. We should also be aware of the extremely timely papers by Cohen(13-15) that have appeared recently in Health Physics. Table 8 lists twenty categories out of 54 reported by Cohen(15) in descending order showing the average loss of life span for various conditions of life as extracted from various population statistics and industrial data. Note that the life span shortening associated with radiation exposure from reactor aperations assumes that all power generation is nuclear.

Statistics formulated by the National Safety Council should also be familiar to us so that they can be transmitted to the public during the course of our local public information programs. Table 9 shows the number of deaths attributed to various conditions for the calendar year, 1977, the latest available. Note the number of radiation deaths during that year was zero. As you might suspect, the number of radiation deaths year after year is consistently zero. The reason, of course, is that the radiation exposures that we experience industrially are so very small and radiation accidents are very rare.

Table 9. Deaths in the U.S. due to various causes (1977).

Cause of Death	Number
Heart Disease	718,850
Cancer	386,686
Stroke	181,934
All accidents	103,202
Pneumonia	49,889
Auto accidents	49,510
Suicide	28,881
Homocide	19,968
Falls	13,773
Fire	6,359
Cataclysm (Tournado, flood, etc.)	202
Radiation	0

One set of NSC statistics bears particular scrutiny. Figure 3 is redrawn from the summary table of the National Safety Council showing both the number of deaths per year and the annual death rate attributed to automobile accidents. Early in this century automobile fatalities were relatively high but dropped precipitously during World War II. They climbed again for former heights until the 1973 Arab oil embargo and the subsequent institution of the 55 mph speed limit. As Figure 3 shows, there was a precipituous drop in automobile fatalities coinciding with the inception of the 55 mph speed limit. We have saved nearly 10,000 lives per year with this lower speed limit.

Figure 3. Total Deaths and Death Rate
From Automobile Accidents

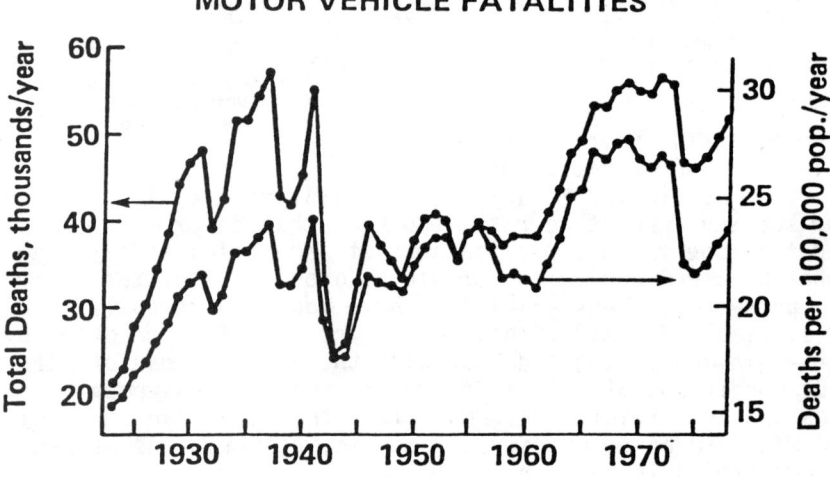

There is an interesting observation to be made from these traffic fatality statistics. If one assumes that prior to 1973 the average automobile speed was 65 mph and that since that time it has been 55 mph, a dose response relationship is possible. From the two ordered pairs of dose (mph) and response (automobile deaths) we can demonstrate the astounding fact, as shown in Figure 4, that automobile deaths follow a threshold type relationship. Consequently if we legislate a maximum speed of 25 mph, the approximate threshold dose value, no automobile deaths would be expected.

Figure 4. Motor Vehicle Induced Lethality apparently follows a linear threshold dose-response relationship.

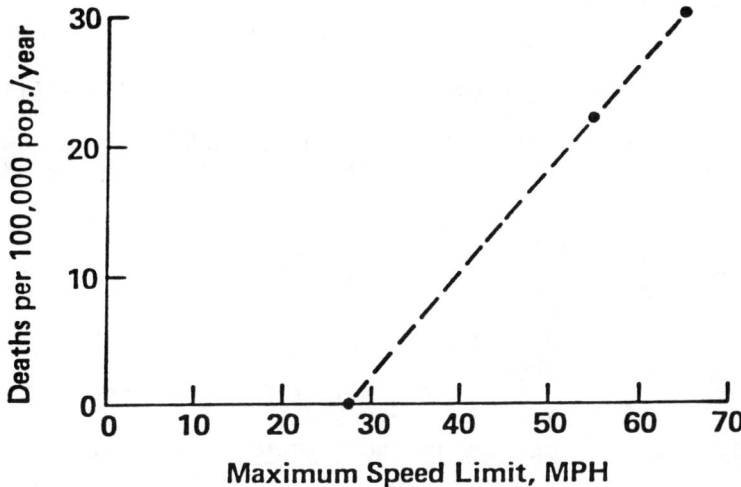

REFERENCES

1. *Syllabus and Problems in Physics for Radiology Residents*, AAPM-ACR revised ed., 1973.
2. V. Arena, "*Ionizing Radiation and Life*", The C.V. Mosby Co., 1971.
3. D.J. Pizzarello, "*Medical Radiation Biology*", Lea & Febiger, 1972.
4. J.I. Fabrikant, "*Radiobiology*", Year Book Medical Publishers, Inc. 1972.
5. E. Hall, "*Radiobiology for the Radiologist*", Harper & Row, 1973.
6. G.V. Dalrymple, "*Medical Radiation Biology*", W.B. Saunders Co., 1973.
7. E.L. Travis, "*Primer of Medical Radiobiology*", Yearbook Medical Publishers, 1975.
8. *The Effects of Population of Exposure to Low Levels of Ionizing Radiation*, NAS-NRC, 1972.
9. *Report of the United Nations Scientific Committee on the Effects of Atomic Radiation*, New York, 1962.
10. *Report of the United Nations Scientific Committee on the Effects of Atomic Radiation*, New York, 1964.
11. *Ionizing Radiation: Levels and Effects*, New York, 1972.
12. ASRT Guide
13. B.L. Cohen, The BEIR report relative risk and absolute risk models for estimating effects of low level radiation" *Health Physics* 37: 509, 1979.
14. B.L. Cohen, Laws of Statistics Ignored by Statisticians, *Health Physics* 35:582, 1978.
15. B.L. Cohen, *Health Physics* 36:707, 1979.
16. *National Safety Council, Accident Facts*, 1979 Edition.

A RADIATION RISK EDUCATION PROGRAM - NATIONAL

Prepared by

William S. Properzio, Ph.D., Director, Division of Training and Medical Applications, Bureau of Radiological Health, 5600 Fishers Lane, Rockville, Maryland 20857

INTRODUCTION

One of the four objectives outlined by the organizers of this symposium was to provide the participants with "an understanding of the accepted dose evaluation procedures and the methods for relating dose to a risk/benefit evaluation." As my contribution I have been asked to outline some of the education programs at the national level that contribute to this goal.

Radiation risk must be kept in mind in any clinical decision but should not be the primary focus of educational efforts at the Federal, state or clinical level. Instead of radiological risk, primary emphasis should be placed on clinical benefit. The risk of any individual diagnostic examination is usually very small, often in the order of one in several thousand. For an examination that is medically needed the benefit is almost always greater than the risk. Thus, the idea of performing a benefit/risk evaluation for an individual patient is usually unrealistic. The real question is if the examination is medically warranted. If the examination is likely to have an influence on patient management then the small risk of long term biological effects is almost automatically outweighed.

If we focus our attention on clinical benefit instead of radiological risk, we find our efforts directed toward answering questions such as:
- Is a particular examination appropriate for this patient? Will it provide useful information? Will the results of the examination effect treatment or outcome? PATIENT SELECTION
- Was the examination performed properly so that the requisite diagnostic information can be obtained? EXAM CONDUCT
- Was the physician able to correctly evaluate the diagnostic information? INTERPRETATION
- Does the patient have a realistic understanding of the role of radiology so that he or she will neither demand unnecessary examinations or refuse those that are appropriately prescribed? Is the patient providing the attending physician or radiological staff with needed information (i.e., indication of previous examinations, pregnancy status, etc.) CONSUMER EDUCATION

A fundamental understanding of radiation biology and risks is important in the development of appropriate action and educational efforts in the areas of patient selection, exam conduct, interpretation and consumer education, but risk reduction should not become understood as the sole target of these efforts.

PUBLIC UNDERSTANDING AND ATTITUDES

The attention that has been directed to events such as human exposures during the nuclear weapons tests in Nevada, the study of exposed workers at Hanford, Washington and Portsmouth, New Hampshire, the events at Three Mile Island, Pennsylvania (TMI), and a host of others has created an atmosphere of public awareness and concern regarding the effects of ionizing radiation. Although all of these efforts occurred in the non-medical application of radiation, an inevitable spillover of concern into the clinical area has occurred. On one hand we see an increased public demand for the reduction of medical radiation exposure, demands which are seldom tempered with an understanding that medical radiation exposure is an intentional administration of radiation to the patient as opposed to the unintentional by-product exposures received in a nuclear reactor or other occupational situation. Countering this wish to decrease exposure is the desire of the patient to receive every advantage of current medical science. The patient often feels the physician has not done his job if every test available has not been run.

We as knowledgeable and responsible professionals must direct some effort to the effective communication of facts so that clear and logical decisions can be made by physicians and physicists, government officials and the public. The responsibility of the professional to educate others has received increased editorial attention. In a recent article in Science (1), Roy suggests that scientists (and in the field of medicine that must be extended to include physicians in clinical practice) has a responsibility "...to devote part of their intellectual energies to inform their fellow citizens about their own field... ." The article goes on to point out that the public reaction to a known or imagined risk can be defined by the "3P" risk equation. That is:

$$\text{Perception} \quad \text{Probability} \times \text{Propaganda}$$

Webster defines propaganda as "the spreading of ideas, information or rumor for the purpose of helping or injuring an institution, a cause or a person." Clearly we all have a stake in making sure that the public receives accurate information instead of slanted progaganda that will assist in developing a realistic picture of radiation and its place in medicine and industry.

For those in direct contact with an incident such as TMI, this need to serve as a source of information becomes immediately evident. William Weidner, Chairman of the Department of Radiology at the Hershey Medical Center in Hershey, Pennsylvania, outlined direct impact a nuclear incident, even devoid of patient care responsibilities, has on a department of radiology. In a paper delivered at the 1979 meeting of the RSNA, Weidner (2) pointed out that a medical center must play a key role in the event of such an occurrence. Two key areas of responsibilities were 1) a source of information and advice for the medical staff, and 2) public relations, dealing with the press, public inquiries, private industry and state government agencies.

As each of us approaches this task of information dissemination it is important to analyze the individual or group one is trying to communicate with. We do this to some degree, but often not to the extent we should. Each audience presents a different challenge and although it is not possible to develop a single descriptive profile for each, some general observations are in order.

In dealing with professional colleagues it is important to have technical points clearly outlined. The interest of this target audience is to understand the technology and how it relates to clinical practice. Although this presents a challenge, we usually handle this with the least degree of emotional concern since we are dealing in a comfortable scientific/academic atmosphere.

Communication with the press and the general public often present a much greater challenge. Representatives of the press are usually interested in accurately reporting the facts but want these facts to be simple, clear and to the point. If you are not able to present your points in a clear and direct way the reporter will often make the simplification for you, often resulting in unintentional misquotations and/or distortions of the facts. Effective communication with the general public, for which there is often nothing general that can be identified, is difficult. To the public the subject of radiation is complex, but they have, without doubt, heard or read enough to form an opinion. They are often questioning and skeptical with regard to the motives of the speaker; are we pro- or anti-nuclear, and can they believe the facts we present to them?

Examples of how all these elements; the radiation expert, the press and the public, come into play can be seen in stories we hear and read in the news every day. An example is an article that appeared on February 14, 1980, in the Washington Post, titled "Nuclear Agency Probes Leaks at Calvert Cliffs." It described the investigation into two leaks of Xenon-133 from a power reactor in Maryland. A Nuclear Regulatory Commission (NRC) spokesperson pointed out that although workers were evacuated from an auxiliary building on both occasions, the leaks were "extremely low" and posed no health hazard. This same NRC expert was quoted as saying the exposure received by the workers (which was estimated to be 0.008 mrem) was 30,000 times less than the radiation from a chest x ray.

One must question what the real situation is and what effect it will have on even seemingly unrelated issues. For example, what attitude will this report build in the individual who may be asked to undergo a needed chest x ray in the near future? Will he or she agree to undergo a procedure that has a purported hazard 30,000 times greater than that for which a reactor would evacuate its operational personnel? Did the NRC spokesperson know that the average entrance exposure for a chest x ray is about 22 mR and not the 240 mR that could be calculated from the article, or was this a misquote on the part of the reporter? Did the NRC spokesperson know that there is no easy direct comparison between a probable whole body immersion in a radioactive gas and a collimated/limited body exposure from a diagnostic x-ray beam?

The examples are numerous, the questions they raise are endless, but the point is clear that we must all attempt to communicate the facts, that which is known as well as that for which we still do not have a clear scientific understanding.

USER EDUCATION PROGRAMS

The Bureau of Radiological Health (BRH) continues to place its major program efforts in the area of diagnostic radiology. The regulatory route has been employed to assure the availability of equipment that meets acceptable standards of performance. These regulatory programs are directed to the manufacturer. In dealing with the user (physician, physicist and technologist) a nonregulatory educational approach has been used. The Bureau's goal is to assist the medical community in improving the clinical benefit of radiological procedures.

Quality Assurance (QA) has been a major area of emphasis. Federal/state QA programs such as DENT (Dental Exposure Normalization Techniques) and BENT (Breast Exposure Nationwide Trends) has provided assistance to facilities that do not have adequate physics support to identify and correct problems with techniques. Exam specific QA programs for other procedures would seem to be an area for future activity. The Bureau has published a general recommendation (3) for QA programs for all diagnostic x-ray facilities. The recommendation suggests that each facility should evaluate its operation and establish a QA program directed to its particular needs. Similar guidance is currently underdevelopment for nuclear medicine.

The Radiological Health Sciences Learning Laboratory (RHSLL) developed under contract and available for purchase from the American College of Radiology is directed to physician education. This training tool is broken into three elements targeted at the areas of patient selection, examination conduct and interpretation. The interpretation phase is accomplished through a collection of approximately 1400 clinical case files. Continuing efforts are being made to improve the system. New cases are continually added to the film file. An entirely new section dealing with physics is presently under development by the contractor in association with selected American Association of Physicists in Medicine (AAPM) physicists.

A major new effort has been launched to aid in the development of patient referral criteria in diagnostic radiology. Following the recommendations of a national conference (4) on the subject held in 1978, the Bureau has initiated a number of program efforts. We view our role as that of a facilitator or catalyst to assist the medical community in the proposal, clinical evaluation and implementation of referral criteria. To this end the Bureau has assisted, through contract, the establishment of a number of expert physician panels to propose selection criteria for a number of x-ray exams. The draft criteria proposed by these experts would be tested where necessary in clinical practice. Professional society review would be sought prior to implementation. A number of research grants have also been awarded to collect clinical data that will aid in future referral criteria development.

The role of the technologist in medical radiology has come under increased attention in the last few years. Eleven states now have technologist licensure programs. It has been estimated that 40 to 80 thousand x-ray operators, up to one-half the work force, have received only on-the-job training. For a number of years the United States Congress has proposed various bills that would establish licensure requirements for operators, but none as yet have been passed. The current public concern for radiation may lead to a change in this status. Presently one Senate and three House bills are under consideration. The impact of nationwide licensure on technologist performance cannot be fully predicted. The Bureau, on the other hand, has always assumed that adequate education will influence better performance. The development of training slide/ tape packages, videotapes and publications has been one focus of our efforts.

A Bureau contract with the American Society of Radiologic Technologists (ASRT) has just completed the development of a self-assessment educational unit. This program targeted at the working technologist consists of a self-test taken by the individual to identify areas of weakness. A series of 19 self-study educational manuals are available to the technologist. A program promoting the use of this tool by certified and noncertified technologists is soon to be announced by the ASRT.

CONSUMER/PATIENT EDUCATION

The role of the consumer/patient in radiology is rapidly being identified. The attitude that "the doctor always knows what is best and I as a patient have no direct role to play in my health care" is rapidly becoming an attitude of the past. The individual now wants to understand and contribute to his or her health care.

The goal of a consumer educational effort should be to develop a realistic view on the part of the individual of what radiology can contribute to his/her health care. The patient should not have unrealistic expectations of benefits from an x-ray exam. We all know of individuals who feel that they have not received appropriate care if one or more diagnostic procedure is not ordered by the physician. On the other end of the spectrum, patients should not refuse appropriately ordered exams based on unrealistic fears. The patient will also benefit if a knowledgeable interface with the physician can be developed. The individual can often identify other exams that have been carried out that may provide information to the physician. Communication by patients of conditions such as a potential pregnancy are also important to the physician. The BRH has just received the results of a survey of consumer attitudes about x rays. The survey (5) was carried out under contract by a public research firm that made phone contact with approximately 1150 individuals 18 years of age or older. Some of the preliminary results are interesting.

Attitudes Regarding X-Ray Exams:

o   Approximately 70 percent agree that "x rays should be taken whenever the doctor orders them."
o   Twenty percent agree that "the better a doctor is, the more x rays he orders."
o   Seventy-seven percent agree that "a good use of x rays is to reassure the patient or the doctor that nothing is wrong."
o   Almost 30 percent would still want an x ray even if the "doctor told (them) that the information from an x ray... would not make any difference in (their) medical treatment.

Communication Between Patients and Physicians

o   Ninety-two percent think that patients should ask doctors why an x-ray exam is suggested. But 60 percent think that most patients do not ask. Over 40 percent of these respondents thought the reason that most people don't ask is because most people "think the doctor knows best."
o   One-third of the respondents would ask for an x ray even if the doctor didn't suggest one.

Current Knowledge Level

o   Only nine percent felt that lead shielding was most important for abdominal x rays; 5 percent thought it was most important for dental x rays; 9 percent for chest x rays; and 60 percent felt "it's equally important for all x-ray exams."
o   Sixty percent felt that pregnant women should go ahead and have an x ray if the doctor explains why its needed. Twenty percent felt she shouldn't and 20 percent didn't know.
o   Over 74 percent think that x rays are sometimes taken when they're not medically needed.
o   Seventy-five percent think people should keep a record of their x rays so they can tell the doctor about earlier x rays; 65 percent so they can tell if they've had too many x rays; and 63 percent so they can add up the radiation they've received.

A report of Federal radiation program activities (6) issued in June 1979 identified a need to increase consumer education efforts. To implement this directive the BRH has launched an intensified program. The effort will utilize various printed materials, slide/tape packages and media public service announcements. Efforts are being made to identify other governmental (Federal and state) and private sector groups who can act as multipliers in distribution of the materials.

The basic messages that will be emphasized in the effort are:

o   don't decide on your own that you need an x ray;
o   don't insist on an x ray;
o   if your doctor orders an x ray, ask how it will help with the diagnosis;
o   tell the doctor about any similar x-ray examinations you have had;
o   ask if gonad shielding can be used for yourself or for your children; and
o   tell your doctor if you think you are pregnant before having an x-ray examination.

REFERENCES

1. R. Roy, Sci. 201, 132 (1980).
2. W. A. Weidner, The Impact of a Nuclear Crisis on a Radiology Department. Radiol. Soc. of N. Amer., Atlanta (November 1979).
3. FDA, Quality Assurance Programs for Diagnostic Radiology Facilities; Final Recommendation, Federal Register, 44:71728-71740 (December 11, 1979).
4. FDA, National Conference on Referral Criteria for X-ray Examinations, HEW Publication (FDA) 79-8083 (1979).
5. Chilton Research Services, A Survey of Consumer Attitudes about X rays, FDA Contract Report (December 1979).
6. F. P. Libassi, Report of the Interagency Task Force on Health Effects of Ionizing Radiation. Office of the Secretary, HEW. (June 1979).

DISCUSSION - RISK EVALUATION AND REDUCTION

L. Wagner: To within what accuracy do you feel you can estimate fetal dose from fluoroscopy and radiography exams when a question arises regarding a particular patient?

S. Bushong: We have not done an error analysis but suspect it is within ± 25-50% and this, we think, is sufficient for most situations. If the calculated dose exceeds 5 rads, we conduct a measurement exercise with TLD's throughout a simulated examination series.

Dr. Goff: Did the NCRP #52 data using skin exposure measurement include scatter or not?

Dr. Bushong: The data represents exposure in air.

Dr. Goff: What do you do to include fluoro spot film exposures in fetal dosage estimates and how do you relate the measured table top (in air) data to the fetal dose?

S. Bushong: We measure fluoro table top and spot film exposure and use the NCRP (BRH) data to estimate fetal dose.

S. Brahmavar: Please clarify the impression that dose from diagnostic x-ray exposure study done with CT is far less than from conventional x-ray study. For example, in CT if dose is 0.5R/slice, then study with 8 slices is nearly 4 R/study. If repeated with contrast, it is additional 4R/study; total of 8R/study. Thus far, more than in conventional x-ray study.

S. Bushong: If the lens dose/slice in CT were 0.5 each, one can correctly assume that only during one slice will the primary beam intercept the lens. Therefore, with and without contrast, the lens dose would be 2 rads.

E. Gregg: There seems to be an avoidance of listing the average absorbed dose in various organs which is of importance for risk calculations. Use of the surface dose only may lead to errors in risk estimates.

S. Bushong: This type data should be made available for most diagnostic procedures. The organ dose index suggested by Rosenstein and Laws is a good start. (Rosenstein, M., "Organ Doses in Diagnostic Radiology", HEW Pub. 768030, May, 1976.)

E. Webster: (Comment addressed to S. Bushong) In your text you note that radiation cataract produced by x-rays has a (simple dose) threshold of about 200 rads. With fractionated radiation, the threshold is considerably higher. Since doses to the lens of the eye received occupationally should be maintained below 5 rads per year and are usually below 1 rad per year, there seems to be no reason to invest in protective glasses or goggles which you note are now available. This would appear to be an unnecessary precaution and expense. Secondly, you also implied in your talk that a single film badge should be worn above the lead apron (e.g., at the collar). I believe, as is stated in NCRP Report 57, pp. 65-66, that a single badge should be worn under the apron, preferably at waist level, since it is far more important radiobiologically to monitor the trunk exposure (leukemia, lung, liver, and breast cancer) than the eye or thyroid exposure. Thyroid cancer appears to have a high incidence following radiation, but has a very low mortality. Moreover, the neck dose, if the only recorded dose, will give a grossly misleading estimate of the important trunk dose. Therefore, if the neck (thyroid) dose is monitored, a second badge should be worn at the collar, in addition to the waist badge.

T. Fields: Comparison of x-ray diagnostic exposure versus nuclear medicine exposures should consider non-uniformity of distribution, fractionation time, and purpose of study of dynamic versus static imaging.

J. Kereiakes: I fully agree, there is non-uniformity of dose distribution for the nuclear medicine exposures compared to the diagnostic x-ray exposures. There is also dose protraction for the nulear medicine exposures compared to the diagnostic x-ray exposures.

E. Webster: In 90% of radioisotope procedures, Tc99m is used and with these procedures, 75% of the dose is delivered in 12 hours or less. This is not a high degree of protraction compared with the protraction for I-131. However, even with Tc99m, the average dose rate is perhaps 50 times lower than that for a typical series of x-ray exposures which are spread over about 15 minutes in a typical examination. (Comment related to earlier point made by Ted Fields, Chicago.)

E. Gregg: The tendency to recommend dose reduction without consideration of the dependence of diagnostic accuracy is to be depreciated.

J. Kereiakes: There has to be a compromise between the dose reduction and the desired diagnostic accuracy.

S. Bushong: In view of Wednesday's discussions, can't we consider the high dose rate in x-ray and low dose rate in nuclear medicine to be equal (protraction-wise) since they are both low < 10 rads and considered for low dose effects?

J. Kereiakes: The variations seen are lesser effects for the low dose rates in nuclear medicine as compared to the high dose rates for x-ray procedures. For example, it was indicated yesterday that the group in Cincinnati reported on the effects in the thyroid for Iodine-131 as being approximately 50 times less than the effects for x-ray radiation. The present thinking is that this difference be given as a range of 20 to 50 times less in effect. However, differences between the two types of radiation also involves the non-uniformity of uptake of the thyroid tissue by Iodine-131 versus the uniform irradiation by the x-rays.

E. Webster: I am concerned that, in general, the whole-body doses and those to some specific organs, such as bone marrow and spleen, are higher than those deliverd by routine diagnostic x-ray examinations. Typical bone marrow doses, e.g., from 15 mc, of Tc99m--diphosphonate used for bone scans, are several hundred millirads (Table 8, Kereiakes). The dose to the spleen from 12 mCi of Tc99m - red cells is evidently 15.6 rads. I believe that these doses should be reviewed in terms of the usefulness of the examination in comparison with those delivered in x-ray procedures. In the latter, only a part of the marrow is irradiated, whereas in nuclear medicine it is the entire marrow. Can these doses be reduced?

J. Kereiakes: There is a tendancy in nuclear medicine for physicians to further improve the image observed by administering higher administered activities. There is a feeling that lower administered activities can be used and that these doses can be reduced.

D. Keys: All of the radioisotope dose calculations have been for whole organs, considering uniform distributions. What maximum doses are we talking about considering point calculations and non-uniform distribution?

J. Kereiakes: There is some indication that maximum doses and minimum doses may vary as much as 10-fold when one considers point calculations in tissue (thus indicating the non-uniform distribution of the radioactive material).

F. Miraldi: I wish to compliment you on your fine compilation of dose data. Since many of the patients we see have markedly altered physiology and/or anatomy compared to "Standard Man", we can look forward to similar estimates for some of the more common problems seen in clinical practice.

J. Kereiakes: The data that I have presented here for children essentially involves, in some cases, patients with disease. We do need more information concerning the uptake and removal of the radiopharmaceutical in patients with altered physiology and/or anatomy. We are attempting to collect such data.

L. Klonowski: What recommendations are there for the pregnant nuclear medicine technologist? Dr. Bushong, for x-ray techs, recommends (1) no fluoroscopy (2) no portables (3) two personnel monitors. What sort of protection recommendations should be applied for the nuclear medicine tech and if the pregnant tech shows excessive concern, should she be permitted to work in the nuclear medicine department?

J. Kereiakes: The information included in my presentation indicates that a major portion of personnel exposure comes from the actual imaging procedure. Protection recommendations for a pregnant nuclear medicine technologist would definitely be the use of distance and the possible use of lead screens and a lead apron (since a majority of the procedures use technetium-99m). If the technologist shows excessive concern, then serious consideration should be given to minimizing her workload in the nuclear medicine area.

T. Agard: Although it is generally recognized that I-133 gives less patient doses than I-131, is not the major problem in its common use still based on lack of availability, since it is cyclotron-produced?

J. Kereiakes: Iodine-133 is cyclotron-produced. It is available on certain days during the week. It would thus be a matter of procedure scheduling to be able to include its use in the laboratory.

F. Miraldi: You show a much larger gonadal dose to 10-year-olds than to adults, even though there is a dose-administered adjustment. What are the main reasons for this?

J. Kereiakes: The gonadal doses are higher primarily because of the geometry of the organs in the younger age groups compared to the adults.

S. Hancock: What are your ideas about the use of syringe shields during injection of patients, considering the difficulty of injecting with the syringe shield?

J. Kereiakes: The difficulty in injecting using the syringe shield is, of course, dependent on the experience of the individual involved. It is also much more difficult when injecting pediatric patients. The Nuclear Regulatory Commission (NRC) requires the use of syringe shields, unless a laboratory has made measurements with and without using syringe shields and can show that the exposure to the extremities of personnel not using syrnge shield is comparable or less than using a syringe shield.

S. Gianelus: What amount of radiation for a diagnostic procedure is considered to be non-significant vs a significant risk? Assume an adult patient.

S. Bushong: Non-pregnant adult = maximum of 50 R.

W. Kendall: It should be noted that extensive efforts to reduce shielding may not be cost-effective if you require non-standard lead thickness. Also, it should be noted that you should also consider potential future use for a room.

S. Bushong: You're right about the first point. Lead thinner than 2 lbs/ft^2 will cost more than 2 lbs/ft^2 thickness. Available, useful thicknesses are 2, 2 1/2, 3, 4, 6, and 8 lbs/ft^2. I disagree with the second point unless you have definite info regarding future use. It doesn't cost much more to retrofit new lead-lined sheet rock than it would have earlier. You really only lose the cost of original sheetrock.

E. Webster: I have two comments for Dr. Bushong. With regard to the developmental abnormalities appearing in children irradiated in utero during the A-bombing (as discussed by Lee Russell), it is important to clarify again the statement that some microcephaly was observed in Hiroshima at relatively low absorbed doses (10-19 rad in air). In this city, 20% of the dose was due to fast neutrons. Thus, a dose of 10 rad was 8 rad gamma plus 20 rem neutrons (RBE = 10). However, the RBE at the 2 rad level for neutrons is more likely to be about 30, so that the dose level was probably about 68 rem (60 + 8). This reconciles the Hiroshima experience more closely with the Nagasaki experience, where no cases of micorcephaly were observed below 150 rads (air dose).

The second comment relates to ethical considerations in connection with an "abortion policy". NCRP Report No. 54 contains, on p. 11, a very telling illustration of the harm that would result from performing abortions in cases where the risk to the fetus is low. It is known that the siblings of leukemic children have a significant probability of also acquiring leukemia--about 1 in 700. An abortion policy for the siblings of leukemics would therefore result in 699 health fetuses being aborted for each leukemia case aborted. This is clearly an unacceptable policy. I believe abortion should only be seriously considered if the risk of cancer or malformation is comparable with the normal risk of abnormality in a live-born child, which is about 1 in 10. I believe dose for this degree of risk is much higher than 5 or 10 rads and probably closer to 50 rads more.

Thus, it would never be necessary to abort a fetus which has been subjected to diagnostic levels of radiation.

T. Agard: What concerns me very much about your (W. Properzio) approach to the education of the consumer/patient is that the figures being quoted by BRH officials about possible cancer incidences will scare the public away from taking examinations that they really need and the end result could be more deaths from the lack of necessary use of x-rays than the questionable reduction in cancers due to over use.

W. Properzio: The intent of the FDA consumer education program is to provide the consumer/patient information needed to develop a realistic view of what medical x-rays can provide. Two basic messages are directed to this goal, namely: 1) Don't decide on your own that you need an x-ray. 2) Don't insist on an x-ray.

The quotation of possible biological outcomes for low-level radiation exposures where an exact understanding of biological effects is still unknown must be used with caution. The BRH has used possible projected effects for public health planning purposes, but is not a component part of our consumer education efforts.

S. Hancock: What impact do you think it would have on public opinion and attitude of media people if we inform the press when we have meetings of this sort so they can cover the meeting, interview a spokesman of the AAPM, and see that we are concerned about the problem of the effects of radiation exposure?

W. Properzio: I feel that medical physicists should make every effort to inform the press of the technical facts regarding ionizing radiation. The identification of key speakers at an educational symposium to meet with the press is often an effective tool. This allows natural experts to directly communicate with the local press.

J. Ovadia: What is the availability of John Villforth's article in FDA Consumer (Dec./Jan.), which was picked up by the Chicago Tribune (coupled with a reference to John Cameron)? In his message to the public (end of paper), six recommendations are made. They do not include a recommendation to keep a record of x-ray exposure. This appears reasonable in view of Gregg's earlier estimate that about 15,000 x-rays give an exposure leading to a doubling of natural cancer incidence.

W. Properzio: The FDA Consumer is an agency publication. Its availability may be limited but can be obtained by subscription from the GPO (or through FDA). The publication is also available in many public libraries. The recommendation to keep a record of diagnostic x-ray exams is one we (FDA) believe will be helpful. It is an aid in meeting the recommendation that the patient inform the physician about any similar x-ray examinations they may have had.

E. Gregg: Many public warnings do not emphasize or deliberately neglect the fact that diagnostic accuracy may improve with number of films. The work of Garland detecting coin lesions in the lung--1 reading, 25% error rate; 2 readings, 14% error rate; three readings, 8%. The emphasis on over-exposure neglects this positive aspect.

W. Properzio: Yes. The point is well made and must be kept in mind as a balancing factor to our concerns for lowering exposure to the patient.

J. Kim: I commend the "tempered" approach by Dr. Properzio and BRH to enlighten the public. I feel some of us may tend to over-react against the over-reaction by the public on radiation risks by over-emphasizing the large benefit/risk ratio. Those of us who have been reading and following the reports and research journals know that benefit of applied radiation far outweighs the risk. The small risk also seems long-term, however. Those of us, the physicists in particular, who run around with ionization chambers and do not know the subtle and complicated biological consequences really should not go around wearing the mantle of someone else's expertise. Instead, we should bring the outstanding experts to explain to us and the public what they know about, say, low-dose effects. The jury is still out on low-dose effects. We may serve best by sharing the facts and ignorance without alarming the public or provoking the media.

W. Properzio: I agree with Dr. Kim regarding our responsibility to "share the facts and ignorance". In our role of medical physicists we should not speculate on yet unproven and often controversial biological effects. Instead, we must attempt to communicate the facts, that which is known as well as that for which we presently do not have a clear scientific understanding.

R. Cooke: To improve the communcation between the physicist and the general public, a group of Health Physicists in the Chicago area has been operating a toll-free (800) telephone number for individual members of the public to call with questions. The "Radiation Effects Information Hotline", as it is called, started operation in September, 1979, for the State of Illinois and expanded to surrounding states in March, 1980 and has been quite successful in improving communcation of factual information to the public. Questions of any kind dealing with radiation may be addressed to (800) 942-9440 for Illinois, and (800) 323-1364 outside Illinois (Wisconsin, Iowa, Indiana, Michigan, Ohio, Minnesota, Tennessee, Kentucky).

S. Bushong: This is an outstanding program. It should be supported and utilized.

M. Gaulden: (Comment to E. Gregg): Although it is difficult at present to prove that mutagenesis and carcinogenesis are related, biological evidence for some relation is strong. The vast majority of carcinogens have also been shown to be mutagens. Most tumors have been demonstrated to be clones, i.e., to be derived from a single cell, which means that the change leading to neoplasia, most probably a mutation, occurred in that cell. In man, 200 genes have been indentified that involve susceptibility to neoplasia: about half of these genes are dominant in expression.

At low doses of radiation, a linear dose-response of neoplasia would be expected if mutation were involved; data for such a response in man have been examined (J.M. Brown, 1977. The shape of the dose-response curve for radiation carcinogenesis. Extrapolation to low doses. Radiat. Res. 71:34-50). It is now generally accepted that two phenomena are involved in carcinogenesis: an initiating event in a single cell and promoting events that foster over a long period of time the growth of the neoplastic cell, e.g., hormones. Because the growth of a neoplastic cell may in some individuals also be prevented, in fact the cell may be eliminated by immune factors, one would be surprised to find a strict linear dose-response of carcinogenesis. Also contributing to the difficulty of relating the frequency of mutations to that of neoplasia is the long latent period of most radiation-induced tumors, which means that some individuals may die of other causes before tumor formation can be detected.

M. Gaulden: (Comment to S. Bushong): I do not agree that elective scheduling of abdominal x-rays and nuclear medicine procedures for women of reproductive age cannot be used by the radiology department of a large hospital. We have used it at Parkland Memorial Hospital in Dallas for over 10 years. That is a 1,000-bed, city/county hospital that does about a quarter of a million x-ray examinations and 10,500 nuclear medicine procedures a year. Once the elective scheduling methods had been worked out and became routine, no difficulties have been experienced with using it (M.E. Gaulden & R.C. Murry, 1980. Medical radiation and possible adverse effects on the human embryo. In Radiation Biology in Cancer Research, R.E. Meyn & H.R. Withers, Eds., Raven Press, N.Y., pp. 277-294).

M. Gaulden: (Comment to J. Kereiakes): There are, to my knowledge, two cases demonstrating unequivocally that Tc99m labeled compounds cross the placental barrier. Winter, et al, (1979, Radionuclide fetal imaging. Eur. J. Nucl. Med. 4:309-311) have imaged the bladder of a 31-week-old fetus with 3 mCi of ^{99m}Tc-pyridoxylideneglutamate administered to the mother. Although the level of radioactivity detected in the 22-hour scan of the maternal liver was much reduced when compared to the 6-hour scan of the maternal liver, that in the fetus was increased in the 22-hour scan. This raises the question of whether the fetus can eliminate the labeled compound as readily as the mother; if not, the fetus will receive a higher dose of radiation than would be calculated on the basis of the radiation emitted by maternal organs. The second case is a recent one in our laboratory (Datz and Gaulden, unplublished) in which the epiphyses of a 30-week-old fetus were imaged two hours after ^{99m}Tc-MDP (10 mCi) was given to the mother for a pre-op bone scan (biopsy of a breast mass revealed malignancy).

III. Medico -- Legal Responsibilities

STATE AND FEDERAL REGULATION OF RADIATION RISK
Joseph M. Nanus
and
David K. Lacker
Texas Department of Health
Radiation Control Branch
1100 West 49th Street
Austin, Texas 78756

There is currently a sentiment in the public sector which borders on hysteria concerning ionizing radiation. The events at Three Mile Island (TMI) and the often distorted media coverage of that situation have added to the already existing apprehension concerning ionizing radiation to produce this level of concern. One national weekly magazine begins its television commercial to sell subscriptions with a picture of TMI on the magazine cover and the voice of the announcer intones "A nuclear nightmare...". This is not the kind of copy intended to inspire a rational objective review of the problems and pseudo-problems of the uses of ionizing radiation. We are already beginning to see some of the fallout from this situation.

Even before TMI, there were some 17 agencies in the federal sector that had regulations which affect the nuclear industry. In addition to these, there are usually several agencies in each state involved in ionizing radiation regulation. Here in Texas there are at least four agencies that have some dealings or regulatory input concerning ionizing radiation.

Most of these agencies, both at the federal level and in the states, do not address medical irradiations. There are three primary agencies that have regulations affecting medical uses of radiation; the Bureau of Radiological Health (BRH) of the U. S. Department of Health and Welfare, the U. S. Nuclear Regulatory Commission (NRC), and the various state radiation control agencies.

BUREAU OF RADIOLOGICAL HEALTH

The Director of the Bureau of Radiological Health, John C. Villforth, in testimony before the subcommittee on Oversight and Investigations of the Committee on Interstate and Foreign Commerce of the U. S. House of Representatives identified four areas associated with the use of medical radiation which the Bureau considers unresolved issues. Mr. Villforth said these areas are sources of unnecessary radiation exposure.[1]

The first of these areas is inadequate or faulty equipment. I think we can agree it is essential for an x-ray machine to operate properly if we are to avoid unnecessary radiation exposure during an examination. Equipment malfunctions may be the cause of repeat examinations due to inconsistent exposure. This leads to poor quality x-ray films and unnecessary repeat exposures. Inadequacies in the equipment frequently fail to provide accurate and convenient methods of restricting the x-ray beam to the area of interest or the image receptor size. Such inconveniences often result in failure to use any beam limitation.

The second area Mr. Villforth addressed was poor techniques on the part of equipment users. Patient exposure can vary widely for the same procedure from facility to facility. The Bureau's National Evaluation of X-ray Trends (NEXT) Program which is designed to estimate the exposures to patients from standard radiologic examinations, has found up to a 200-fold difference in exposure from one facility to another or even from one machine to another in the same facility. Such differences must be laid at least partially at the door of the x-ray unit operator. A lack of adequate quality assurance in processing of film is a second possible cause for this 200-fold difference.

A third area of concern voiced by Mr. Villforth concerned unnecessary x-ray examinations - x-ray procedures that are not medically useful. Mr. Villforth defined such unnecessary x-ray examinations to include repeat examinations. In his testimony Mr. Villforth used a figure of 30 percent for the number of x-ray examinations that fall in this category.

Several reasons have been given for these unnecessary examinations. Repeat examinations have already been mentioned. Add to this the concern about possible future malpractice litigation, a lack of scientific data concerning when x-ray examinations are indicated by the clinical picture, a possibility of economic benefit, consumer demand, and finally screening examinations of symptom free individuals and you begin to see that 30 percent is probably not an unreasonable figure.

Mr. Villforth pointed out that elimination of these examinations would result in a savings to the medical consumers of $2 billion annually.

The last area covered in Mr. Villforth's testimony was that of insufficient consumer-patient awareness. Patients can sometime pressure the physician into ordinary unnecessary x-rays that have little or no clinical value. Some patients seem to hold unreal expectations of the value of x-ray examinations. On the other side of the coin, they may be so apprehensive as a result of what they have heard or read through the popular media that they resist having even medically useful and needed x-ray examinations.

THE STATES

State radiation control agencies must be divided into at least two groups insofar as they interface with the two federal programs. There are currently 26 Agreement States which have assumed a majority of regulatory authority from the NRC concerning use of radioactive material in the particular state. The remaining 24 states are nonagreement states and do not regulate use of radioactive materials, but lease this authority vested in the NRC.

The states each have programs in radiation control and protection. Some states' programs are voluntary and radiation protection activities are accomplished by persuasion while others are regulatory, having regulations which prescribe certain minimum standards of radiation protection. The state authorities, in general, have much the same concerns as those expressed by Mr. Villforth. In addition, they are aware of the problems of health care delivery in remote, low population areas. Each state has problems which they, at least, consider unique.

The program directors of the several states are members of a body incorporated as the Conference of Radiation Control Program Directors, Inc. The Conference was formed with several stated objectives; these include exercising leadership with radiation control professionals and consumers in radiation control development and action. Also, encouraging and promoting cooperative enforcement programs with federal agencies and between related enforcement agencies in each state. In order to promote radiological health in all its aspects and phases, the Conference encourages interchange of experience among radiation control programs and seeks to collect and make accessible to all radiation control program directors such information and data as might be of assistance to them in the proper fulfillment of their duties. The Conference seeks to promote and foster uniformity of radiation control laws and regulations, to encourage and support programs which will contribute to radiation control for all, and to assist members in their technical work and development.

The Conference has fulfilled its objective concerning the uniformity of radiation control regulations by its continuing attention to the Suggested State Regulations for Control of Radiation. These regulations are under continuous revision to address the latest state of the art in radiation use and protection. Task forces of Conference members aided by federal advisors from the BRH, the U.S. Environmental Protection Agency and the NRC have each of the several parts of the Suggested State Regulations under constant review. They are also frequently in contact with nongovernmental professionals in the area of interest of the particular Task Force.

Some of the areas of task force consideration that affect the medical radiation area are:
Program Criteria
    Part A. Criteria for Adequate Radiation Control Program - X-ray
    Part B. Criteria for Radioactive Material - Radioactive Material
Efficacy of Applications of Radiations in the Healing Arts
Nationwide Evaluation of X-ray Trends (NEXT)
State Credentialing Program for Allied Health Operators
Suggested State Regulations for the Control of Radiation
Public Health Impact of Nuclear Medicine Practice
Quality Assurance in Diagnostic X-ray
Personnel Dosimetry

NUCLEAR REGULATORY COMMISSION

The third primary agency in the medical radiation area is the

U.S. Nuclear Regulatory Commission (NRC). The NRC is limited by the Atomic Energy Act of 1954 to regulation of radioactive materials that are products of reactor operation, called by-product materials, special nuclear materials, and source materials. The Act, by omission, does not authorize regulation of naturally occurring or accelerator produced radioactive material (NARM). The NARM vacuum of regulation at the federal level is viewed uneasily by a number of federal agencies. Several have exhibited an interest in filling this gap and continually search their legislation in an attempt to ferret out statutory authority.

The NRC has assumed a stance aimed at radiation protection for the users of radioactive by-product materials and for workers in the area, as well as for the public.

In addition to the foregoing three agencies of government, a fourth entity must be considered, the White House. On October 23, 1979, President Carter announced a series of administrative initiatives aimed at low-level ionizing radiation. The President approved the establishment of a Radiation Policy Council to advise on broad radiation policy, to coordinate federal activities that use or control the use of radiation, to resolve problems of jurisdiction, to recommend legislation, to ensure effective liaison with States and Congress, and to provide a forum for public input. This Council will be chaired by the administrator of the Environmental Protection Agency and will include high-level officials from the other relevant agencies.

The President also directed that during the preparation of his FY-1981 budget request, there be included in the research budget a sound research program on the long-term health effects of low-level radiation. An Interagency Radiation Research Committee, chaired by the director of NIH, will review the kinds of research needed and the quality of research in this area supported by the federal government.

In addition, a task force already established to examine criteria for compensation for civilians exposed to unusual radiation hazards was given the additional assignment of assessing criteria for workers and veterans. [4]

It is difficult, at this point to predict what effect these groups will have on medical use of radiation, but the increased emphasis on input from the consumer-patient could cause significant changes in federal radiation regulatory policies.

BRH RESPONSE TO CONCERNS

The four sources of unnecessary radiation exposure cited by Director Villforth in his testimony have resulted in creation of a number of programs by the BRH. Probably the most visible, and best known program (though not always the best understood) is the manufacturers performance standard for diagnostic x-ray equipment which took effect on August 1, 1974. This standard is subjected to constant examination to adequately provide for technological innovations. Currently work is in progress to promulgate a new regulatory amendment for computed tomography systems.

With properly functioning machines, the next link in the chain of service delivery is the x-ray unit operator. Without a properly trained operator, repeat examinations may constitute a large portion of the unnecessary exposure received by the public.

The BRH is aware of the need for a basic minimum standard of qualification for operators of x-ray units. They have been active with the Conference of Radiation Control Program Directors in seeking to develop such a minimum standard. In addition, they have published a call in the Federal Register for comments concerning a voluntary credentialing of allied health radiation machine operators.[6] The results of this call have not yet been published.

In another program, aimed at exposure reduction through elimination of poor techniques, the BRH has, with the help of state radiation control programs, instituted several quality assurance projects. Two such projects are the Dental Exposure Normalization Technique (DENT) project and the Breast Exposure: Nationwide Trends (BENT) project. In each project, special thermoluminescent dosimeter cards are mailed to users of dental and mammography equipment with explicit instructions for a test exposure to x-rays. The thermoluminescent dosimeters are then returned to the states for evaluation. Follow-up visits by state personnel are made to facilities where higher than normal exposures are obtained. These visits allow pinpointing of problems and suggested corrective actions.

Still another program, directed at reducing repeat procedures, is a quality assurance effort being fostered by the Bureau. Final recommendations for quality assurance programs in diagnostic radiology facilities were issued in the Federal Register of December 11, 1979. These recommendations suggest the basic aspects of such programs, but recognize that programs will vary greatly from facility to facility depending on the size, type, and need of the particular facility.

The Bureau's recommendation is that any quality assurance program should contain:
1. Responsibility and authority for the overall quality assurance program.
2. Written desired performance specifications for the equipment before purchasing new equipment.
3. A routine quality control monitoring and maintenance system incorporating state-of-the-art procedures.
4. Standards of acceptable image quality established.
5. Means for two levels of evaluation:
    (a) First level, the results of the monitoring to evaluate the performance of the x-ray system,
    (b) Second level, means for evaluating the effectiveness of the program itself.
6. Provisions for keeping records on the results of the monitoring techniques.
7. A quality assurance manual should be written.
8. Provisions for appropriate training for all personnel with quality assurance responsibilities.

9. Consider the establishment of a quality assurance committee.
10. Quality assurance program be reviewed to determine whether effectiveness could be improved.[5]

The Bureau has recently completed work on a consumer-awareness program. This program will be advertised to and through high schools, members of the American Hospital Association, county agricultural agents, and the various state regulatory programs. The program is a multimedia approach including a slide-tape presentation, posters, and TV and radio spots on what the consumer can do to be an informed partner in the health care delivery system. For further information on this program, the state radiation control agency should be contacted.

One final area of interest is the Bureau's investigation of the feasibility of establishing recommended ranges of patient exposure for various x-ray examinations. The Bureau is currently attempting to develop a system that can relate image quality for a particular x-ray examination to patient exposure. There exists some five years of experience with an approach of this nature to radiation exposure reduction: the State of Illinois has used exposure guides on four standard projections for table top exposure values per radiograph since 1974. (See Table I)

Table I Illinois Exposure Ranges

	Should not exceed	Shall not exceed	Patient Size
AP Abdomen	350 mR	500 mR	22 cm 14 x 17 field
Lateral Lumbar Spine	1,000 mR	1,400 mR	30 cm 14 x 17 field
AP Cervical Spine	100 mR	140 mR	12 cm 8 x 10 field
AP Skull	200 mR	400 mR	21 cm 10 x 12 field

STATE RESPONSES

Although the Bureau of Radiological Health recommends many programs and changes, the States are generally the agencies which implement the projects. For example, the BENT project is being taken to the consumer by 45 state programs. In addition, 38 states and local governments are pursuing the DENT project. The Bureau also contracts with 34 state radiation control agencies to provide on-site inspection of x-ray units subject to the manufacturers performance standard.

The Illinois dose limit concept is an area where a state program has been the guiding light and the Bureau proposal is a reaction to the apparent success of that concept.

The Conference of Radiation Control Program Directors (CRCPD) has been in the forefront of development of concepts and programs for radiation control and protection. The Task Force on Quality Assurance of CRCPD has developed a guide for state radiation control programs to implement statewide programs on quality assurance (QA). This guide is a "how to" cookbook. It spells out what QA is, why it should be implemented, program implementation methods, measurement parameters, implementation costs, and evaluation procedures. In short, a total program outline is provided.

Another task force working on credentialing of allied health radiation operators has completed work on a basic minimum standard for diagnostic x-ray operators. It is currently developing an implementation document and suggested legal terminology and regulatory guidance. Nine states and Puerto Rico already require credentialing of x-ray machine operators who apply radiation to human beings.

The document "Suggested State Regulations for Control of Radiation" (SSRCR) is an up-to-date, viable document as a result of constant review and revision by the task forces of CRCPD. Each part of SSRCR has a task force assigned to review and update it, as necessary.

The part of the Suggested State Regulations dealing with the use of x-rays in the healing arts and veterinary medicine has been amended to incorporate most of the same standards placed on manufacturers of x-ray equipment, but applies them to the user of the equipment. Not all states have adopted this approach, but I expect these amendments to become more universally applicable with the passage of time.

The U.S. Nuclear Regulatory Commission provides an advisor to each Conference task force dealing with parts of the Suggested State Regulations that affect radioactive material or its users. This advisor provides information concerning changes in the NRC regulations and can keep the members of the task force informed of those items the NRC considers "items of compatibility".

State regulations, in agreement states, must be compatible with the regulations of the NRC. This does not mean identical, however. There is a great diversity in the regulations of the 26 agreement states, but the intent of the various parts is compatible. Individual states have different methods of operation, often dictated by the state's enabling legislation, but the result of the regulations is the same.

The NRC does not require compatibility on all parts of the regulations, but even when compatibility is not involved, a change in NRC regulations does have a great effect on thinking in state programs.

The NRC, for some time now, has been trying to extricate itself from the medical realm. By agreement with the FDA, they no longer look at efficacy, dosage, or use of radiopharmaceuticals. This allows for broader use as determined by the medical expertise of the nuclear medicine physician. In response to this broader freedom, however, the amount of training and experience required for a physician to be authorized to use radioactive materials in the practice of medicine has increased significantly.

The NRC also has attempted to implement the As Low as Reasonably Achievable (ALARA) concept in the medical community. The purpose here is to being the exposure of all handlers of radioactive material, in the medical workplace, down to the level already maintained by 90 percent of those doing the work and reporting exposure levels to the NRC. This proposal originally had an implementation date of March 4, 1980, but due to significant meaningful criticism by the medical community the implementation date was withdrawn and the document is currently under revision.

The letter which first went out to NRC licensees in September 1979, required that licensees develop and implement a specific action program to maintain occupational radiation exposure levels ALARA. The NRC set an action and reporting level for medical licensees at 500 millirem per year. The NRC would have required submission of written justification for exposure levels exceeding the 500 millirem level. A committee for overview of exposures would also have been required.

A new date for implementation on this document should be coming out soon. What changes will be effected in the document cannot be predicted with any degree of certainty. The NRC did note strong objections to reporting exposures less than 1.25 rem, though little objection to in-house action. In addition, as you might well expect, few of the NRC licensees were enthusiastic about instituting another committee for review of exposures. These may be two of the primary areas modified.

The thing to note in this situation is that the NRC is prepared to listen and to modify its position based on rational objections and coherent expression of these objections. The ALARA concept is coming. It will be implemented. But reasonable, rational input from the medical community can have and already has had an impact on the program.

NONIONIZING RADIATION

The foregoing comments have been directed toward ionizing radiation used in medical practice. A very brief overview follows of regulations and programs concerned with nonionizing radiation in three areas of medical practice.

There are approximately 30 states that have enabling legislation permitting exercise of some type of control of nonionizing electromagnetic radiation (NER). Several states require registration of laser devices. Two types of lasers that could pose a significant hazard if misused or operated too close to the eyes are photocoagulators and surgical lasers. Both types of lasers are Class IV and could cause significant biological damage if not properly used.

The lasers used for patient alignment in radiation therapy are Class II, having very low power densities. Injury would be possible only if a person stared into the device for an extended period of time.

Diathermy units, using ultrasound and microwaves, are used in medical practice for deep heat treatments. Units operating at 2450 megahertz are being reviewed by the BRH to determine what regulatory consideration should be applied.

Diagnostic ultrasound energy density levels are on the same order as energy densities found to be threshold levels for microwave biological damage. The BRH is seeking to determine if injury might result from abuse or misuse of these devices. Here too, the Bureau is looking at regulatory action.

Generally there is an attitude that, in the near future, permissible exposure levels are very likely to be lowered by an order of magnitude for NER in the 10 megahertz to 400 megahertz range. A document prepared jointly by the U.S. National Bureau of Standards and CRCPD titled "Requirements for an Effective National Nonionizing Radiation Measurements Program", was presented to a Senate Committee on March 15, 1980. In it was a reference to an Environmental Protection Agency decision memorandum dated April 9, 1979. This decision memorandum indicated a limit in the 0.1 mW/cm^2 to 1 mW/cm^2 range is under consideration for NER frequencies between 30 MHz and 1 GHz. This guidance may take effect by the later half of calendar year 1981.

If, in fact, such guidance is issued it will be binding only on Federal agencies. The report goes on to say, however, that it would also serve as a model for private applications and could, at some later date, be promulgated as a proposed exposure standard.

It is reasonable to expect mandatory, federally imposed, broadly applicable, personnel protection standards to be promulgated during the next few years.[3]

There is a constant push, particularly from the informed private sector, to lower permissible exposure rates in both ionizing and nonionizing radiation fields. Professionals need to be aware of this and move now to meet these demands even before they are added to regulatory packages.

As stated before, there is a public concern bordering on hysteria about radiation. This concern must be met by information. Radiation needs to "go public". For so many years, we have failed at public relations. The public will not allow radiation to remain a mystery. Until the public is informed and educated, they will continue to demand more and more regulation to protect themselves. If their fears are not allayed, the public will continue to seek more and more regulation, even if regulation reaches the extent of prohibition.

1. John C. Villforth, "Unnecessary Exposure to Radiation from Medical and Dental X-rays. Hearings before the Subcommittee on Oversight Investigation of the Committee on Interstate and Foreign Commerce, House of Representatives, Ninety-Sixth Congress, First Session, July 24 and 31, 1979", U.S. Government Printing Office, p. 70-79.
2. Task Force on Quality Assurance, Maury Neuweg, Chairman, "Quality Assurance in Diagnostic Radiology - A guide for state program implementation", Conference of Radiation

Control Program Directors, 1979.
3. National Bureau of Standards in cooperation with the Conference of Radiation Control Program Directors, Inc., "Requirements for an Effective National Nonionizing Radiation Measurements Program", U.S. Government Printing Office, March 1980, p. 12-15.
4. Office of the White House Press Secretary, Press Release, October 23, 1979.
5. "Quality Assurance Programs for Diagnostic Radiology Facilities; Final Recommendation", Federal Register, Tuesday, December 11, 1979, p. 71728 & 71740.
6. "Notice of Intent to develop recommendations on voluntary national standards for qualifications of medical radiation technologists", Federal Register, Tuesday, March 13, 1979, p. 14637 & 14638.

OFFICIAL AAPM RESPONSE TO
ALARA
(AS LOW AS REASONABLY ACHIEVABLE)

Robert G. Waggener, Ph.D
President, American Association of Physicists in Medicine
Professor, University of Texas
Health Science Center at San Antonio, Texas

INTRODUCTION

ALARA is a concept that evokes strong responses in the radiological community and other segments of our society. Many members of the scientific and medical communities are violently opposed to ALARA and see it as an unwarranted intrusion of government into the affairs of the institutions and individuals who work with radiation. Other individuals hold that it is a completely justifiable government action in that it will decrease the average annual dose in the United States thereby saving lives and engendering better health by reducing the number of injuries from ionizing radiation. The latter viewpoint is generally held by individuals who work for the government or are consumer advocates. A third and more cynical viewpoint is held by some radiation workers who view it as an opportunity for personal gain, both economic and professional, by increased need for the services of qualified experts.

Regardless of the individual viewpoint, it appears that ALARA is going to occur. The only questions seem to be, when and in what form? Implemented in its most extreme form, ALARA could be a red-tape nightmare that could effectively severely restrict the use of radiation in medical institutions. The greatest fear in the radiological community is that ALARA instituted by the Nuclear Regulatory Commission (NRC) for radioisotope licensees will be expanded state agencies to include X-ray equipment. A more benign form of ALARA could simply result in continuation of the "status quo" for most medical institutions.

Many individuals in the radiological community who work in medical institutions feel the profession has done a good job in keeping radiation exposure of workers to a reasonable minimum. They fear that the _average_ radiation dose received by workers will become an upper limit under the ALARA concept and that it is possible in many cases for exposures to exceed the ALARA limit as it is presently construed. One conceivable interpretation is that all radiation workers who receive a dose in excess of the average radiation dose are in violation of the ALARA concept. This interpretation of the ALARA concept could effectively reduce the Maximum Permissible Dose to Radiation Workers by a factor of ten. In other words, because the average dose to radiation workers has been held substantially below the Maximum Permissible Dose, radiation workers will now be penalized for their good efforts in the past.

In an effort to beneficially influence the implementation of ALARA several members of AAPM, led by George Callendine, have developed and submitted to the NRC an alternative Model Program for Maintaining Occupational Radiation Exposures at Medical Institutions ALARA. This model program is a revision of the original NRC ALARA document.

AAPM REVISED MODEL PROGRAM FOR MAINTAINING OCCUPATIONAL RADIATION EXPOSURES AT MEDICAL INSTITUTIONS ALARA

(Licensee's Name)

(Date)

I. Management Commitment

   a. We, the management of this (medical facility, hospital, etc.) are committed to the program described in this paper of keeping exposures (individual and collective) as low as reasonably achievable (ALARA). In accord with this commitment, we hereby establish an administrative organization for radiation safety and develop the necessary written policy, procedures and instructions to foster the ALARA concept within our institution. The organization will include a Radiation Safety Committee (RSC)[1], a Radiation Safety Officer (RSO), and a qualified medical radiation physicist* (at least in a consulting capacity). We are also committed to following the guidance provided by U.S. Nuclear Regulatory Guides 8.10 and 8.18 when practical.

   b. We will perform a formal audit annually to determine how exposures might be lowered. This shall include reviews of operating procedures and past exposure records, inspections, etc., and consultations with the radiation protection staff or outside consultants. A brief summary of the audit will be prepared covering the scope of the review and the conclusions reached.

   c. Modifications to operating and maintenance procedures and/or to equipment and facilities will be made when they will significantly reduce exposures and can be accomplished at reasonable costs. We will be able to demonstrate that improvements have been sought, that modifications have been considered, and that they have been implemented where practicable. Where modifications have been considered but not implemented, we will be prepared to describe the reasons for not implementing them.

---

1. Private practice physician licenses do not include a RSC.
* Definition: Qualified Medical Radiation Physicist: An individual who is certified by the American Board of Radiology in the appropriate disciplines of Radiological Physics, including Diagnostic, Therapeutic, and/or Medical Nuclear Physics; or an individual who demonstrates equivalent competence in the disciplines. The qualified medical radiation physicist can also serve in the role as the Radiation Safety Officer.

d. In addition to maintaining doses to individuals as far below the limits as is reasonably achievable, the sum of the doses received by all exposed individuals will also be maintained at the lowest practicable level. It would not be desirable, for example, to hold the highest doses to individuals to some fraction of the applicable limit if this involved exposing additional people thereby significantly increasing the collective radiation dose received by all involved individuals.

II. Radiation Safety Committee (RSC)[2]

   a. Review of Proposed Users and Uses

   1. The RSC will thoroughly review the qualifications of each potential authorized user with respect to the types and quantities of radioactive materials and uses for which he has applied to assure that the user will be able to take appropriate measures to maintain exposure ALARA.

   2. When considering a new use of byproduct material, the RSC will review the efforts of the authorized user to maintain exposure ALARA. The user should have systematized procedures to ensure ALARA, and should have considered the use of special equipment such as syringe shields, rubber gloves, etc., in his proposed use.

   3. The RSC will ensure that the user justifies his procedures and that they will result in ALARA doses (individual and collective).

   b. Delegation of Authority

   1. The RSC will delegate sufficient authority to the RSO for enforcement of the ALARA concept.

   2. The RSC will support the RSO in those instances where it is necessary for the RSO to assert his authority. Where the RSO has been overruled, the Committee will record the basis for its action.

   c. Review of ALARA Program

   The RSC of our medical facility will perform an annual review of all radiation safety programs. This review will be performed independently of that performed by managment.

---

[2] The RSO on private practice physician licenses will assume the responsibilities of the RSC under Section III.

1. The RSC will encourage all users to review current procedures and to develop new procedures where appropriate to implement the ALARM concept.

2. The RSC will review all known instances of deviations from the ALARA philosophy. Information in support of the review will normally be supplied by the RSO.

3. The RSC will evaluate our institution's overall efforts toward maintaining exposures ALARA. This evaluation will include the efforts of the RSO, authorized users and occupational workers, as well as those of management.

d. Public Statement of Commitment by the RSC to ALARA

All pertinent elements of our institution will be informed of the RSC's commitment to the ALARA concept.

1. The RSC will ensure that employees are aware of the RSC's commitment to the ALARA philosophy.

2. The RSC will demonstrate its commitment to the ALARA concept through the methods employed in its review of proposed users and uses.

III. Radiation Safety Officer (RSO)

a. Periodic Review and Audit of the Radiation Safety Program for Compliance with ALARA Concepts. (This is the key element in any ALARA program.) Frequent reviews of procedures will be conducted.

1. The RSO will review and audit, on a regular basis (at least annually), the effectiveness of his own radiation protection program in maintaining doses (individual and collective) ALARA.

2. The RSO will review exposures of authorized users and occupational workers to determine that their exposures are ALARA.

3. The RSO will review radiation levels in unrestricted and restricted areas and releases of effluents to unrestricted areas to determine that they are at ALARA levels.

b. The RSO's Education Responsibilities for an ALARA Program

1. The RSO will schedule briefings and educational sessions to inform workers of ALARA program efforts.

2. The RSO will assure that authorized users, occupational workers and ancillary personnel will have been instructed in ALARA philosophy and know that management, the RSC, RSO and the medical radiation physicist (MRP)* are committed to implementing the ALARA concept.

c. Cooperative Efforts for Development of ALARA Procedures

Individuals who must work with ALARA concepts will be given opportunities to participate in formulation of the procedures that they will be required to follow.

1. The RSO will be in close contact with all users and workers in order to develop ALARA procedures for working with radioactive materials.

2. The RSO will establish procedures for encouraging, receiving, and evaluating the suggestions of individual workers for improving health physics practices.

d. Reporting and Reviewing Instances of Deviation from Good ALARA Practices

1. The RSO will investigate all known instances of deviation from good ALARA practices; and, if possible, determine the causes. When the cause is known, the RSO will propose changes in the program to maintain exposures ALARA.

2. The RSO will report all significant known instances of deviation from ALARA concepts to the RSC for review.

IV. Medical Radiation Physicist

a. Since the ALARA concept involves consideration of radiation exposures in the clinical medical environment, the professional judgement of a qualified medical radiation physicist is necessary. He will function as the expert radiological protection advisor to the institution.

b. Functions

1. The MRP will be available for consultation with the RSC, the RSO, the authorized user(s) and the occupational worker(s), as necessary.

2. The MRP will perform a semi-annual review as outlined in Section VII below.

---

* The MRP can also serve as the RSO.

3. The MRP will report to the RSC on actions recommended as a result of his review.

4. The MRP will suggest to the RSC specific actions to strengthen the ALARA program.

V. Authorized Users

   a. New Procedures Involving Potential Radiation Exposures

   1. The authorized user will consult the RSO and RSC before using radioactive materials for a new procedure.

   2. The authorized user will consider all procedures thoroughly before using radioactive materials to ensure that exposures will be kept ALARA. This may be enhanced throught the application of trial runs.

   b. Responsibility of the Authorized User to Those He Supervises

   1. The authorized user will thoroughly explain the ALARA concept and his commitment to maintain exposures ALARA to all of those he supervises.

   2. The authorized user will ensure that his occupational workers are trained and educated in good health physics practices and in maintaining exposures ALARA.

   3. The authorized user will be responsible to the radiation safety concerns of the individuals that he supervises.

   c. Continuing Review of ALARA Concepts by the Authorized User

   1. The authorized user will continuously review his procedures to ensure that his ALARA program is optimal.

   2. The authorized user will maintain contact with the RSO to ensure that he is aware of and employs the most current methods to maintain exposures ALARA.

VI. Occupational Worker

   a. What the Occupational Worker Must Consider About ALARA

   1. The worker will implement ALARA procedures developed by the authorized user and the RSO.

2. The occupational worker will know what recourse is available if he feels the ALARA concept is not being promoted on the job.

3. The occupational worker will understand the ALARA concept, and will review both his own working conditions and those of his fellow workers with respect to implementation of the ALARA concept.

VII. Implementation of Actions to Insure ALARA Doses

The implementation of the ALARA program will be reviewed at least semi-annually by the qualified medical radiation physicist. Based on his review, he will determine if and what further actions are, in his professional judgement, necessary to implement, maintain, and strengthen the ALARA program appropriate to the institution, and make written recommendations.

Documentation of these recommendations and any actions taken will be maintained on file by the institution, and will be available for inspection by the NRC.

LIABILITY FOR RADIATION EXPOSURE
FROM THE VIEWPOINT OF THE PRACTITIONER

Vincent P. Collins, M.D., J.D.
9200 Westheimer, Houston, Texas 77063

ABSTRACT

A mounting concern for environmental radiation hazards spills over into an increasing fear and mistrust of medical uses of radiation. This situation sets the stage for an increasing recourse to litigation particularly in the area of low level radiation exposure. Knowledge that the initial exposure is unfelt, that the injury may be long-delayed in appearance, and that the injury is nonspecific, only feeds the apprehension of the public. Over centuries of experience, courts have evolved rules of law for the decision-making process that call for definitions of "proof" and "truth" that differ from those of science. A series of legal cases involving radiation injuries are presented to demonstrate the evolution of applicable legal mechanisms. The earliest cases leaned to strict application of the elements of negligence, proof of injury, causation and fault. These requirements relaxed gradually to minimize the burden of proof of the injured plaintiff. Elements of anxiety were recognized as compensable. A requirement of informed consent replaced a need to prove negligence. The element of fault, becoming increasingly difficult to prove with the complexity of delayed effects and statistics of probability, is dropped in the doctrine of "product liability" or "strict liability". This may be a necessary solution to allow compensation of an innocent injured party where fault may be impossible to prove and where, in fact, it may not exist.

INTRODUCTION

Nuclear warfare, nuclear reactors and nuclear waste constitute a mounting menace in the minds of a very vocal portion of the public. This spills over into fear and distrust of medical uses of radiation in nuclear medicine, diagnostic radiology and radiotherapy. Fear and distrust do not a law suit make, but they do set the stage, and the radiation medicine practitioner or any other person utilizing radiation has a mounting susceptibility to liability for claims of radiation injury.

Unique backgrounds of history and technology have shaped the development of law and medicine producing funds of knowledge and patterns of thinking that are not shared. The surging importance of radiation in medicine, industry and economics makes this a very important field of law. Our concern is for one small aspect of this broad field, the liability of the radiation medicine practitioner. Some understanding of this problem may best be offered in brief in a series of legal cases illustrating the evolution of the current basis of liability. To select from hundreds of pertinent cases and to present in barest abstract, calls for the admonition of

Alexander Pope,

> "Drink deep, or taste not the Pierian spring:
> There shallow draughts intoxicate the brain,
> But drinking largely sobers us again."

(A glossary of key words and concepts of legal argument is appended.)

ILLUSTRATIVE LEGAL CASES

1. Sweeney v. Erving (U.S. Supreme Court, 1913)

This early case is of historical interest as the first instance of radiation injury to reach the Supreme Court of the United States. A jury verdict for the defendant was affirmed by both appellate and Supreme Courts.

The injury was a burn sustained by Mrs. Sweeney as a result of repeated diagnostic exposures to demonstrate a rib fracture. The patient's employer had warned her that "the x-ray was dangerous," but Dr. Erving, "a specialist in the use of x-ray, had assured her that he and his wife, who was his assistant, had never had an accident in the thousand or more exposures made by them.

The charge was negligence. Injury and causation were shown but the element of fault was lacking. Expert witnesses testified that the examination was "in accordance with the practice of careful and prudent x-ray operators". The court found no evidence that the danger of injury was forseeable, that Dr. Erving knew it might happen, or that he should have advised her of the possibility of such an injury. Lacking this, the basis for negligence was not established.

This decision seems bound by strict observation of legal principles that characterized many of the decisions of the time, rather than any obligation to provide a remedy for the patient's injury. There seems also to be a deference to the physician and expert medical witnesses that has gradually been dissipated with charges of "a conspiracy of silence".

2. Coover v. Painless Parker, Dentist (Calif., 1930)

The report of this case states only that the injury was sustained "as a result of over exposure in the taking of dental x-ray photographs", with no note of the circumstance that might explain how it could have happened. It does describe a third degree burn that appears to have healed with some atrophy, scarring and telangiectasis.

This is a straightforward legal injury. However the possibility of cancer is raised, and a physician testified, "---a cancer may develop in this region --it is common". To the objection that this is "wholly conjectural and uncertain", the court holds that "---this predisposition in itself is come damage----which must be held to a real and not a fanciful element of damage".

This is a thoughtful appraisal of the problem offered in 1930 that might be considered equally applicable 50 years later and is in line with current decisions allowing "damages for future injury".

3. Ferrara v. Galluchio   (New York, 1958)

Mrs. Ferrara was treated by Dr. Galluchio for bursitis and suffered a radiation burn of the shoulder. Liability for the burn is not contested. However, Mrs. Ferrara was seen by a dermatologist for care of the skin lesion and he cautioned that she should be seen periodically because of the possibility of developing cancer. This precipitated the development of an anxiety neurosis and cancerophobia. The court awarded additional compensation for the cancerophobia.

There is a strong dissent by Judge Froessel that this decision "introduces into law a new field of damages for cultivation by plaintiffs and affording countless opportunities for fraudulent, unverifiable claims".

Such claims have indeed proliferated and in the present atmosphere of mounting apprehension related to nuclear energy, nuclear waste, pre-natal and genetic injury, and carcinogens, anxiety neuroses are likely to receive favorable consideration in the courts. Tort law has allowed recovery for "interference with peace of mind" provided there was accompanying physical injury, but we may anticipate some relaxation of this requirement.

4. Natanson v. Kline   (Kansas, 1960)

In the course of post-operative radiation following mastectomy for breast cancer, Mrs. Natanson sustained a radiation injury, "--the skin, the flesh and the muscles beneath her left arm sloughed away and ribs of her left chest were so burned they became necrotic or dead". From this language in the report, one may sense a resolve that this patient must have a remedy for her injury.

There was much testimony as to radiation physics and dosimetry that could only confuse the Court. There is a clue in the report as to the reason for the injury, that even the participants overlooked. There was evidently a seroma in the axillary region which, as a sterile inflammatory process, might well augment radiation effect to a degree that a customary dose could result in the necrosis described.

"--where the physician or surgeon has failed to point out the probable consequences of the course of treatment, he may be subjected to a claim of unauthorized treatment". Thus the requirement of "informed consent" was introduced and a mechanism of recovery became available, that would overcome the impossible burden of proving negligence in the face of a "conspiracy of silence" or testimony and evidence of a technical nature beyond the court's comprehension.

5. Wilkinson v. Vesey (R.I., 1972)

In 1952, radiation therapy was given to a mediastinal tumor without a biopsy. In 1972, by the court's report, -
"At trial time Winifred's medical-surgical box score listed eight operations, numerous skin grafts, the removal of seven ribs the clavicle and the sternum. Her heart had been moved and is cushioned and supported by muscle taken from the left arm. She had had innumerable and lengthy hospitalizations".

From the court's description of the patient's plight, there is an evident resolve to find a legal route to relief from this burden of injury. Here injury and causation are clear but to establish fault in an act of 20 years ago would be difficult. Lack of informed consent has up until this time required expert testimony as to the custom in the community. This presents difficulty after twenty years but the court will find a way. It abolished the requirement of expert testimony and leaves to the jury the determination of what a physician should have told his patient 20 years earlier.

The court holds that there was no necessity for expert testimony since the jury could determine, without recourse to a showing by the plaintiff what the "medical fraternity" in the community tells its patients, the reasonableness or unreasonableness of the extent of a physician's communication with a patient.

6. Arevalos v. Serra Memorial Hospital (Calif.,1974)

A 13 year old girl was scheduled for an I-131 uptake and thyroid scan with an intended dose of 100 μCi but received, by error, a dose of 100 mCi.

No further clinical details are available and the legal proceedings are not reported since the case was not appealed, but a settlement of $225,000 was allowed for: 1) loss of thyroid function and 2) "risk of future injury", specifically, cancer of the thyroid, leukemia and damage to offspring.

Ablation of thyroid would be a prompt, apparent and permanent injury. Of particular interest and significance is allowance of damages for "risk of future injury". This is not greatly different from the allowance for "predisposition" in the Painless Parker case and the "cancerophobia" in the Galluchio case, and, as in both of these cases, there is an evident physical injury to support the possibility of liability to low level exposures where the "no threshold" concept means a statistical increase in the risk of future injury.

7. Martinez v. Univ. of Calif. (N.M., 1978)

The plaintiff was employed in the University of California facility at Los Alamos for 30 years "exposed to radioactive materials and other toxic chemicals" (unspecified). He developed a "form of cancer in one eye" (not further described) and an anxiety neurosis, "--a total physical disability, by reason of an occupational disease,---unable to perform any work for remuneration or profit". Thus an anxiety neurosis, induced by a fear of radiation, was held to be a compensable occupational disease. There is a sound precedent for this in the "Acrophobia Case" (Texas, 1955). Here compensation was allowed for a workman's neurosis that developed as a result of collapse of a scaffold eight stories above the ground from which a co-worker fell to his death. There was a strong dissent to this decision in 1955 because the "disability (was) due to his mental condition, the failure of his mind to function properly" without a clearly physical component to the injury. In today's climate of fear of radiation, any unwanted exposure however minimal, may be presented as a basis for a compensable injury by personnel, patients, family or the general public with expectation of a sympathetic hearing in court.

8. Neuberg v. Michael Reese Hosp. (D.C. Illinois, 1978)
   Dubin v. Michael Reese Hosp. (App. Illinois, 1979)

Both of these cases represent suits based on cancer of the thyroid developing in patients who had had irradiation for tonsillitis as children in the period 1947 to 1951 when such treatment was being extensively used at Michael Reese Hospital and in many other centers.

These cases illustrate two points of interest for our purpose. First, that courts do reach contradictory opinions on the same available evidence and outcome may depend less on the facts of the case than on the human aspects of counsel's presentation, jury's reaction and an individual judge's opinion. Second, the cases are notable for introduction of a legal mechanism new to radiation injury, the theory of strict liability or product liability.

Application of the product liability, strict liability or liability without fault, to x-ray is an innovation that may find wide application. Originally applied only to the sale of food and based on implied warranty, it was later extended "to cover the sale of any product which, if it should prove to be defective, may be expected to cause physical harm to the consumer or his property. The purpose of imposing strict liability is to insure that the costs of injuries resulting from defective products are borne by those who market such products, rather than by the injured persons, who are powerless to protect themselves". There was some precedent for its application in medical litigation, in that a 1970 decision (Cunningham) held blood to be a 'product' rather than a service and subjected a hospital to strict liability in providing transfusions.

In the Neuberg case a district court held that the doctrine of products liability was not applicable. However, the Dubin case states: "We do not agree with the Neuberg court in its refusal to extend the doctrine of products liability to the defendents supply of x-radiation, because it was incidental to the rendering of a service". This court holds x-radiation to be a product and sees no reason to apply the doctrine of strict liability to cases involving whole blood---but to require proof of negligence involving z-radiation."

DISCUSSION

The essential problem addressed in this presentation is the occupational hazard of the physician utilizing radiation in his practice for diagnosis or treatment.

Over the years since the announcement of Roentgen's discovery of the x-ray, the courts have had a broad experience in litigation involving radiation. For the acute exposures and even for late effects, rules of law are applicable as for any other dangerous agent. It is the unique characteristics of low level radiation exposure that strain the experience of the courts in the matter of personal injury. 1. The claimed exposure may be unknown or unnoticed so that the time of occurrence, duration and dose may be uncertain at best. 2. There may have been prior or intervening exposures to radiation, including necessary medical examinations, that could be alternative or contributing causes. There are likely to be other environmental or habitual hazards as possible etiologic factors. 3. The delayed appearance of radiation effects makes recall or confirmation of the exposure occasion vague. The latent interval may well exceed the statute of limitations, although this will vary from state to state. 4. When radiation comes to court it brings savants of physics, biology and mathematics who offer their truths to judges and juries who are in the main unprepared to deal with such esoteric information.

Decision-making in the face of uncertainty is a problem common to medicine and law. In medicine decision can wait, or even must wait, until enough evidence becomes available. In law the parties are entitled to a decision that may not be deferred indefinitely as may be a final diagnosis in medicine.

The court's dilemma is to choose between alternatives that will be unfair to one party or the other. 1. The plaintiff is an innocent victim and needs relief, but the defendant is not at proven fault, and should not have to accept the burden of damages. This is the older attitude as illustrated in Sweeney v. Erving and the dissents to the decisions in Ferrara v. Galluchio and Natanson v. Kline. 2. The plaintiff is injured but the defendant is better prepared to bear the burden as a cost of doing business, - better a possibility of fraud than an innocent injury without a remedy.

In recent years there has been a trend to recognition of a social responsibility to shift the burden of injury from the injured party to the shoulders of society generally, by insurance, by legislation or by legal decisions that circumvent older rules of liability. Workmen's compensation was an early and worthy legislative effort that modified tort law by relieving the injured workman of the need to prove negligence on an employer's part.

Then courts developed the doctrine of informed consent that avoided the need to prove fault or causation in complex medical situations. This was a new tort, neither battery (the result of an act) or negligence (which by definition is unintentional). Even here, the original requirement of expert testimony as to custom (Natanson v. Kline) was abandoned and left to the jurors' opinion (Wilkinson v. Vesey).

The most recent device to assure recovery for the injured plaintiff is to extend the doctrine of strict liability, or product liability, from food products and cosmetics to blood transfusions and now to claim of radiation injury. Here radiation is held to be "a form of electricity", a product rather than a service. The Dubin court holds that "the purpose of strict liability is to insure that the cost of injuries resulting from defective products are borne by those who market such products rather than by the injured persons, who are powerless to protect themselves".

It does seem clear that the social climate, reflected in current legal decisions, is to have society spare the individual the burden of innocent injury, and even to chance fraud to achieve this end. This being so, there is merit to "no fault" liability. It may be enough that the defendant be liable in damages for something that chance or statistics dictates must happen, without at the same time bearing the opprobrium of fault.

* * * * * * *

GLOSSARY

LIABILITY
    Subject to the consequences of rules of law or equity to make satisfaction, compensation or restitution for a wrong.

INJURY
    Any wrong or damage done to another, either in his person, rights, reputation, or property.

DANGER
    The <u>possibility</u> of injury. This is inherent to a given situation and there is no liability for danger as such. Dangerous activities are required and condoned by society. Dangerous procedures are made feasible by the careful conduct of the actor.

RISK
> The <u>probability</u> of injury. It is in the power of the actor to increase and decrease this probability by care, or lack of it, in a given circumstance. This is the basis for liability.

DUTY
> The obligation to meet the expectations of another as to his person, his possessions and his actions, such as are recognized by custom, by law, or by agreement. There is no duty unless there is an identifiable person with a right to receive the obligation.

RIGHT
> That which a man is entitled to have, or to do, or to receive from others, by custom, by law, or by agreement. There is no right unless there is an identifiable person with a duty to satisfy the desire.

CORRELATIVE
> Having a mutual or reciprocal relation, in such sense that the existence of one necessarily implies the existence of the other. (Left and right, up and down, duty and right).

TORTS
> This is the study of a continuously evolving area of law which has to do with the rights, wants, and desires of the individual. When these are recognized in law (and this is a state of mind, restrained by the past, and urged by the future), one who interferes with their realization will be liable.

TORT
> This is the offense. It has four essential components. A legal injury must be proven. There must be a duty which one party owes another. There must be a violation of this duty. The injury must result from such violation.

INTENTIONAL TORT
> The types are Assault, Battery, Interference with Peace of Mind and False Impriosonment.

UNINTENTIONAL TORT
> This is negligence.

NEGLIGENCE
> Arises when a duty of care between two parties is breached by act or omission that is at odds with what a reasonable and prudent person would do. It is necessary to prove the injury, the act, and that the act caused the injury. The act was not intended to cause the injury, but the injury was forseeable, and the act entailed an unreasonable risk.

FAULT
   Any deviation from prudence, duty or rectitude; any shortcoming or neglect of care, of performance resulting from inattention, incapacity, or perversity.

ARGUMENT
   An effort to establish belief by a course of reasoning.

PROOF
   The conviction or persuasion of the mind of a judge or jury, by the exhibition of evidence, of the reality of a fact alleged. (Anything you can get judge or jury to believe).

REFERENCES

1. Sweeney v. Erving 33 S. Ct. 416 (1913).
2. Coover v. Painless Parker 418 S.W. 2d 572 (1930).
3. Ferrara v. Galluchio 152 N.E. 2d 249 (1958).
4. Natanson v. Kline 354 P. 2d 670 (1960).
5. Wilkinson v. Vesey 295 A. 2d 676 (1972)
6. Arevalos v. Serra Mem. Hosp. L.A. Sup. Ct., June 10, 1974.
7. Martinez v. Univ. of Calif. D.C., 1st Judicial District County of Rio Arriba, N.M. 5 April, 1978.
8. Neuberg v. Michael Reese Hosp. D.C. Ill. 1978, No 78 C 3844.
9. Dubin v. Michael Reese Hosp. 393 N.E. 2d 588 (1979)

AN ANALYSIS OF THE PHYSICIAN'S PROFESSIONAL LIABILITY FOR IRRADIATION OF THE FETUS

Jim M. Perdue
Perdue, Turner and Berry, Attorneys at Law
Houston, Texas 77002

INTRODUCTION

The advent and subsequent sophistication and extension of x-ray techniques for diagnosis and treatment has heralded medical and legal issues that transcend those normally presented in the usual medical negligence case. Principal among these is the physician's liability for radiation injuries to a fetus being carried by the patient submitting to diagnostic or therapeutic x-ray.

Injury to an adult by x-ray may not be immediately apparent. Indeed, the most devastating results to the adult exposed to excessive doses of x-ray may be delayed and highly unpredictable. Even when significant and demonstrable injury or disease appears following x-ray, there will probably be serious medical debate, if not an insurmountable burden of proof, facing the adult who was subject to excessive or negligent doses of radiation. As significant and complex a legal challenge as is presented in these cases, it waxes a dull finish compared to the mirrored image of liability for x-ray injury to the fetus. Volatile, Gordian medical and legal principles and concepts blend with a touch of ecclesiasticism to reflect back more questions than answers in an area of medical practice encountered daily by many physicians and all too commonly by pregnant women.

An evaluation of professional liability in the utilization of x-rays on a female patient of childbearing age must be predicated on a basic understanding of the biological effects of radiation. These effects, either somatic or genetic, depend on a number of factors; the principal ones are the quantity of radiation received and the area of the body exposed. The greater the dose of radiation, the larger the area of the body exposed, or the more sensitive the parts of the body involved, the greater will be the damage. Further, a dose-time relationship must be taken into account. Generally, the equivalent dose given in a single exposure rather than fractional over a period of time will be significantly more deleterious.[1] These topics are fully developed in earlier chapters in this volume.

The author wishes to acknowledge the research and writing contribution of Andrea Schwartz, without whose assistance this article would not have been accomplished.

I. LEGAL PRINCIPLES

A. THE "EARLY" LAW

At common law, the unborn child was not yet a "person" to whom a duty of care existed, and therefore no cause of action would lie on his behalf for prenatal injury. This judicial position was first given explicit expression by Justice Holmes in a decision of the Massachusetts Supreme Court, Dietrich v. The Inhabitants of Northampton.[2] This case was cited and relied upon heavily in numerous cases denying relief for prenatal injuries for some sixty years. Acceptance of the concept was further fortified by its adoption by the RESTATEMENT OF TORTS §869 which stated, "A person who negligently causes harm to an unborn child is not liable to such child for the harm."

During this state of the art, two lawsuits arose dealing with the question of prenatal injuries caused by irradiation, Smith v. Ruckhardt[3] and Stemmer v. Kline.[4] in the former, a physician negligently diagnosed a pregnancy as a tumor of the womb and administered 6 one-half hour x-ray treatments over a period of 3 months. The child was born with profound mental retardation and was crippled. The child lived to age thirteen, but died subsequent to the commencement of the suit. Similarly, Stemmer v. Kline involved a suit against a physician who, without availing himself of any one of several tests available, and after a manual examination, erroneously assumed that the pregnancy was a tumor and treated it with x-ray. The child was born a microcephalic of severely subnormal intelligence, without skeletal structure, sight, speech, hearing, or the power of locomotion. In accordance with the rule laid down in Dietrich, both cases were denied as a matter of law.

B. THE "NEW" RULE

Although Dietrich spawned an impressive line of precedent,[5] it was finally supplanted in 1946 by a case enunciating what is commonly referred to as the "new rule." A decision of the District of Columbia district court, Bonbrest v. Kotz,[6] relied heavily upon the much-quoted dissent of Justice Boggs years earlier in Allaire v. St. Luke's Hospital,[7] and made a dramatic departure from precedent in allowing recovery for a prenatal injury. In 1900, Justice Bogg's dissent expressed the view that a viable child is one who is capable of sustaining life independent of its mother, and therefore should be entitled to an independent cause of action for injuries. The court followed suit in Bonbrest, and boldly pronounced that precedent, or the lack thereof, should not be dispositive in determining liability:

> The absence of precedent should afford no refuge
> to those who by their wrongful act, if such be
> proved, have invaded the right [of] both the
> mother and child . . . The common law is not a
> void and sterile thing, and is anything but
> static and inert.[8]

Since 1946, Bonbrest has been recognized as the accepted rule establishing the potential liability for both physicians and other negligent tortfeasors regarding injuries prenatally sustained. Generally, a child can now maintain a tort action for prenatal injuries negligently inflicted or, if he dies as a result of such injuries, an action will lie for his wrongful death. The right to recover for personal injuries suffered before birth by a surviving child belongs to the child, not to the child's parent. Virtually all the jurisdictions have now adopted the "new rule." Texas was the die-hard in casting aside the old rule, but finally did so relatively recently in the case of Leal v. C.C. Pitts Sand & Gravel Co.[9] The rule substantially broadens the physician's duty with respect to pregnant women; he now owes a duty to two persons instead of one.

C. THE QUESTION OF "VIABILITY"

It is significant that Bonbrest extended its ruling only so far as prenatal injuries to the viable fetus. It left open to prolific dispute the question of whether a wrongful death action will be sustained for the child who aborts or is stillborn. A number of courts have been called upon to decide whether the parents of a fetus that died in utero may recover under wrongful death statutes. This decision may be predicated on the definition of "person" in the wrongful death statute of the particular jurisdiction. However, another source of reluctance in allowing the action is the problem of proving causation--the difficulty of the proof increasing the earlier the injury occurs in gestation. The normal miscarriage rate is disproportionately high in the first trimester. The underlying policy reason residual in that judicial line of authority which emphasizes the dubious causal connection in the case of a previable fetus is merely an amplification of the same fear which long ran through the cases denying recovery for any prenatal injury itself. The concern is that recovery would often be based on mere conjecture and speculation and thus the door would be opened to fictitious claims.

It is interesting to note that the very case which expressly overruled the fetal radiation case of Stemmer v. Kline virtually argument for argument, Smith v. Brennan,[10] addressed this concern directly and at length. It dismissed the fear of opening Pandora's box by pointing out that fictitious suits abound in all fields of law, and the judiciary is accustomed and adept at ferreting them out. More importantly, this court sought to align legal theory with the matured state of scientific knowledge in the field of antenatal pediatrics. It first noted that fetal age is not always the sole measure of viability and thus there would be no way of determining whether or not a fetus was viable at the time of injury.

This consideration is particularly applicable to fetal radiation cases because some x-rays, particularly x-ray treatment for disease, are typically given over a period of time that might encompass what would be estimated to be both nonviable and viable stages. If there is damage, how can we determine in which stage of gestation it occurred? In this regard, the viability limitation thwarts the establishment of causation.

Restricting recovery to the viable stage is further out of keeping with the medical research which has unequivocally emphasized that the crucial stage of intrauterine development during which the fetus would be most radiosensisitve is the first trimester, long before viability. Therefore, we are confronted with something of a legal/medical Catch-22, which has the potential of working a grave injustice: A person may recover for a prenatal negligently inflicted abortion, deformity, or mutation if the injury occurred during the viable stage of gestation, but almost all these injuries occur BEFORE viability. Thus, it is forseeable that the viability limitation which is already on the wane in most jurisdictions will necessarily have to be eliminated in the remaining jurisdictions in order to comport with medical knowledge regarding injury to the fetus. Texas, in the 1971 case of Delgado v. Yandell,[11] granted that a cause of action exists for prenatal injury at any prenatal stage, but added the proviso that the child be born alive.

This case points out the overlapping problem of whether an action can be maintained for wrongful death if the child is stillborn as the result of the injury. The argument advanced by most courts which have answered this question in the negative[12] is that such an infant is not a "person in being," a semantic squabble shared by the proponents of the viability rule. As Professor White perceived over twenty-five years ago, the argument that such an infant is not "in being" simply does not accord with physical fact.[13] A stillborn child represents a living entity which has died.

Just as with the aborted fetus, the stillborn infant shares a knotty problem of causation in fact, in addition to proximate cause. Unless there is a patent mechanical indication of cause of death such as strangulation by the umbilical cord, the phenomena of miscarriage and of being stillborn are both idiopathic. Further, it is widely accepted that a deformed embryo is often the cause in itself of spontaneous abortion. This knowledge further complicates the causation picture for the fetus which has been irradiated and subsequently aborts. How can we distinguish whether the abortion was due to a deformity prior to any x-ray exposure or whether it was attributable to the radiation absorption? Thus, there exists an inherent stumbling block to proving a causal connection between radiation and the miscarried or stillborn fetus. To exacerbate this legal problem by defining the parameters of prenatal injury as exclusive of nonviable and stillborn fetuses could well render the hurdle insurmountable. This reality has prospective implications for the trend of tort law regarding prenatally sustained injuries, especially those resulting from in utero radiation.

D. ANALYSIS AND DISCUSSION OF PRESENT LAW
ON X-RAY INJURY TO FETUS

The barriers of viability and live birth notwithstanding, the landmark ruling of Bonbrest has fathered a plethora of successful litigation granting relief for negligent prenatal injury claims. These include the tortious acts of physicians and other people who breach a duty of care to the pregnant woman involved. Many of these cases have emanated from motor vehicle accidents[14] resulting in miscarriage, premature delivery with consequent deformity, or death to the fetus from the impact itself. Actions based on injuries have also been effectively maintained for contraction of diseases due to unsanitary premises[15] or contaminated food,[16] resulting in either premature delivery or ultimate deformity.

Since the Bonbrest decision expanded the physician's duty to include the fetus as well as its mother, there have been a host of malpractice actions affording recovery for prenatal injuries. Although several involve negligent x-ray utilization, it is remarkable that only one case, Salinetro v. Nystron,[17] has dealt specifically with injury to the fetus by irradiation. The Salinetro action failed on the issue of causation. Pursuant to insurance recovery for an accident, the plaintiff was required to submit to x-rays of her back and abdominal area. Although the woman was not yet aware of her approximate one month pregnancy, the physician did not inquire whether she was pregnant or the date of her last menstrual cycle. When her pregnancy was later discovered, the plaintiff's obstetrician advised her to undergo a therapeutic abortion because of the possible damage to the fetus from the x-rays and, in fact, the pathology report stated that the fetus was dead at the time of the abortion. However, the court concluded that the physician's failure to question the plaintiff about any pregnancy, or the possibility of such, was not the cause of her injury because she would have replied in the negative had he asked.[18]

This decision seems ill-considered since it apparently takes no cognizance of scientifically based recommendations on refraining from x-ray of the abdominal or pelvic regions of a woman who has not been almost certainly established not to be pregnant.[19] A large body of medical authorities advocate deferring x-ray, in the absence of a critical and urgent need to proceed, until it can be adequately determined that a woman in the reproductive years is not pregnant. If the onset of menses has not occurred within 10 days prior to x-ray, it cannot be safely assumed that a woman is not pregnant.[20] Although the plaintiff in the Salinetro case would have responded to any inquiry that she was not pregnant, she also would have replied in the negative if asked whether her last menstrual cycle had begun in the last 10 days, or for that matter, in the last 6 weeks!

Thus, if legal theory is to be in accord with medical perspective on the safety in the use of x-rays, the duty of the physician would be considerably expanded from that set forth in Salinetro. It would be incumbent upon a physician to ascertain any possibility

of pregnancy, and would accordingly fall below the standard of care to subject a woman not "proven" to be free from pregnancy to x-rays. If a woman neither uses an oral contraceptive, nor an intrauterine device, nor has been surgically sterilized, nor has experienced the commencement of menses within the last 10 days, then the physician cannot safely dismiss the possibility of pregnancy for the purpose of administering an x-ray.[21] In keeping with this duty, it is highly <u>inconclusive</u> if a woman such as the plaintiff in <u>Salinetro</u> would, <u>if questioned</u>, reply that she was not pregnant. <u>The burden is upon the physician, not the patient</u>, to make an analysis of the possibility of pregnancy. Thus, the physician in <u>Salinetro</u> may be viewed as falling far below the standard of care by:
 (1) Not inquiring about pregnancy or the date of the last menstrual cycle.
 (2) Not deferring the x-ray, regardless of the plaintiff's lay opinion that she was not pregnant, when we would have discovered that the last onset of menses had exceeded the 10 day limit by several weeks.

 The <u>Salinetro</u> decision also seems to fly in the face of the implied standard of care relied upon in the legion of cases allowing recovery for negligence which results in prenatal injury. In no judicial holding has the alleged tortfeasor been exculpated on the basis of ignorance of the woman's pregnancy. In fact, judicial evolution post-<u>Bonbrest</u> is replete with cases allowing recovery before the child was viable.[22] It would then follow that in a great number of these cases (particularly those dealing with the injury in the first trimester) the woman would appear <u>not</u> to be pregnant. Those decisions comport with the thin-skull doctrine. . . the tortfeasor takes his victim as he finds him. <u>Salinetro</u>, on the other hand, represents a selective blindness to this doctrine of tort law.

 Once the <u>Deitrich</u> barrier to recovery for prenatal injury was removed, it appeared that the time was ripe for recovering for injurious irradiation of the fetus. Were <u>Smith v. Luckhardt</u>[23] or <u>Stemmer v. Kline</u>[24] litigated today, it could be predicted that relief would now be granted since the only bar to recovery in those cases was stated to be that which was raised by <u>Bonbrest</u> in 1946. It is remarkable that only one case, <u>Salinetro v. Nystrom</u>, dealing with irradiation of the fetus, has reached the appellate level. The paucity of litigation in this area leaves us without a case affirmatively stating under what conditions recovery will indeed be allowed for prenatal injury from negligence in irradiating the fetus. However, we may extrapolate from the prenatal injury cases cited, and the ones to follow involving physicians, that irradiation of the fetus is a potential area for recovery. There is, additionally a line of cases involving injury by x-ray, albeit not to the fetus, that indicate that the judiciary is disposed to grant relief for injury by negligent irradiation.

 In several cases, the courts have found physicians liable for malpractice in connection with negligent care before birth, resulting in a child being born with physical or mental defects. In <u>Libby v. Conway</u>,[25] a 3 year old girl was accorded damages for serious brain damage incurred during delivery. The mother's attending physician, as well as two nurses and the anesthetist, pushed with considerable force on the mother's stomach while she was in the delivery room. A specialist called by the defendant-physician testified that the injury was due to pressure upon the skull during delivery.

An obstetrician in <u>Brooks v. Serano</u>[26] was held liable for a fractured left humerous sustained by the infant by negligent manipulation during the course of a breech birth. Another obstetrician in the case of <u>Seattle-First Nat'l Bank v. Rankin</u>,[27] was held answerable in damages to a child who was born with cerebral palsy and brain damage resulting both from the negligent treatment of the mother while the fetus was <u>in utero</u> and from a negligent delivery. It was alleged that the <u>mother suffered from a serious</u> anemia during pregnancy, and that the physician negligently failed to discover the condition and take proper steps to correct it. It was further alleged that the physician also negligently failed to ascertain the pelvic measurements of the plaintiff's mother, thereby not realizing that a normal delivery would probably be impossible to perform and that consequently he negligently failed to perform a cesarean section soon enough. It was further alleged that the physician negligently attempted to deliver the plaintiff transvaginally with forceps and, as a proximate result of the foregoing negligent acts, the plaintiff suffered permanent damage.

Similarly, the physician in <u>Larrabee v. United States</u>[28] was found liable for the plaintiff's blindness, which was found to be the proximate result of a negligent use of forceps in delivery. In <u>Norland v. Washington General Hospital</u>,[29] a quadriplegic plaintiff successfully brought an action against the obstetrician for rupture to his spinal cord occasioned by application of excessive force in effecting emergence of the head in the course of a breech delivery.

Of even more moment to our purpose in assessing the potential liability for fetal irradiation are the relatively recent precedents which have extended forseeability and thus duty to persons <u>before</u> their conception. Significantly, these three sunrise cases involved the liability of each of the entities of the health care triumvirate: The drug company, the physician, and the hospital.

In <u>Jorgenson v. Meade Johnson Laboratories, Inc.</u>[30] the mother sustained an alteration of her chromosome structure as a result of oral contraceptives prior to the conception of twin daughters. This alteration in the chromosome structure was established as the proximate cause of Mongoloid deformity in the fetus during the developmental period. One twin lived with this deformity and the other died after 3-1/2 years.

This expanded scope of duty was applied similarly in <u>Park v. Chessin</u>.[31] There, the parents as legal representatives of a child who survived for 2-1/2 years, successfully brought an action to compensate for the malpractice that proximately caused the wrongful conception, and consequently the pain and suffering. It was alleged that the mother had had a former child a few years earlier who died shortly after birth as the result of a polycystic kidney condition. The doctors, without testing the parents for chromosomal or genetic makeup, advised the mother that a future pregnancy would not result in the birth of a congenitally defective child. Upon such advice, she became pregnant and gave birth to the plaintiff in 1970. Contrary to the doctors' assurances, this child too had a polycystic kidney condition from which she died after 2-1/2 years. The physician's duty extended to this preconception negligence because the child's deformity was foreseeable, foreseeability being the touchstone of negligence and one basic criterion in determining duty.

Perhaps the farthest reaching extension of preconception negligence was recognized as calling for compensation in <u>Renslow v. Mennonite Hospital</u>.[32] The plaintiff's mother, 9 years before her birth (when the mother herself was only 13 years of age), was negligently transfused with Rh-positive blood, which was incompatible with her Rh-negative blood. Her mother had no knowledge of an adverse reaction from the transfusion and did not know that she had been improperly transfused or that her blood had thereby been sensitized. The defendants, however, discovered they had administered the incompatible blood, but at no time notified the plaintiff's mother or her own parents.

The resulting sensitization of the mother's blood allegedly caused prenatal damage to the plaintiff's hemolytic processes, which put her life in jeopardy and necessitated her induced premature birth. As the ultimate result, the plaintiff suffered permanent damage to her brain, her nervous system, and various organs.

The court in <u>Renslow</u> emphasized foreseeability, not even entertaining the notion that a 9 year gap in time between the act and the injury made the foreseeability factor in any way attenuated.

> It was foreseeable that this 13 year old girl would grow up, marry, and become pregnant. Upon the happening of this event, the defendant-hospital were chargeable with the knowledge of what she and her child would encounter as a result of the wrongful transfusion of blood.[33]

Thus, the physicians breached their standard of care not only by the negligent injurious transfusion, but also by failure to inform the plaintiff's mother of her heightened risk of giving birth to a deformed child due to reaction of her blood to Rh incompatibility. By breaching this duty to the plaintiff's mother, they breached a duty to safeguard against foreseeable prenatal injuries to the plaintiff herself.

II. PREDICTION AND PREDILECTION

These preconception decisions have implications for the demise of the theory of exculpation in the <u>Salinetro</u> case of fetal irradiation. If a physician has a duty to protect against foreseeable injuries to a fetus not even conceived at the time of his actions, then, a fortiori, he has a duty to a fetus which <u>has already been conceived</u>, but whose existence is simply not manifestly apparent without injury. Since it is highly foreseeable that x-ray will possibly damage or kill an embryo, there is a duty to protect against that risk being actualized by being <u>affirmatively</u> on guard for <u>possible</u> pregnancy. Thus, <u>Salinetro</u> simply does not square with the preconception injury cases, which seem to be more attuned to medical reality. Those latter three decisions hold the physician to a duty commensurate with the expectable standard of medical expertise. Medical science has developed various indicators and techniques that can mitigate, or better still, prevent prenatal injury and the physician's legal duty should logically entail utilizing that sophisticated knowledge.

Secondly, these preconception precedents present an entirely new question concerning liability for x-ray diagnosis. The fetus might well recover from alteration of the chromosomal makeup of its parent sustained years before its conception, but ultimately resulting in a mutation during its development which may become manifest in that fetus or, more likely, in his own offspring.

Among the recent cases which have found the physician liable for negligent injury by x-ray, albeit to the person himself as opposed to the fetus, one case poses by implication another prospective facet of the duty required in administering x-rays to pregnant women. The case itself, <u>Green v. Hussey</u>,[34] did not involve a pregnant woman. Instead, it involved a woman with breast cancer who had undergone surgery. Subsequent to the surgery and without first obtaining the plaintiff's informed consent, the physicians embarked on a series of cobalt and x-ray treatments, which damaged her severely. The appellate court agreed with the plaintiff's contention that she was entitled to know the foreseeable results before the treatment was undertaken if reasonable medical practitioners of the same school, in the same or similar circumstances, would have told the patient of such risks. This duty of obtaining informed consent was recognized in Texas in <u>Wilson v. Scott</u>,[35] expressing that a surgical patient has a legal right to be informed of the hazards of the treatment, the inverse hazard of foregoing the treatment, and any alternatives.

The doctrine of informed consent is quite likely to be litigated in conjunction with x-ray treatment that results in damage. Although x-ray treatment is not an operation per se, it does involve tantamount hazards in many cases. Certainly, a pregnant mother has an especial need to have advance knowledge of potential damage to the fetus; as the situation now exists, the mother is often presented with a <u>fait accompli</u> and the dilemma of either undergoing a therapeutic abortion or risking damage to her infant, the latter choice inevitably involving months of anxiety if she does take the pregnancy to term.

Since injury disproportionately befalls the woman who does not yet know she is pregnant because of the first trimester radiosensitivity of the fetus, it would appear that informed consent might prevent this unfortunate coincidence to a large extent. The physician might inform the mother of the advisability of the alternative deferment of x-ray diagnosis until her next menstrual cycle or until she can be tested for pregnancy. This policy of informed consent for x-ray diagnosis of pregnant women would include the normal discretion not to disclose the hazards when such knowledge itself would be deleterious to the patient. However, this variable will probably only be present when the use of x-rays is critical and cannot be deferred, such as when a patient has been in an accident possibly involving fractures, or when the patient must receive x-ray treatment for disease.

There is a conceivable final twist to the question of informed consent and irradiation of the fetus. If the mother is informed of the risks, proceeding nevertheless with the x-ray diagnosis, would a child who is later born with a deformity or deficiency have a cause of action against the mother, instead of the physician?

REFERENCES

1. Debakan, J. Nuc. Med, 471, 473 (1968).
2. 138 Mass. 14, 52 Am. Rep. 242 (1884).
3. 299 Ill. App. 100, 19. N.E. 2d 446 (1939).
4. 128 N.J.L. 455, 26 A.2d 489 (1942).
5. Gorman v. Budlong, 23 R.I. 169, 49 A. 704 (1901). Nugent v. Brooklyn Heights Railway Co., 154 A.D. 667, 139 N.Y.S. 367 (1913); Buel v. United Rys. Co.of St. Louis, 248 Mo. 126, 154 S.W. 71, (1913); Lipps v. Milwaukee Electric Ry. & Light Co., 164 Wis. 272, 159 N.W. 916 (1916); Drobner v. Peters, 232 N.Y. 220, 133 N.E. 567 (1921); Stanford v. St. Louis-San Francisco Ry. Co., 214 Ala. 611, 108 So. 566 (1926); Magnolia Coca-Cola Bottling Co. v. Jordan, 124 Tex. 347, 78 S.W.2d 944 (1935); Newman v. City of Detroit, 281 Mich. 60, 274 N.W. 710 (1973); Berlin v. J.C. Penney Co. Inc., 339 Pa. 547, 16 A.2d 28 (1940)
6. 65 F. Supp. 138 (D.C. D.C. 1946).
7. 184 Ill. 359, 56 N.E. 638 (1900).
8. 65 F. Supp. 138 at 142.
9. 419 S.W.2d 820 (Tex. 1967).
10. 31 N.J. 353, 157 A.2d 497 (1960).
11. 468 S.W.2d 475 (Tex. Civ. App.--Fort Worth, 1971) writ ref'd n.r.e. per curiam, 471 471 S.W.2d 569 (Tex. 1971).
12. See Hogan v. McDaniel, 204 Tenn. 235, 319 S.W.2d 221 (1958); Drabbels v. Skelly Oil Co., 155 Neb. 17, 50 N.W.2d 229 (1951); Prates v. Sears, Roebuck & Co., 19 Conn. Supp. 487, 118 A.2d 633 (1955); Amann v. Faisly, 415, Ill. 422, 114 N.E.2d 412 (1953); Stegall v. Morris, 363 Mo. 1224, 258 S.W.2d 577 (1953).
13. White, La L Rev, 12, 383 at 395 (1952).
14. Williams v. Marion Rapid Transit Corp., 152 Ohio St. 114, 87 N.E.2d 334 (1949); Shepard v. Midland Mut. Life Ins. Co., 152 Oh. St. 6, 376 Pa. 497, 103 A.2d 681 (1954); Von Elbe v. Studebaker-Packard Corp., 15 Pa. D. & C.2d 635, 106 P.L.J. 219 (1958); Puhl v. Milwaukee Auto Ins. Co., 8 Wis.2d 343,99 N.W.2d 163 (1959); Sinker v. Kneale, 401 Pa. 267, 164 A.2d 93 (1960); Marlow v. Krapek, 20 Mich. App. 489, 174 N.W.2d (1969); Miller v. Highlands Ins. Co., (Fla. App.) 336 So. 2d 636 (1974).
15. Dillon v. S.S. Kresge Co., 36 Mich. App. 603, 192 N.W.2d 661 (1974).
16. Cavanaugh v. First Nat'l Stores, Inc., 329 Mass. 1970, 107 N.E.2d 307 (1952).
17. 341 So. 2d 1059 (Fla. App. 1977).
18. Id. at 1061.
19. Hammer-Jacobsen, Dan Med Bull, 6, 113,120-121 (1959) Russell and Russell, Rad, 58, 369 at 373 (1952) Swartz and Reichling, JAMA, 329, 1907 at 1908 (1978).
20. Id.
21. Swartz and Reichling, JAMA, 329, 1908.

22. Stokes v. Liberty Mut. Ins. Co., 213 So. 2d 695 (Fla. 1968); Tucker v. Howard L. Carmichael & Sons, Inc., 208 Ga. 201, 65 S.E.2d 909 (1951); Hornbuckle v. Plantation Pipe Line Co.,212 Ga. 504, 93 S.E.2d 727 (1956); Daley v. Meier, 33 Ill. App.2d 218, 173 N.E. 2d 691 (1961); Womack v. Buckhorn, 384 Mich. 71, 187 N.W.2d 218 (1971); Smith v. Brennan, 31 N.J. 353, 157 A.2d 497 (1960); Gleitman v. Cosgrove, 49 N.J. 22, 227 A.2d 689 (1967); Kelly v. Gregory, 282 A.D. 542, 125 N.Y.S. 2d 696 (1953); Re: Scanelli, 208 Misc. 804, 142 N.Y.S. 2d 411 (1955); Sinkler v. Kneale, 401 Pa. 267, 164 A.2d 93 (1960); Von Elbe v. Studebaker-Packard Corp., 15 pa. D. & C. 2d 635, 106 P.L.J. 219 (1958); Simmons v. Weisenthal, 29 Pa. D. & C.2d 54 (1962); Sylvia v. Gobeille, 101 R.I. 76, 220 A. 2d 222 (1966); Seattle-First Nat'l Bank v. Rankin, 59 Wash.2d 288, 367 P.2d 835 (1962).
23. 200 Ill. App. 100, 19 N.E.2d 446 (1939).
24. 128 N.J.L. 455, 26 A.2d 489 (1942).
25. 192 Cal. App.2d 865, 13 Cal. Rptr. 830 (1961).
26. 209 So. 2d 279 (Fla. App. 1968).
27. 59 Wash.2d 288, 367 P.2d 835 (1962).
28. 254 F. Supp. 613 (D.C. Cal. 1966).
29. 461 F.2d 694 (Ark. 1974).
30. 483 F.2d 237 (10th Cir. 1973).
31. 88 Misc.2d 222, 387 N.Y.S.2d 204 (1976).
32. 67 Ill.2d 348, 367 N.E.2d 1251 (1977).
33. Id. at 1258.
34. 127 Ill. App.2d 174, 262 N.E.2d 156 (1970).
35. 412 S.W.2d 299 (Tex.1967).

LIABILITY FROM THE VIEW OF THE MEDICAL PHYSICIST

Robert J. Shalek
The University of Texas System Cancer Center
M. D. Anderson Hospital and Tumor Institute
Houston, Texas

The treating physician is held broadly responsible for the adequacy of medical treatment, but with the passage of time, case law has lifted some of that responsibility and placed it upon others in instances where it would not be reasonable or possible for the treating physician to have personal knowledge of the details of some component of diagnosis or treatment. For example, the anesthesiologist in controlling anesthesia, the pathologist in reaching a diagnosis from tissue specimens, the pharmacist in filling drug prescriptions, the unsupervised nurse on the ward administering drugs and the hospital in providing functioning apparatus likely would be held responsible if they failed to perform to an expected standard of care and injury to the patient was due to that failure. By analogy the medical physicist particularly in relating to radiation therapy, performs radiation measurements and calculations which are seldom reviewed totally by the treating radiotherapist. Reliance upon the physicist for the scientific and technical aspects of the fulfillment of a radiation dose prescription is the common practice in the United States. It is not surprising that medical physicists have been named as defendants in suits involving the possibility of the delivery of more radiation than intended. To the author's knowledge none of these suits have come to trial and thus there is no case law for specific guidance. Conceivably, miscalibration of the amount of radioisotope administered to a patient, the incorrect measurement or calculation of a radiation dose to a fetus in an abortion decision or negligent radiation overexposure to personnel or the public also could result in liability for the medical physicist.

That liability is assumed by the physicist's employer if the physicist was acting in the course of his employment. However, the employer could attempt to recover his losses by suing the employee. A consulting physicist takes full responsibility for his actions since there is no employer standing behind him.

LEGAL EXPOSURE OF MEDICAL PHYSICISTS COMPARED TO THAT OF PHYSICIANS

Perdue (1) has discussed eleven theories of liability which may be applied by a patient against a physician. These are listed in Table I with an additional (last) entry. Also, those theories which conceivably might be applied against a physicist are marked. Negligence is by far the most likely action against a physicist but strict liability and res ipsa loquitur are possible theories.

TABLE I

THEORIES OF LIABILITY

	PHYSICIAN	PHYSICIST
Negligence	X	X
Battery	X	
Lack of Informed Consent	X	
Abandonment	X	
Fraud	X	
Contract to Cure	X	
Malicious Prosecution	X	
False Imprisonment	X	
Strict Liability	?	X
Unauthorized Disclosure of Confidential Information	X	
Experimental Medicine	X	
Res Ipsa Loquitur (the thing speaks for itself)	?	?

Negligence. A physicist may be negligent if he makes a mistake resulting in injury to a patient. The mistake may be an error which the physicist would recognize immediately or the mistake may result from a lack of understanding by the physicist of generally accepted practices by the profession. More formally, the elements of negligence are (2):

    a. A duty, or obligation, recognized by law, requiring the actor to conform to a certain standard of conduct, for the protection of others against unreasonable risks.

    b. A failure to conform to the standard.

    c. A reasonably close causal connection between the conduct and the resulting injury constituting what is known as "legal cause" or "proximate cause".

    d. Actual loss or damage resulting to the interests of another.

Some considerations of how these elements apply to medical physicists follow:

    a. The duty applicable to medical physicists without doubt would be a national standard of care similar to that required of medical specialists rather than a community standard of care sometimes applied to general practitioners.

Thus medical physicists would be expected to have knowledge of international and national protocols and codes of practice in areas of activity where codes exist. In areas of activity where codes do not exist a knowledge of the literature and usual standards elsewhere would constitute the standard of care.

    b. Whether a failure to conform to the standard of care has occurred is judged by the requirement that "ordinary" care be employed. Ordinary care is that which would be employed by an ordinary, reasonable medical physicist under like circumstances. He would be expected to employ the learning and skill of a physicist in good standing in the profession, provided the standards of the profession are not unacceptably low. This definition of the standard of care seems comfortable and forgiving, however, in the authors limited opportunity for observation, an unintended or ignorant mistake admitted or proved is not forgiven. Thus an arithmetical error by a physicist which results in harm to a patient would not be excused even if that physicist made only one error in 100,000 calculations. An argument that everyone and even computers make errors would not avail. A system sufficient to detect accidental errors should have been in place.

    A mistake due to inadvertence or ignorance is culpable but an error of judgment is not. For example, a physician is not negligent if he has gathered and understood all of the diagnostic information which an ordinary, prudent physician would have required and then makes a mistaken decision for treatment which other like physicians might have made upon the same information. Similarly, medical physicists have some latitude of professional judgment, through it is generally more narrow than that of physicians. For example, some complex dose calculations in radiation therapy require approximations which can be done in different ways with somewhat different results. There may be no recognized standard way. In such instances a reasonable though not the best approximation would be a matter of professional judgment not likely cuplable in a negligence action.

    c. A reasonably close causal connection between the conduct and resulting injury, or proximate cause, is easily stated as above, but may be difficult for a planitiff to demonstrate. In addition to biological variabity between patients there is expected morbidity attendant to some medical procedures. On the other hand there are communication pitfalls for physicists when there is confusion caused by multiple participation of different professionals. There may be errors in physics of insufficient magnitude to cause the observed results together with questionable judgments by the physician. The problems in communicating such complexites to a court and jury are formidable. Experienced lawyers say that it is difficult to minimize any error admitted or proved especially when jargon obfuscates the issue. The Radiological Physics Center has shown by physics review visits to about 250 institutions that systematic errors in physics, usually small and often compensatory, occur at almost every institution. (Please see the other contributions to these proceedings by this author). Thus, small errors could become the focus of a suit where there was clearly a poor clinical result but no other negligence evident. Fortunately, the acceptable criteria of $\pm$ 5% in the accuracy of fulfilling radiation dose prescriptions in radiation therapy adopted in interinstitutional clinical trials is widely accepted and provides a barrier to the over emphasis of small errors. However, this concept is sometimes difficult to communicate to lawyers and likely more so to jurors who want to deal with absolute accuracy and to give significance to very small radiation dose differences.

    d. The last element of negligence is actual damage to the patient such as physical disability, medical expenses, loss of earnings, loss of earning capacity, and pain and suffering. These considerations in an action against a medical physicist would be similar to those against a physician.

Strict Liability. Strict liability as applied in civil law is liability without a showing of fault. If there is injury to another due to ultra hazardous activities such as using explosives or harboring wild animals there may be liability without a demonstration of negligence. A developing area of strict liability concerns consumer product liability assumed by manufacturers. Medical physicists sometimes provide equipment or devices for use by physicians and technicians. If that device fails or causes an inappropriate procedure to be performed, conceivably the physicist could be sued on the basis of strict liability. For example, if a physicist supplied a tray for holding secondary lead blocks used for shaping radiation fields and if the tray broke resulting in injury to a patient, the physicist might be a defendant in an action based upon strict liability rather than negligence.

    Physicists might acquire liability by modifying a manufactured product which then fails as a result of the modification. Suppose a physicist intending to attach a redundant timer to a radiation machine changes the circuitry. And suppose that an exposure is not terminated due to failure of the circuitry resulting in an overexposure to a patient. The physicist might well have acquired liability which otherwise would be imputed to the manufacturer.

Res Ipsa Loquitur. Res ipsa liquitur, or the thing speaks for itself, is a cause of action in which the plantiff does not know what happened, but has an injury which ordinarily would not happen except for negligence. Damage to a part of the body not under treatment is an example of such injury. The conditions necessary for the application of res ipsa loquitur are (2): (a) the event must be of a kind which ordinarily does not occur in the absence of someone's negligence; (b) it must be caused by an agency or instrumentality within the exclusive control of the defendant; (3) it must not have been due to any voluntary action or contribution on the part of the plaintiff. If the plaintiff can show that it is more likely than not that these conditions pertain, it has the procedural effect of shifting the burden of going forward with the evidence from the plaintiff to the defendant. This cause of action is rarely used, but might be employed in instances where the defendant has more knowledge of the events than the plaintiff. In such an action there would likely be many defendants since blame is not localized to a person or action. A medical physicist as one defendant would want to be able to document that pertinent machines were functioning correctly and that measurements, calculations, and procedures were adequate.

LEGAL EXPOSURE OF MEDICAL PHYSICISTS COMPARED TO THAT OF PHARMACISTS

In some activities the role of the medical physicist resembles that of a pharmacist. Each assumes responsibility in the proper fulfillment of prescriptions given by physicians and each has a duty to raise questions about a prescription if it does not accord with usual practice. A pharmacist may be held liable for delivery of the wrong drug (3, 4), for delivery of one patient's prescription to another, even though the drugs were correctly labeled (5), and subject to punitive damages for not revealing a mistake (6). The extent of the pharmacist's responsibility and therefore liability is under active discussion by pharmacists (7). Most writers agree that pharmacists should screen patient's drug profiles for drug interactions and be willing to advise patients generally on drug questions. When a physician gives a drug prescription which the pharmacist believes will be harmful to the patient, the pharmacist has a duty to challenge the physician's order. If the pharmacist and the physician cannot resolve the disagreement, a hospital pharmacist should consult higher hospital authority and a community pharmacist could dispense the drug to the physician rather than the patient in order to shield himself from liability (8).

The above discussion applicable to pharmacists, by analogy, supports the view that medical physicists (a) are responsible and liable for errors in their work, (b) may be exposed to a charge of gross negligence and liable for punitive damages if they fail to inform the treating physician of an error upon discovery and (c) have a duty to inform the treating physician if they believe a treatment prescription by him may be injurious to a patient and if they are employed by a hospital to inform the hospital if the physicist and physician cannot reach agreement. A landmark Illinois case in 1965, Darling v. Charleston Community Memorial Hospital, held a hospital liable for failure to review treatment approved by a physician. In this instance the physician on emergency call set a broken leg.

The patient complained of pain and the protruding toes became dark not long after the cast was set. The same physician treated the patient ineffectually for several days. Finally the cast was removed, but it was too late to save the leg harmed by interference of the cast with the circulation of blood. In the patient's suit against the hospital the appellate court concluded that a verdict of negligence against the hospital was supportable on either of two bases: (a) the hospital failed to have a sufficient number of trained nurses on duty who could have recognized the progression of a gangrenous condition..... "it became the nurses' duty to inform the attending physician, and if he failed to act, to advise the hospital authorities so that appropriate action might be taken." or (b) (the hospital) "failed to require consultation with or examination by members of the hospital surgery staff skilled in such treatment..." Thus in this instance the hospital was held responsible for medical treatment and employees of the hospital were expected to protect their employer from liability even to the extent of going to hospital authorities if the attending physician failed to take appropriate action. Darling is an important case because it holds that the hospital has responsibilities for patient treatment and is contrary to the long held view that the physician is solely responsible for medical treatment. However, as in any case, this is a holding for the parties and circumstances presented. The extend of the hospital's liability for medical treatment will be elaborated in other cases, statutes and administrative rules.

SUGGESTIONS FOR REDUCING LEGAL RISK

Know Protocols and Codes of Practice. A medical physicist is expected to know those things which an ordinary, prudent medical physicist would know about the work he performs. It is not enough to be conscientious if one is ignorant of the standard practices of the profession. If the profession itself is lax in its standards, a court may define higher standards. Thus a medical physicist should be willing to question whether usual practices are adequate in his situation. An example discussed by Hart (9) involves a workmen's compensation award (10) to the widow of a worker who died of myoblastic leukemia. Though the worker had received radiation exposures well below the maximum permissible dose the court reasoned from testimony that "there is no 'threshold' or 'safe' dosage of radiation because at the present stage of scientific knowledge it cannot be ascertained exactly what effects radiation has on the human body." Workman's Compensation cases are easier for the plaintiff to win than civil cases, but this holding may be a warning that limiting employees' exposures to the legal Maximum Permissible Dose may not be a barrier against liability in the current state of public consciousness about radiation.

Records. Records should be identified, dated, and be done in a clear and routine way (11). Such records will be accorded more respect as evidence than ad hoc scribblings. The period of time that records should be retained is not easily answered in a categorical way. For hospital use, physics records should be retained at least as long as other patient records. For legal use, the records should be retained at least for a period exceeding the statute of limitations for bringing a tort (e.g. negligence) action. In some states the statute of limitations is 2 years from the event. In other states the statutory period will be initiated when the patient knew or should have known of the injury.

Assuming Someone Else's Liability. Medical physicists often see patients repeatedly. In an effort to be cheerful, a physicist might be tempted to say something which the patient could interpret as a promise of cure. An unfilled promise can be a basis for a suit.

The possibility of voiding a manufacturer's warranty and responsibility for the safe performance of a machine should be considered before making alterations upon a machine. An example is discussed above.

Separate Attorney. If a medical physicist is named as a defendant it is well to have his attorney advise him even though his employer assumes responsibility and hires an attorney. The interests of the hospital and the physicist are not necessarily identical.

What Must Be Told When a Legal Situation Arises. Questions should be answered truthfully and evidence should be preserved. However, it is not necessary to volunteer information to an adversary or to answer questions which are not asked.

Consultation and Verification. It is common practice by pathologists to seek review by other pathologists when a diagnosis is difficult. Such action is evidence against a negligent diagnosis. Medical physicists can take analogous precautions by asking for independent verification of key elements in their procedures. As an example, mailed thermoluminescent dosimeters from an independent source can serve this purpose in the therapeutic and diagnotic use of radiation.

CONCLUSION

The negligent performance of professional duties is the most probable type of legal action against a medical physicist. A mistake resulting from ignorance or inadvertence is an example; an error in professional judgment is not negligence if an ordinary, prudent physicist in the same situation would have made the same decision. A physicist or any hospital employee has a duty to protect his employer from liability even to the extent of reporting to the hospital medical practices which could harm the patient. Suggestions for reducing legal risk include recommendations for professional knowledge, record keeping and outside verification of important elements of operating systems.

REFERENCES

(1) J. M. Perdue, The Law of Texas Medical Malpracitce p. 1-20, Houstan Law Review, Inc., Houston, 1975.
(2) W. L. Prosser, Law of Torts p. 143 and 214, West Publishing Co., St. Paul, 1971.
(3) Duensing v. Huscher, 431 SW 2d 169 (1968).
(4) Boeck v. Katz Drug Co., 127 P2d 506 (1942).
(5) Davis v. Katz and Bestfoff, Inc. 333 So. 2d 698 (1976).
(6) Burke v. Bean, 363 S.W. 2d 366 (1962).
(7) Simmons, J. C., J. Am. Pharm. Assoc. 17, 730, (1977).
(8) R. F. Steeves and F. T. Patterson, Am. J. Hosp. Pharm. 26, 404,(1969).
(9) J. C. Hart, Health Physics 23, 343 (1972).
(10) Besner v. Walter Kidde Nuclear Laboratory et al 265 N. Y. Sup. 2d 312 (1965)
(11) E. J. Norton, Jr., So Med J. 60, 439 (1967).

DISCUSSION - MEDICAL-LEGAL RESPONSIBILITIES

S. Gianelos: Is Texas an agreement state? If so, Title 10, Parts 19.13, 10.401 require, at the request of a worker, an annual exposure report shall be given to him/her. I know of one state where it is mandatory to issue annual exposure reports whether asked for or not. What does Texas require, at the request of or as a mandatory requirement?

J. Nanus: Texas is an agreement state. Texas has the requirement for annual exposure reports at request of worker and, upon termination, provided exposure < 10% of MPD. Also, if Rhode Island has it mandatory by its regulation, you can ask for an exception; otherwise, you have to compy with it.

E. Webster: (Comment to R. Waggener) The effective action level (Level 2 at which something should be done) in the current NRC ALARA document is essentially 1/4 of the MPD, i.e., 1.25 rem per year. This is expressed as 310 mrem per quarter.

J. Fitzpatrick: Please discuss (addressed to both J. Perdue and V. Collins): (1) The Karen Silkwood case and (2) recent VA acceptance of Nevada Test Site Radiation Exposure as cause of ex-soldier's leukemia--from standpoint of precendents (and future judgments and ultimate cost to nation).

Perdue: The vast majority of the damages found in the Karen Silkwood case were comprised of punitive damages. It will be interesting to see whether the appellate courts allow the amount of this verdict to stand on appeal. In Texas, we hear often of million dollar judgments being rendered, but the media does not report when the appellate courts reduce those judgments by way of remititure or reverse those judgments completely. On the question of precedent, the court's normally adhere quite vigorously to the doctrine of state decisions. However, there are principles of law which, while they have long and established history, should probably be discarded, given new social and scientific facts and conditions.

Collins: (1) Re: Karen Silkwood case - Available information is from lurid accounts in press and popular magazines. The claim of deliberately causing the death of Silkwood by running her car off the highway is no more bizarre than the account of her life story. The case is on appeal and eventually a believable report may be available.

However, the case should alert all of us to the likelihood of increasing claims of radiation injury, both accidental and deliberate, real and contrived. Judges, attorneys, and juries are ill-prepared to cope with radiation and it will require that science and medicine come to court as expert witnesses prepared to cope with the responsibility to educate.

Re: Nevada test site radiation exposures--Claims of leukemia or other forms of cancer will bring to bear law, science, and personal conviction in unpredictable mix to produce decisions in individual cases. Where a government agency is the defendant or a party to a claim of injury for a large number of individuals, some device comparable to workmen's compensation may evolve where the requirments for proof and negligence are modified by legislation. The solution must be a balance between society's commitment to compensate an innocent victim and reasonable precaution to minimize the risk of fraud.

Kendall: What duties or responsibilities does the patient have?

Perdue: Both the law and the jury expect and demand that the patient be responsible. Indeed, it has been my experience that juries tend to penalize patients more than they deserve when there is the slightest showing that the patient was not responsible in seeking medical attention or in following the physician's orders. So, both as a practical and legal matter, the patient does have responsibilities and his responsibility depends and varies on the facts of each given medical/legal case.

Kendall: If the patient refuses the x-ray, does the MD have the right to withdraw from the case?

Perdue: Of course a physician has the right to withdraw from the treatment of a patient at any time. The only caveat is that the physician must not withdraw "untimely" such as to constitute an abandonment. The physician must be sure that at the time of the withdrawal he gives the patient reasonable opportunity to make arrangements for future, adequate medical care. If the physician gives the patient this opportunity, then he would not be guilty of an abandonment and he may legally withdraw from the case.

R. Shalek: I'd like to ask Dr. Gaulden at what dose she recommends th erapeutic abortion when radiation exposure to the fetus has occurred in the third trimester?

Dr. Gaulden: That is a very difficult question in that one does not feel comfortable, in view of the paucity of data at lower doses, with giving a cut-off dose. In general, I recommend serious consideration of risks at doses between 15 and 20 rads. Each case must be considered on an individual basis and a number of factors must be taken into consideration, not the least of which is the hazard to the mother of the abortion itself.

V. Collins (Comment to J. Nanus concerning the statement that "30% of x-ray examinations are unnecessary"): Percentage expressions are deceptive. If 1 of 3 is unnecessary, is this 33.3% of exams or a 50% increase over justifiable? Consider breast biopsies-4 of 5 (80%) to 9 of 10 (90%) are negative and therefore unnecessary as proven by the pathologist's report of "no cancer". However, it is hard to tell which is positive or negative before biopsy. More importantly, if a surgeon maintains his record of NO mistakes--by biopsy of only obvious or sure things--then he is missing some.

It is even more difficult or hazardous for Mr. Villforth to recognize an unnecessary examination in Luling, Texas, as viewed from Washington, D.C.

INDEX

Aging, 83-86

ALARA, 293-299

Ankylosing spondylitis, 63-64, 68

Anxiety neurosis, 304

Background radiation, 15, 41-42, 56, 74, 166

BEIR III, 1, 11, 12, 14-16, 18, 55, 69-70, 73

Benefit-risk evaluation, 262-265

Bross papers, 74

Burden of injury, 305

Burden of proof, 309

Bureau of Radiological Health, 283-284, 286-290

Cancer, 21-22, 26-29, 66, 81-83
 -bone, 62, 68, 74
 -breast, 56, 62, 70-72
 -childhood, 62, 73
 -exposure in utero, 73-74
 -incidence, 73
 -Jewish effect on, 70
 -leukemia, 62-64, 68, 74-75, 85, 86
 -lifetime risks, 67
 -lung, 70-71, 74
 -lymphoma, 74
 -mice, 56
 -multiple myloma, 74

Cancer (cont.)
 -neoplasia, 85
 -rats, 60
 -risk estimates, 66, 68
 -solid, 63-65
 -statistics, 164

Cancerphobia, 302

Carcinogenesis, 61, 163-165

Cell Sterilization, 160-162

Chromosomal aberations, 57-58, 78-81, 161
 -dicentric, 57
 -sub-lesions, 60
 -translocations, 80

Consumer education, 271

Death from various causes, 263

Demonstrable injury, 309

Dermatologists, 256

Diagnostic radiology
 -benefits, 170-173
 -cancer risk from, 167
 -CT, 119-120
 -dose evaluation, 105-122
 -entrance exposure, 111-113
 -gonad dose, 115-116, 168
 -GSD, 116-117, 168

INDEX (cont.)

Diagnostic radiology (cont.)

- lens dose, 113-114

- mamography, 118-119

- mean marrow dose, 114

- occupational exposure, 121-122

- organ dose, 113

Dose fractionation, 4, 111

Dose protraction, 33, 36-37, 45, 82, 111

Dose rate effect, 3-4, 6, 23, 28, 55, 58-60

Dose response curve, 56-57

- linear, 23, 63, 65, 68, 70, 83, 105

- linear quadratic, 57, 63, 65, 67, 68, 70, 78, 82

- quadratic, 57, 68, 83

Down's syndrome, 79

Dual radiation action, 60

Fallout, 41-42, 75

Fetus, 33

- diagnostic exposure, 228

- sensitivity, 73-74

Future injury, 302-303

Genetic burden, 10-11

Genetic effects, 78, 162-163

- frequency of disorders, 163

- low level irradiation, 1-19

Genetically significant dose (GSD), 15, 116-117

Hiroshima, 14, 26, 33, 37-38, 45-46, 62-63, 70, 72, 227

Human abnormalities

- cataracts, 224

- CNS, 37, 39

- embryonic death, 224

- growth retardation, 37, 46, 224

- mental retardation, 38-39

- microcephaly, 37-39, 46, 224

Informed consent, 302-303, 306, 317-318

Intrauterine irradiation, 37-39

Irradiation effects on human tissue, 87-88

Latent period, 63

Legal exposure, 325-326

Legal injury, 301

Legal risk, 326-327

Legal terms, defined, 306-308

LET

- high, 57, 71, 82

- low, 57, 62, 78, 82

Liability

- for irradiation of fetus, 309-318

- view of practitioner, 300-308

INDEX (cont.)

Liability (cont.)
  —view of medical physicist, 321-327
  —without fault, 304

Life span shortening, 83-86, 263

Malpractice, 313

Mancuso Report, 74

Medical irradiation, 89-90

Microdosimetry, 61

Motor vehicle fatalities, 264

Multigeneration irradiation, 10

Mutations, 161-162
  —dominant, 6, 7, 8, 10
  —recessive, 2
  —skeletal, 13-14

Nagasaki, 14, 26, 38, 45, 62-65, 71-72

Negligence, 301, 322-324

Neonate, 33, 42-43

Neutrons, 63, 88, 170

"New rule", 310

Non-ionizing radiation, 290-291

Non-stochastic effects, 87-89

Nuclear medicine
  —administered activity, 127-128
  —dose evaluation
    —physical factors, 129-136
    —physiological factors, 126-129

Nuclear medicine (cont.)
  —patient dose, 136-151

Nuclear Regulatory Commission, 285-286

Organogenesis, 36

Patient selection, 267

Phenotypic damage, 6-9

Portsmouth Naval Shipyard, 74-75

Postnatal irradiation, 42-43

Pregnant women
  —counseling, 230-240, 244
  —estimating risk, 230-240
  —risk of 1 rad, 233
  —use of diagnostic radiation, 242-245
  —use of therapeutic radiation 242-245

Preimplantation, 34

Product liability, 304-306

Public information program, 260-261

Rad, 107-108

Radiation biology, 255

Radiation in daily life, 253

Radiation teratogenesis, 223-245

Radiation therapy
  cancer induction, 156

INDEX (cont.)

Radiation therapy (cont.)
- dose evaluation, 157-158
- genetic risk, 156
- growth impairment, 156
- organ damage, 156
- teratogenesis, 241-242
- tolerance dose, 155

Radiologists, 86, 254

Radionuclides in pregnancy, 40-41

Radioprotective chemicals, 85

Radium dial painters, 86

RBE, 58, 61, 64

Regulations, 283-291

Rem, 109

Rep, 108

Repair, 3-4, 58

Res ipsa loquitur, 324-325

Risk education, 253-273

Risk estimation, 21-31
- direct method, 13-14
- doubling-dose method, 12-13, 80-81
- effect of model, 57

Risk reduction
- diagnostic radiology, 177-189
- nuclear medicine, 193-213
- radiotherapy, 216-221

Roentgen, 106-107

Safety
- interstitial radiation therapy, 258
- nursing instructions, 259

Sensitivity patterns, 34-37

SI units, 105-106

Skin erythema dose, 106

Somatic effects, 4, 21, 89

Specific energy, 60

Specific locus method, 2-6

State radiation control agencies, 284-285

Statistical requirement, 56

Stem cell, 2, 4, 21

Strict liability, 304, 306, 324

Study population, 56

Supreme court, 301

Synergistic effects, 37, 45

Ten-day rule, 185

Two-hit model, 66

UNSCEAR, 11, 12, 14, 17, 78

User education, 270

U.S. population exposure, 30, 166

Viability of fetus, 311

Whole body exposure, 62, 83-86, 110